Kwai River Christian Hospital:

Voices from the First 60 Years

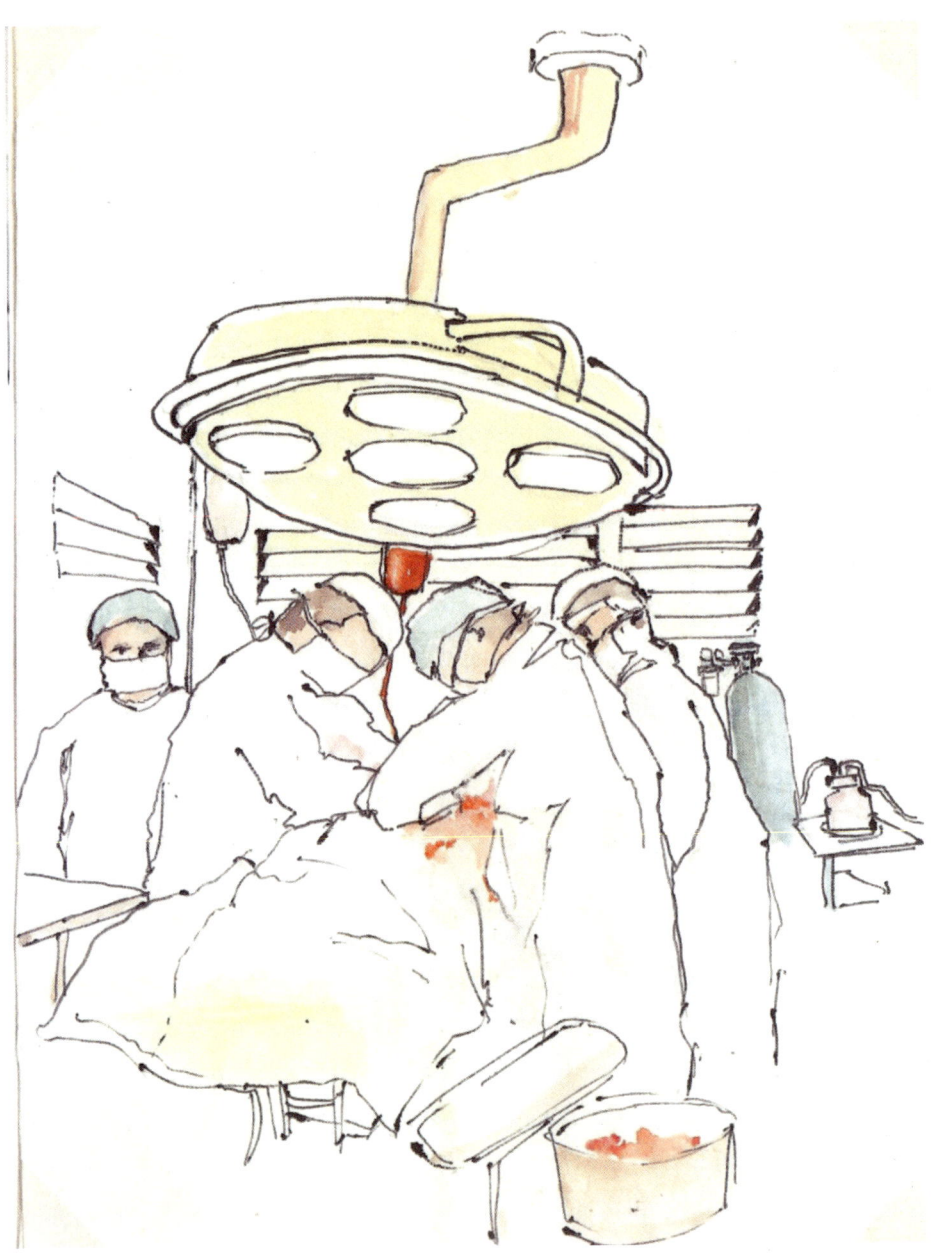

Surgery at the Kwai River Christian Hospital

(The watercolor on this page and on the front cover are by Mr. Myint Oo, nurse aide from Burma in the late 1970's)

Kwai River Christian Hospital:

Voices from the First 60 Years

Edited by

Philip McDaniel, MD

ISBN 978-1-09832-884-9

Published by BookBaby, Pennsauken, NJ

Author's email: krchphil@gmail.com

Dedication

To Douglas Corpron, MD and Winifred Dodge, RN
who brought modern medicine to Sangkhlaburi District

and

To all the nurses, aides, lab techs, chaplains, pharmacy staff, office
personnel, laundresses, janitors, and gardeners who have faithfully
served at the Kwai River Christian Hospital

Table of Contents

Part 2

Memoirs on Expat Family Life

Part 3

Hospital History in Photos   269

Acknowledgements

Many thanks to all my friends and colleagues who contributed memoirs. I have enjoyed reading your remarkable stories!

Doug Corpron, Paul Dodge, John Freeman, Jan Vertigan/Yawan: you all contributed photographic images. Thanks for that. Karl Corpron, son of Dr. Doug Corpron, kindly digitized many of his dad's slides from the early days of the Kwai River Christian Mission.

Jit and Jan Yawan were able to identify individuals in some of the old photos and provide important historical details.

Many thanks to my sister Carol Licht and to my wife, Melba McDaniel, for proofreading the text.

Foreword

Mud, Murder, and Malaria!

My brother Dr. Phil McDaniel has compiled the fascinating recollections of many of the people who founded and staffed a remote mission hospital on the border between Thailand and Burma beginning 60 years ago. Possessing a pioneering spirit and deep compassion forged from faith, these were men and women who set aside the comforts of home and family in order to erect a jungle hospital for a population still reliant on village spirit doctors.

Mud! Having made the decision to locate the Kwai River Christian Hospital on the banks of the Ranti River, a tributary of the famed River Kwai, the intrepid founders soon discovered that one of their biggest challenges was the deep mud that swallowed Land Rovers up to their axels during the monsoon season, making travel long, dangerous, and uncomfortable in the sweltering heat. Founder, Doug Corpron, describes what it was like to forge swollen streams with their seven children in a jeep with the top off, once even overturning in their vehicle, scattering not only the kids but also 12 big containers of eggs!

Murder! The courage it took to stick it out in this remote mission station is underscored by the account of my sister-in-law, Melba McDaniel, who describes the time a local woman was murdered, together with her children, by bandits who had heard about two bars of gold she had recently acquired and recklessly bragged about. In actual fact, the gold was being kept in a safe in Phil and Melba's bedroom together with all the payroll money for the employees of the mission hospital. I can only imagine how vulnerable Melba may have felt knowing the thieves had yet to claim their intended loot!

Malaria! This disease was experienced personally by many of the contributors to this book. It was also a major part of inpatient and outpatient medicine and one of the most frequent causes of death. The medical work relied heavily on nurses who worked alongside the physicians, including an exceptionally courageous and dedicated missionary nurse, Winifred (Winnie) Dodge, who helped Dr. Doug Corpron open the remote mission station in 1961. Her letters home capture the stamina and faith that was often demanded by the challenges she faced! In a single day she might home school her sons, train a nurse's aide, assist in surgery, host visitors from abroad, study one of the several languages used in the area, all while attending sick patients. Numerous times she had to take over the entire medical work when Dr. Corpron was away on trips. During her fourth pregnancy—while the Corprons were on furlough—she shouldered the medical work while uncertain who would be around to deliver her when her time came! She ended up delivering at home on the mission compound, assisted by a visiting missionary nurse-midwife.

Finding nurses and doctors willing to staff KRCH was a big challenge. So, it was an enormous blessing when Phil and his wife, Melba, committed to serving there. Thailand was always part of Phil's DNA. I have often wondered what our grandfather, Dr. Edwin Bruce McDaniel, would have thought if he could have known that one day both his son, Edwin Bailey McDaniel, and grandson, Philip McDaniel, would follow in his footsteps to become missionary physicians in the same country where he had served! In 1902 when Edwin and his wife, Ellen, stepped off the boat in Bangkok, the country still went by the name Siam. Their service was in the southern part of the country where they worked principally to help patients suffering with leprosy.

Our dad, the youngest of six children, came to the States for high school, college and medical school, and never ceased yearning for the day when he'd return to Siam to live and work among its people. Our mom, Charlotte, used to joke that he was more Thai than the Thai. After a lifetime of fulfilling work, notably in the area of family planning, he died in Chiang Mai in his early 80s. As Phil recounts, his medical career in Thailand overlapped with our dad's by almost 20 years and on many occasions, Dad came to KRCH to help out. Altogether, these three generations of our family form a century of service in Thailand.

The Kwai River Christian Hospital was the perfect fit for Phil's personality and skill set. He rose to the challenge of inadequate equipment by being resourcefully inventive. He met fatigue and relentless heat with perseverance. In the face of inadequate staffing and uncertain future funding, he prayed. He appreciated the local culture and was respectful towards the different ways people sometimes approached healing. His childhood gave him ease with the Thai language and he genuinely loved the lush hill country and rivers that surrounded the hospital. His 23 years of medical mission work reflect the gentle humility and steadfastness befitting a follower of Jesus.

Phil and I, along with our siblings, Ed and Julie, all attended a small mission school in Chiang Mai. Dr. Doug and Helen Corpron's son, Bill, lived in the boarding house and was one of my five classmates. Bill used to expound on the virtues of Yakima, Washington—the Stateside location the Corpron family called home. Apparently, his rhapsodizing sunk in, because many years later I moved to Yakima with my husband and our three children. One of the joys of living here has been the opportunity to connect with Doug (who has outlived Helen) whenever Phil and Melba come to visit. The two doctors have spent long hours swapping stories about the hospital—surgeries done by lantern light with flying termites falling into the operating field and the infamous operating table that gradually sank lower and lower as the operation proceeded. There is something gratifying about the doctor who founded the hospital being able to reminisce with the doctor who later picked up the work and poured his heart into the hospital for 23 years to keep it going, believing so strongly in its mission.

This compilation is a wonderful tribute to the pioneers who established the small hospital at the edge of the jungle. The bridges it has formed between different ethnicities and faiths are no less significant than the famous bridge that takes its name from the Kwai River. Sick and injured people with nowhere else to safely turn are still carried for hours by their friends, arriving in makeshift sarong slings between bamboo poles. No wonder displaced Karen soldiers lined up on an island in the river to salute Dr. Doug Corpron as he and his family passed by in their boat when heading to the States for the last time.

These memoirs are evidence of God's faithfulness in the midst of the mud, murders, malaria and other challenges that surrounded the first sixty years of a little mission hospital set into the same jungles that took the lives of thousands of POWs forced to build the Siam-Burma "Death" Railway a mere fifteen years before this story begins.

Carol McDaniel Licht, June 2020

Preface

"If we do not record the history of the early work there, the opportunity may be lost forever." That was the voice of Dr. Doug Corpron talking to me over the phone in the summer of 2018. Doug had had a similar conversation in a visit with Rev. Paul Dodge and wife, Winnie Dodge, RN a few months previously. Paul and Winnie (in February 1961) had been the very first missionaries to move onto the grounds of what would become the Kwai River Christian Mission (KRCM). Dr. Douglas Corpron and his wife, Helen, moved onto the grounds the following month. These two pioneering families oversaw the development of a ministry that ultimately included a hospital, a school, a boarding house, and an evangelistic program. Over the years, personnel from the USA, South Africa, Australia, the UK, Thailand, Burma, Japan, Norway, and Singapore have served at the Kwai River Christian Hospital (KRCH).

My time of service as director of the Kwai River Christian Hospital began in 1979 and continued for 23 years. Since my watch formed a bridge between the early days of KRCH and more recent times, I volunteered to put together something by way of a history. This has been done by collecting primary source material such as letters and contemporaneous documents and by asking several long-term former hospital personnel to record memories of their connection to the KRCH. The memoirs vary in length and style and subject matter. For some of the authors, English is a second or third language.

I have divided the book into three parts, not counting the appendix.

Part I includes background by Rev. Paul Dodge plus letters and memoirs of nurses, doctors, and a pharmacist.

Part II comprises memoirs by wives of former doctors. These portray the family life of expat personnel.

Part III uses old slides and photos to paint a picture of what it was like to work (or be a patient) at the Kwai River Christian Hospital in the first 60 years.

I hope these pages bring to life the hospital's purpose statement, "Serving the least on behalf of the Almighty."

Key to Spellings

Thai, Karen, Mon, Burmese, and Lao are languages spoken in the catchment area of the Kwai River Christian Hospital. Each of these languages uses a non-Roman script. Spelling the names of people and places using Roman (English) characters can be challenging. Proper names in this book sometimes contain sounds that are not encountered in English. There are systems for representing Thai sounds with Roman characters. Where there is no single Roman character to represent a given sound, a combination of letters might be employed. The "Royal Thai General System of Transcription" is the official system used by the Thai government for writing Thai words using Roman characters.

In some of the older letters and documents in this book, it appears that the authors improvised their own spellings of proper names. I have generally left these spellings "as is" to preserve the whimsical mishmash of do-it-yourself transliterations. In the 1960's and 1970's Sangkhlaburi District was still the "wild west" of Thailand and English spellings of proper names had not been widely standardized. Some spellings and alternative spellings used in this volume are listed below:

Chiang Mai (Chiengmai, Chiangmai)
Huay (Huai, Huey) as in "Huay Malai", the name of a village
Jewt (Jut, Jute), the name of a Mon patient and, later, employee
Kanburi (Ganburi) contraction for "Kanchanaburi"
Kanchanaburi (Kanjanaburi) a province; also, its principal city
Khwae (Kwae, Khwai, Kwai) Khwae Noi and Khwae Yai rivers
Nithe (Nikki), a village
Pwo (Poe, Po) a branch of the Karen ethnic group
Ranti (Ran Ti, Run Tee) a tributary of the Khwae Noi River
Sangkhlaburi (Sangklaburi) a district; also, its principal town
Sangkhla (Sangkla) contraction for "Sangkhlaburi"
Sgaw (Skaw) a branch of the Karen ethnic group
Sudah (Suda) first receptionist/translator at KRCH
Talako (Telakhon, Telacon, Telacone, Telecone, Telakho,
  Ta-la-kon, Ta-la-ku) a Karen religious sect
Thakhanun (Takanun, Takanoon) a town on the River Khwae Noi
Yakadee (Wiakadee)

A special word about the "River Kwai": There are two rivers Khwae: the Khwae Noi (small Khwae) and the Khwae Yai (large Khwae). The Thai name for these rivers was Anglicized (not very accurately) to "Kwai" many decades ago, and until the latter part of the 20th century seems to have been the most frequent spelling used. However, the spelling "Khwae" more closely represents the sound of the Thai word for these two rivers. Both rivers flow south and east from their origins in a mountainous region near the border with Myanmar. The Kwai River Christian Hospital was built on the north bank of the Ranti River, one of the tributaries of the Khwae Noi River. The famous "Bridge Over the River Kwai"—a railway bridge—crosses the River Khwae Yai in the city of Kanchanaburi. This bridge was part of the "Death Railway" (Siam-Burma Railway) built during World War II which—after crossing the Khwae Yai River—followed the Khwae Noi River up past Sangkhlaburi and then on into Burma. The Khwae Noi joins the Khwae Yai in the city of Kanchanaburi. The confluence of these two rivers is called the Mae Klong River.

"Karen" (pronounced ka-REN) refers to a large ethnic group found on both sides of the Thai-Myanmar border. Two major subgroups of Karen are Pwo (sounds like Poe) and Sgaw (sounds like Sa-gaw), each with its own dialect and manner of dress.

"Myanmar" and "Burma" are both used in this book to refer to the country immediately to the west of Thailand. While "Myanmar" is the official name, "Burma," the old name, is the one that was current at the time of many of the events described in this book. It is also the name used most frequently by ordinary folks in the rice fields and in the marketplaces of Sangkhlaburi District.

The authors of the letters and memoirs collected in this volume were born in six different countries, including South Africa and Australia, where British spelling and punctuation are the norm. In general, I have left spellings such as "oedema" and "anaesthesia" as written by the author even though these may look odd to some American readers. I have mostly used American conventions for punctuation.

Curved brackets ( ) generally contain clarifying information provided by the original author. Information in square brackets [ ] is generally supplemental information provided by the editor, Phil McDaniel.

Map of Thailand
(excluding the deep south)

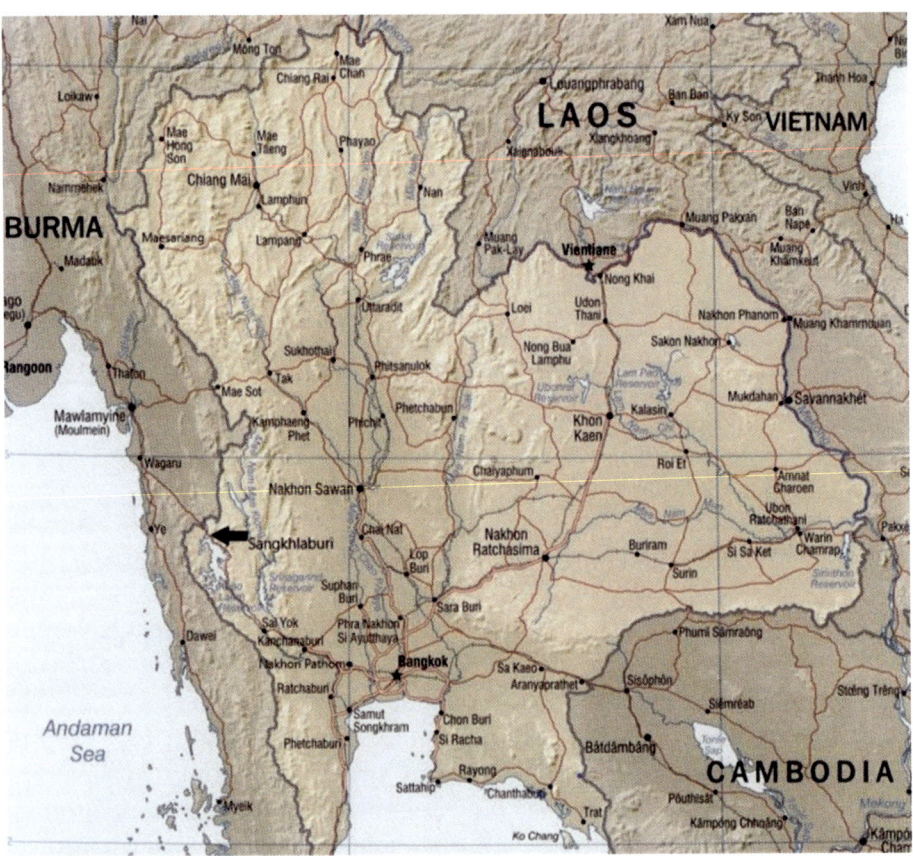

Physical Map of Thailand from "Free Maps of ASEAN Countries" at aseanup.com

Introduction

High fever, teeth-chattering chills, headache, body aches, nausea, vomiting, and cold sweats: these are symptoms typical of malaria. It can also cause seizures, coma, and death. I've often thought that if one was trying to design a disease that produced maximum misery, it would be difficult to come up with one much worse than malaria. Yet in the latter half of the 1900s (and probably for decades before), many of the villagers living in the valley of the River Kwai (River Khwae Noi) had suffered from malaria not just once or twice, but repeatedly. Other causes of misery in the valley of the Kwai were tuberculosis, leptospirosis, dysentery, trauma, and complications of pregnancy.

Prior to the 1980s there were no government hospitals in Sangkhlaburi district or the adjacent district of Thong Pha Phum (pronounced "Tong Pah Poom").

In the early 1960s pioneering missionaries founded a small hospital at the headwaters of the River Kwai and named it the Kwai River Christian Hospital. KRCH was welcomed not only by the villagers of Sangkhlaburi District and adjacent districts but also by patients brought across the border from Myanmar (Burma) for land mine injuries and gunshot wounds. The hospital eventually became a center for treatment of tuberculosis as well as a place patients could go for emergency and elective surgery.

By 1984 Sangkhlaburi District and Thong Pha Phum District each had a government hospital and there was a network of health stations in the villages. However, most of the surgery done in Sangkhlaburi District was still done at the Kwai River Christian Hospital (through 2019), and the hospital was the primary center for referral of refugees requiring more care than could be provided at the two nearby refugee camps.

There have been many mission hospitals in the world. Typically, these have started out as heroic efforts on a shoestring budget. Some have grown to be large teaching institutions. Others have dwindled to nothing for lack of funds, personnel, or equipment. Still others have been given over or taken over by national governments. Time will tell what the future holds for the Kwai River Christian Hospital, which is still functioning at the time of this writing despite a history of shortages of staffing and funding, two closures, and a major relocation.

1

Introduction

Regardless of how things unfold, an account of the humble beginnings of this hospital deserves to be captured in order to document and clarify the past, and hopefully inspire future generations.

This story of the Kwai River Christian Hospital is told in first person accounts by people who actually worked there.

Part 1

Letters and Memoirs of Early

Hospital Staff

Chapter 1

Early History of the Kwai River Christian Mission

By Rev. Paul Dodge

(With excerpts from the letters of wife, Winifred Dodge, RN)

About Paul and Winnie Dodge:

Paul's role at the Kwai River Christian Mission/Kwai River Christian Hospital was multifaceted. He was evangelist, bookkeeper, supervisor of construction, and general troubleshooter.

Winnie was head nurse, trainer of nurse's aides, wife, mother, and homeschool teacher.

Paul and Winnie were the first missionaries to move in at the original campus of the Kwai River Christian Mission.

Period of service for Dodges at KRCM/KRCH: Feb 1961 to June 1968

A Little Background (Prologue)

During the middle of the twentieth century the long-standing debate over mission strategy was heating up. A booklet authored by Earl H. Cressy titled "A Program of Advance for the Christian Movement in Thailand"[1] stressed the need for emphasizing the development of urban churches and Christian institutions. He was heard to say that while it certainly gave one a warm feeling to shake the hand of a tribal person who had become a fellow believer in Christ, the emphasis of Christian missions should focus on the dominant culture of a country rather than on the peripheral ones which had little influence and would eventually die out in the worldwide trend toward urbanization. At the same time, a revolutionary approach was drawing much attention. Its proponent was Dr. Donald McGavran, the professor of missiology at Fuller Theological Seminary and a member of the Disciples of Christ denomination, who published a book titled *The*

Bridges of God.[2] His thesis was that the Gospel spreads dramatically when missions identify and focus on "people movements"— ethnic/cultural groups which tend to adopt change as a group rather than as individuals—and he pointed out the great success of Baptist mission efforts in Burma with the Karen and other tribal cultures as one such example. Moreover, his analysis of the current situation led him to point out the Telakhon sect located in the no-man's-land deep in the jungle along the Thai-Burma border, about halfway between Mae Sod and the outpost of Sangkhlaburi on the Thai side.[3] He added a note of urgency as well, citing the inevitable rush toward the same urbanization which motivated Cressy's call for change, but with the warning that the opportunity would be lost forever if not acted upon soon. It appears that the United Christian Missionary Society (UCMS), which is the overseas mission agency of the Disciples of Christ (Christian Church) denomination, took McGavran's recommendation to heart. They already had some missionaries working in Thailand, working primarily with the Lao Song ethnic group near Nakorn Pathom and had a small hospital in that city. The UCMS leaders contacted the mission board of the American Baptists, whose missionaries had had enviable success with various ethnic peoples in Burma for a century and a half and who also had begun work with the Sgaw Karen who had filtered into northern Thailand in recent decades. The enthusiasm of the UCMS and the long experience of the American Baptists seemed like a logical and Spirit-led combination to explore. Furthermore, the proposal would require more financial undergirding and personnel than either mission could undertake alone, as the logistics of a full-orbed outreach in such a remote area would be significant. As a result, several exploratory trips to various Pwo Karen areas in northern and western Thailand and up the River Kwai by missionaries from both organizations took place in the 1950's.

Missionaries and Karen or Thai church leaders involved in some of these survey trips included: Carl M. Capen, American Baptist Mission (ABM) Secretary; Alfred Q. Van Benschoten, ABM; Thra Thinker, Karen colporteur (1953 trip to Sisawat and Na Suan).

Raymond W. Beaver, ABM, Burma; Aye Myat Kyaw and Mahn Knight, both of the Pwo Karen General Conference, Burma; and Addison Truxton and James Conklin, both ABM missionaries were members of the 1956 trip to areas other than Sangkhlaburi. Ray Beaver wrote "Report of the Survey of Five Pwo Karen Dialects of North Thailand, April–May 1956" which recommended that a simplified version of the script used by the Pwo Karens in Burma be developed for Thailand.

John Sams, Dr. H. T. Chen of the Nakhon Pathom Mission Hospital, Jose D. Estoye and Richard Carlson, both of UCMS were involved in the1956 survey to Sangkhlaburi. Dr. Chen was assured that a hard surface road would be built within 3 years and that food supply and security conditions were good! He also felt that "Buddhist influence is not strong in these parts."

Donald McGavran's "Report to the Board of Managers of the United Christian Missionary Society," September, 1956, after visiting Thailand & Burma, recommended that "There is more than a good chance if we could put a team of three missionary families and six Karen families from Burma into that area we would meet with a great response."

Carl Capen's report of a survey by him and John Sams, Jan. 31– Feb. 22, 1958, expressed his misgivings: "Insofar as the Sangkhlaburi area is concerned, I am inclined to doubt if there would be any general or large-scale response to the Gospel. One reason for my doubts is the Buddhist influence one observes wherever he goes. On the other hand, some remarks we heard would indicate that among these Karens the Buddhist religion does not go very deep."

The Feb. 12–23, 1959, trip included: Dr. Douglas O. Corpron; Dr. H. T. Chen; Victor McAnallen, UCMS; Cecil Carder, ABM; Khru Chamong, Carder's Thai language teacher; Taylor Potter, American Presbyterian Mission (APM) and CCT architect; Jose D. Estoye, UCCP/UCMS; Sra Po Sin, Pwo Karen preacher from Burma.

Their recommendations: (1) As soon as possible personnel to man the "Operation Sangkla" should be appointed… (2) … the buildings and compound should not bind personnel to the station. (3) As much as possible the work and establishments should be integrated into the CCT—maybe a separate Pahk (District) of the Church of Christ in Thailand.

It should be noted that both missions also had missionaries assigned to urban and ethnic Thai ministries, either in Bangkok (the American Baptists) or Chiang Mai (the UCMS' seminary professor) and Nakorn Pathom (the UCMS hospital, school, and church), so they did not view the strategies favored by Cressy and McGavran as being mutually exclusive.

The Sangkhlaburi region probably seemed most attractive because the offices of both missions were in Bangkok rather than in the north and also because the river, made famous by the World War II book and subsequent movie, "The Bridge on the River Kwai," was just a bit farther west from Nakhon Pathom, where the UCMS had established work. Also, Sangkhlaburi, located at the confluence of the three tributaries of the River Kwai [River Khwae Noi] and already about three days' travel by boat from Kanchanaburi was as far as practicable for establishing the mission. It was agreed by all that a medical component would be essential, both to minister to the severe health needs of this malaria-infested area and also to provide for the well-being of the missionary families and staff. Furthermore, it was assumed that married couples would be more likely to commit to long-term service—again, due to the isolation. Providentially, the UCMS already had a doctor (Douglas Corpron and his wife, Helen, a nutritionist, and their three young children) who was interested in the project. Doug had been raised in his early years in China, where his father, also a medical doctor, had founded a hospital which still exists. It is recognized with gratitude by the Chinese government, which has invited Doug or some of his children to be their guests on two occasions celebrating the work of the hospital. The Baptist mission board in turn soon provided a recently appointed couple (Rev. Paul and "Winnie" Dodge and their 2 small children) as the other part of the team. The fact that Winnie was a nurse with considerable experience was no doubt a key consideration, along with the fact that they had ministered in a remote part of Maine. Before long, both couples were involved in intensive Thai language study at the Union Language School in Bangkok. This was to continue almost 2 years.

During this time occasional further survey trips up the River Kwai were undertaken for the purpose of obtaining a suitable location for the mission station. Those taking part in the August 15–25, 1959 trip were Douglas Corpron, Jose Estoye and Victor McAnallen (all from UCMS) and Chester Galaska, Richard Gregory, and Paul Dodge (all from ABM). Eventually, a large site on the banks of the Ranti stream was recommended by Kamnan Thun Sa, the local headman, and was "purchased" for a nominal sum. Later on, we learned that it was available because it was an unofficial burying ground, which was thought by the local people to be haunted! Arrangements were made to have the site cleared of some of the brush and small trees while the two couples completed their Thai language study, which culminated in passing exams for both speaking and writing "proficiency"—which really meant "sufficiency." Doug and Winnie passed their exams for practicing medicine in Thailand (thankfully, these could be taken in English at that time) and Paul did extra study of Buddhism in the Thai language. Daily interactions with Thai people along with volunteer work in various mission enterprises, afforded opportunities for developing colloquial speaking ability. Association with fellow missionaries as well as orientation trips to observe established work provided a sense of being part of a support network. Supplies for the soon-to-come move had to be ordered and packed. Meanwhile, new babies were born in both families! Also occupying our attention was the need to draw up mutually-agreed-upon house plans and get them passed by the Property Committees of the missions. A Thai contractor from Kanchanaburi was recommended who was able to assemble a crew of 25 which was willing to commit to stay until the job was done (they were all "city boys") and the 2 homes, built of wood and elevated on cement posts in order to discourage snakes from easy access, were essentially completed in November of 1960. Furniture, canned goods, and most of our personal belongings were sent up by train and boat by the end of October on the last "rice barge" which could navigate the river before the water level dropped as the dry season began.

Moving in at Last!

Finally, on February 9, 1961, we boarded the 6:20 a.m. wood-burning train at the Thonburi station across the Chao Phraya River which divides that city from the much larger Bangkok. That was an adventure in itself, with hot cinders coming in the open windows now and then and the bustle of the food vendors in the towns where we stopped to pick up more passengers—sometimes along with chickens or other unusual baggage. Of course, we were the freakish standouts, with our three blond kids and all the personal stuff we were bringing with us! But the countryside was beautiful.

Rev. Paul Dodge

Paul, writing to his parents a few weeks after arrival at Sangkhla, reported:

> We arrived on Saturday, Feb. 11, travelling from Bangkok by train one day, boat one day, and our car [mission Land Rover] one day. Doug Corpron came with us to help with the move and stayed a few days unpacking some things and tending to some patients, then took the Land Rover back part-way and left it there, travelling on in a rented boat as far as the railroad. In Bangkok he will buy supplies, pack, etc., then bring his family to stay… We have had plenty of company. Three carpenters are still here finishing up odds and ends. This week we have had another crew of 5 come up to do the wiring and plumbing. I am writing by electric light (we have a generator), but the water is still not pumping… We will continue to bathe in the stream in front of the house and boil the water for drinking. We got the water tower up today and three 400-gallon water tanks set up on it.

The letter didn't mention that the carpenters were sleeping in what was intended to be the boys' bedroom, separated from ours by a partition! We were in a "camping" mode for quite a while, as the 32 boxes of belongings and supplies which we had brought on the train were stuck at the railhead, waiting for a truck to pick them up. The boys, naturally, thought it was a lot of fun getting rides on the elephants which were occasionally routed through our front yard, as well as seeing lots of wildlife right on our property and along the river when we traveled by boat.

Within a month, the Corpron family arrived, and that very evening a Mon man was brought to Doug to see if his life could be saved. He and his friends had been dynamiting for fish (strictly illegal) in another tributary of the Kwai River and a stick of dynamite blew up in his hands, sending his finger bones like shrapnel into his face and chest. He was not only blinded but was barely conscious due to pain and loss of blood. Doug agreed to do his best, unpacked his surgical equipment, and we set up an "operating room" in the storage area on the ground floor of the Corpron house. A work bench was the operating table. Helen Corpron and Paul had to check blood pressure and give transfusions and shots while Winnie assisted Doug in amputating both lower arms and patching him up as much as they could. We all worked on him until 6 a.m. but to no avail. He died the next afternoon, leaving a wife and five children. We wondered if losing this first big case would have an adverse effect on our acceptance by the people in the area, but his wife and neighbors were grateful that such an all-out attempt had been made on a hopeless case. People began coming in increasing numbers—up to 30 or 40 a day—to the small clinic building near the Corpron home with complaints ranging from sore throats to leprosy. Both families were settled in, the well was dug deeper, and the houses had running water. Helpers were hired to take care of the children and do household tasks and gardening, and we began making acquaintances in the area. The mission was underway!

Beginning Stages

A routine was not easily reached, though, especially for the Dodges, as within a few weeks two mission secretaries[4] from the Baptist headquarters in New York came to see the new work. Winnie wrote that Paul had to take them back to Bangkok and then stay for 3 days of Executive Committee meetings; so, she decided to take the boys, too. "It had rained in one section and what normally would have taken 7 hours took 19 hours instead. ... Land Rovers can really take it!" That was just a warm-up for their return trip, which took 8 days! She writes:

We left Bangkok Sunday a.m. and drove a packed Land Rover to

Ganburi [Kanchanaburi] (125 kilometers), planning to put the car

on a railroad flat car but because we had sent a telegram and not

signed the order in person, it wasn't there and we would have to wait 4 days for one! We checked with our mining friend there and found [that] 2 trucks were leaving Tuesday, so we decided to wait and drive all the way with them... Tuesday noon we left for Tha Sao, a 3 to 5 hour drive, but due to rain we spent the night in the jungle and didn't arrive until 4:30 p.m. the next day!!! [Note by Paul: That was the night when we got stuck in the mud and the guide hooked the winch onto a tree. The car lights did not reveal that it was a dead tree—a post, really. It fell onto the car just inches from the windshield and left a permanent dent in the fender. A close call!] Thursday, we started for Thakanun, a 7 to 11-hour drive, but 1/3 of the way there our fan belt broke!! Luckily, we were near a brook and 2 homes, which took us in for the 2 days we waited while our guide walked back to Ganburi for a new one! Saturday p.m. he got back, and we left immediately for Thakanun. We got into Thungna (1/2 way) at 10:30 p.m. Sunday a.m. We left for Thakanun and arrived at 1:45 p.m....and treated a little girl for facial cuts. Left at 4:30 p.m. for Sangkhla and arrived at 10:30 p.m., all tired but well!!![5] We've all gained back weight we lost.

The same letter, dated April 29, 1961 reports:

Yesterday Doug and I did gastric surgery on a 21-yr. old boy with a duodenal ulcer. Paul had to take the B.P. and give Pentothal, so he'll soon be a medical pro too!! We removed his Levine tube [nasogastric tube] today and he's doing very well. Had a little better set up in the clinic this time. Gave him a spinal. It's hard to do surgery with only a doctor and nurse!" (Note by Paul: This, of course, was Jewt, the "Jut" mentioned in Winnie's other letters.)

Not all the patients were local people, however. In a May 1961, newsletter Paul remarked:

As I write this, "Winnie" is over at the Corpron house helping Doug (who is a doctor) deliver Helen's fifth baby. It is 4 a.m.; the sound of our electric light generator will tell people in the nearby villages that something unusual is going on, and they may think it is another emergency case such as the one we operated on all night several weeks ago.

Another excerpt explains the pressure which the approaching rainy season put on our daily activities, not to mention the traveling conditions:

Right now, we are hurrying to stockpile sand and gravel before the river rises, so that in a few months we can begin the construction of the hospital and the hostel for students from outlying villages. We have about a dozen workmen doing this, but they need almost constant supervision.

Recruiting nurses posed a real challenge due to the remoteness and the lawless reputation of the area and its proximity to Burma. In June [1961] John Sams brought a Thai nurse for a three-day visit in hopes that she would augment the two-person medical team, but comments in one of Winnie's letters reveal both disappointment and resignation:

I'm afraid that the R.N. they brought up with the hopes of staying, even though a dedicated Christian, thinks this is a little too remote for her. They had kinda (sic) a hard time coming up. Lots of rain and the water is very swift now. If she wouldn't be happy, she shouldn't stay.

In August of 1961 the Corprons were on a well-earned vacation. Winnie wrote:

Our boatman is going down to meet Dick Worley & "Andy" Yousko and their 2 sons plus 2 Chinese Christians who will be visiting us for 2 ½ days before we go on vacation and mission business meeting. It's been fairly busy with meeting the medical needs and Paul trying to get land cleared and sites chosen so construction of hospital and hostel can begin next month. The boys now have a gibbon monkey ('Honey,' 6 months old) and so they haven't minded the absence of the Corpron children so much. Go with me on calls, too.

The "2 ½ day visit" extended for several more days as the rains were incessant, and the river became very treacherous. Samuel Kho was anxious to get back for business reasons as well as to allay his wife Shirley's fears; so, finally we were able to get a ride on a rice barge which was being towed by a boat with a powerful inboard motor. We all slept as best we could on the rice, but we marveled at the large whirlpools which threatened to cause the boat to lose control. The most impressive sight was the submerged railroad trestle which usually was high above the river level. The train tracks were right at water level! It should be noted that Andy Yousko opted to walk north from Sangkhla with a guide, emerging at Mae Sod a week or so later. His son must have gone with him. The next letter of note is dated Nov. 10, 1961:

We've had 4 fellows visiting us the past 4 days and it's been busy[6]... Paul is very behind on his treasury books... [Construction on] the hospital and hostel is in full progress now… Our piano is stuck at Thakanun till we can get a small boat down to pick it up, as the water has dropped too much for big boats to come up now. Hope we get it soon!

From a September 30, 1961 letter by Winnie to Paul's parents:

Here we have 3 cases of polio!!! Doug has to go back down to Ganburi [Kanchanaburi] Monday to testify at a trial of murder! [Note by Paul: I think that this was the time when Doug nearly drowned on the return trip; Doug can fill in the details.] Paul has been out 2 or 3 times this week on short trips preaching… Last night an elephant got loose while grazing and smashed our fence in 4 places!!!

During 1961 Doug hired Suda Yawan, a local Pwo Karen daughter of a headman and sister of Jit [and Chatree] Yawan, to be receptionist and translator at the little clinic building and later, in the hospital. He also trained Surin—a Mon who had studied in Burma—to do basic lab tests. Several years later, Surin opened a pharmacy in the new Amphur [district seat]. His daughter operates the pharmacy and his son became manager of a local bank. Winnie trained Tryphena Pan, an educated Karen from Burma—and later her sister—to be excellent nurses.

From Paul's Christmas newsletter [late 1961]:

They just left the house a while ago—twelve young adults from this area who are now coming every Sunday in order to learn more about Christ. None of them has made a decision yet: a "decision for Christ" involves a lot more for them than it does for someone in a "Christian" environment. A quick decision might be just as quickly renounced in the face of opposition... But we are grateful for their recent surge of interest, which was sparked by the visit of a very enthusiastic young man who is a recent convert from Buddhism. Peerun has visited several villages in the area, and his straightforward testimony has made quite an impact. We are hoping that he can come and work with us on a regular basis.

We have been studying the Mon language under the tutelage of a young man who owes his life to a stomach operation performed by Dr. Doug Corpron … Now we are beginning to study Karen, the principal native language here. [7]

Blueprints for the hospital and youth hostel have been finished; most of the cement and other materials have been brought up the River Kwai by boat; the logs have been dragged in from the jungle by elephants and will soon be hand-sawn into boards. So, before long we will see more of our dreams become a reality.

From Winnie's December 24, 1961 letter to Paul's parents:

The station had "Open House" last night for the area, and we had 400 to 500 people out to see the mission children portray the Christmas story. Olivepa's wife and 2 daughters sang 2 Christmas carols, then a Thai and Mon group did their tribal dances, and on our new Kodak 16 mm sound projector we showed films in the Thai language (2 religious films, 2 public health, and 2 agricultural). Served Thai and American sweets and Kool-Aid, and many—no, most—saw and heard the Christmas story for the first time in their lives.

Had 25 at our service this morning and 35 last week.

February 8,1962:

Movies tomorrow night again. Average about 200 weekly for them!

Rev. Paul Dodge

A Year of Transition

January 22, 1962, Winnie to Paul's parents:

> Paul has had a cold since his return from Bangkok and this Saturday he leaves again for Karen convention at Musikee, a 3 day walk from Baw Gow in N. Thailand. So, I'll be w/o a husband for 2-3 weeks again!! … Guess I miss regular mail service the most living up here.

February 8, 1962, Winnie to Paul's parents:

> Hostel now has the floors ½ completed and the hospital its mud-cement walls nearly completed, but nearly daily the contractor finds some material they haven't sent enough of, so that's why this quick letter as our boat has to make a trip to Ganburi for reinforcing steel tomorrow and I want to send this with them.

April 5, 1962, Winnie to Paul's parents:

> We have a 12-day old Karen baby and mother staying with us. He developed Tetanus 2 days ago because they cut the cord w/ a dirty piece of bamboo!! He's nearly "over the hump" but still has convulsions and needs gavage feedings.

[Many years later when the Dodges visited KRCM in retirement, the mother introduced her now-grown son to Winnie—a heart-warming experience, as surviving neonatal tetanus under those conditions was a rarity.]

Early History

May 3, 1962, Winnie to Paul's parents:

Next Sunday we are having our first baptism of 3 young men, and there are 3 more young men who, in another 2-3 months, should be ready, too. ... Daily we could use our X-ray machine if we had one. ... In about 9 weeks we will go on vacation and as Dr. Corpron & family fly July 16th for furlough I will carry the medical load. We are hoping to get a nurse or two to help out.

May 1962 newsletter by Paul:

Many villagers are hoping that we will establish a mission school, even though our schooling would cost more. The mission and the CCT are currently studying the matter. ... Our need for another doctor will not end when Doug returns from furlough, for we found that one doctor cannot handle the load locally and get out into the hills, too, and that is really our biggest objective.

May 18, 1962, Winnie to Paul's parents:

The Corprons definitely leave July 16th by air for U.S. and just had a very hard trip returning from vacation—in fact, Doug still hasn't got back as one boat hit a log and now is being repaired. They brought 3 nurses from India who are on vacation, so we have 2 of them staying with us and will be going on sick calls w/ me this afternoon. ... No word yet on any nurse willing to come up and work here, so please pray very soon one may be challenged to. Two boys, learning a language, and doctoring around the clock is just too much for one woman. ... Well, it's been very busy this past month and somehow the Lord has given knowledge and healing, though one little 5-year-old girl died with cerebral malaria.

August 9, 1962, Winnie to Paul's parents while on vacation at Cha-am: "My, how we've enjoyed the variety of fresh fruits and vegetables!"

August 29, 1962, Winnie to her Mom from Bangkok: "We are all fine and anxious to get back to cool Sangkla. Shall travel on Sept. 4th by rice barge, which probably will mean 5 days!"

September 1962, Winnie to her Mom:

It took us 5 days (4 on the rice barge) and I don't think we'll do it again, as too long in such crowded conditions. … Today we slaughtered our last pig, so will have to buy more soon. … The hostel is nearly completed now, and the hospital's 2nd layer of floor cement & paint will complete it except for cupboards. … I'm sending Jut, our young Christian convert whom we did surgery on over a year ago, to Bangkok as he's had another bout of abdominal pain and vomiting.

October 21, 1962, Winnie to Paul's parents:

We are fine, and since last writing 11 U.S. troops came here on a "good-will" visit and we enjoyed them for 2 days. They were young and shocked to find Americans "way out here in the jungle." Seemed to relish the home cookin'. … Two elephants have arrived to haul logs for the building where patients' families will stay. … The rumor is that Nov. 9th a group of U.N. people (10-40 people) will come up to see the Burma border. I've already informed the mayor that I cannot prepare food for them as we will have 3 to 6 visitors ourselves then, as Paul plans to leave on his 4–5-week elephant trip to the Telacon people then.

October 9, 1962, Winnie to her Mom: "Our piano arrived in perfect condition. How I've enjoyed it!"

October 9, 1962, Winnie to Paul's parents:

As I write, Paul has gone to check on wood we purchased. The elephants are arriving to take the fellows on their 4–5-week trip to Umphang beginning Nov. 17th and can carry it here. I'm not sure who will be staying here with me. ... This past week 9 SEATO [Southeast Asia Treaty Organization] officials from Bangkok were here with us. ... Another group of U.N. or something are coming up next week, but doubt if we will see much of them as we will have our own company. I've been busy delivering babies. Had 4 since our return and 3 more due any day.

November 3, 1962, Winnie to her Mom:

Paul got away on his trip the 15th and I've been "holding the fort." ... Really didn't try to celebrate yesterday on Thanksgiving, though did have a can of cranberry sauce opened special. Will make up for it Christmas when Paul is here to celebrate. Supposed to arrive Dec. 15th. ... Jut survived his gastric resection alright but the 19th had an intestinal blockage that required surgery again. He went into shock and though some better the next day, he was having to have special nurses, etc., and I haven't heard since. Pray for him! Our "hoped-for" doctor can't come, as 3 of his 4 older girls have contacted TB!!![8] [Editor's note: It is unclear at this late date what was meant here by "contacted TB": Did the girls have laboratory or x-ray evidence of active TB? That is, had they "contracted TB," or had they merely "had contact with" a known case of TB (with or without skin test conversion)? In any case, the event was of great enough concern to the "hoped-for doctor" to prevent him from coming to help out.]

I'm hoping we can find at least one nurse when we go to Bangkok in January. Yes, the boys are in school—Sherwood 2nd and Glen ready for 1st. … We will be going to Bangkok the day after Christmas, as Conference is in Chiang Mai… Dec. 31st. Not sure yet where this baby will be born. … The hospital and hostel will be finished when you receive this. Just now I have a 24-year-old fellow who was struck by a huge limb, probably breaking his spine, as he's unable to use legs, bowels or bladder. (No X-ray yet!!)

December 15, 1962, Winnie to her Mom:

Just a note to let you know Paul arrived home safe & sound last night about 6:15 p.m. They were unable to convert the Telecon on this trip but felt there were wonderful possibilities and were invited to return in March. … They had a hard time finding elephants to come back by and wanted to see Dr. West (the U.S. Sec. of the Disciples) and Dick Carlson (Field Sec.) who have been here 4 days, so walked all day yesterday the distance it takes 2 days for an elephant to go. Paul lost quite a bit of weight, otherwise is fine.

December 17th (same letter):

Yesterday morning at 9:45 Dr. West, Dick Carlson, and Allan Eubank went back [home], and about 1 ½ hours later in walked Thom, the Karen Baptist Christian (1st Karen university student in Thailand). He hoped to arrive in time to meet them and return to Bangkok. Olivepa and the rest arrived in evening by elephant. All fine. … There will be no medical help here, so that complicates my delivery, etc.

December 17, 1962, Winnie to Paul's parents: "The X-ray installers will be here about the 21st."

January 6, 1963, Winnie to her Mom, from Chiang Mai: "Jewt looked very well when we saw him last week but just today had word he may have to have more surgery."

February 8, 1963, Winnie to her Mom, from Sangkhla:

Jewt is back here and doing pretty well, tho' has had some abdominal pain the last few days. Glen has the chicken pox, just as Sherwood & Forrest did 2 weeks ago. … My cook has gone to the city, so that means added work, and our hospital wash girl quit! Paul gave the generator its bi-yearly cleaning, so we were w/o running water & electricity. … Yes, I've been quite busy medically w/ pneumonia cases (4 since return) and then yesterday had to sew up a Mon man who was hit in the head with the blunt end of a machete by a crazy guy. Paul's considering visiting the Telacon the first week of March if our Baptist nurse can be with me. ... The Land Rover is down in Bangkok being registered and fixed! We moved the "clinic" into the hospital on Feb. 4th, tho' none of our sink drains are finished yet. ... Yes, the boys are back at school and we at Karen language study, too!

Paul has gone to Three Pagodas Pass hunting tonight via Border Patrol helicopter, so I'm alone with the boys. A group of 8 Americans came and wanted him to go, too. [9]

February 15, 1963, Winnie to Paul's parents:

I've no cook now (husband transferred) so things are mighty busy! Guess the 20th a nurse (American Baptist missionary) [10] will join me while Paul goes to visit the Telecone again. ... The boys are all over the Chicken Pox and apparently had no complications. ... Our clinic has been in the hospital since Feb. 4th, so things are more spacious, though hospital isn't finished yet."

Early History

April 9, 1963 Winnie to Paul's parents:

Want to get a letter written today, as the Border Patrol helicopter comes tomorrow and want to send this along. It would be nice if I delivered today so the news could go out tomorrow, but I feel fine and the baby isn't due till the 15th and I'm usually late, sooooo!

Well, the helicopter came today, so this won't get out as fast as I had hoped. Did get to send out Sherwood's test; hope we can finish second grade. However, he still has 60 more lessons. Paul has been sick with a virus this week but is much better today. We just hope that none of the rest of us get it! ... Paul had hoped to baptize Jewt and Surin on Easter but if he doesn't hurry up and get better, he won't be able to. We have had 30 to 35 out the past few weeks. Do wish they could find a replacement for us so the evangelistic work could progress this next year, too, but it looks quite doubtful!! ... Tiger's six puppies are so cute! Don't know what the boys will do when we begin to give them away. "Barkie", our deer, now has long horns but still loves to go swimming with us.

April 29, 1963, Paul to his parents:

I'll scribble off this note to tell you that our 4th boy arrived safely on April 26—10:10 a.m. He weighed in at 8 lbs., 10 oz., and says his name is Brooks Alton. Winnie was in labor all night but didn't have too bad a time. Esther Greenmun is a good midwife and had the situation well under control. Winnie feels good but is still resting, of course. Esther will return to Chiang Mai in a week or so. I'm the only unhealthy one—had flu (or something like it) for the last 3 weeks. I tried to get up too early and had a first-class relapse. Lost 10 lbs. (It will take me the rest of my life to get it back!) I'm just starting to get back into circulation now."

From May 1963 newsletter:

The Telakhon people have been visited twice in the last several months by Paul and some others. The first trip took a full month, and the second one just half that time. A different missionary friend accompanied Paul on each trip and Olivepa, our Karen Christian worker, made both trips in order to help with translating. … The Telakhon people, you may recall, are a Karen religious sect who long have been looking for the arrival of "the white brother." They live in a very inaccessible part of the jungle, surrounded by mountains, so we have been unable to visit them before this. The most direct route we have found so far takes 5 days from Sangkhlaburi, traveling generally northward. ... These people are trying to lead the Karens back to their traditional belief in a creator God. Their ancient legends also tell of a lost "Golden Book of Eternal Life" which "the white brother" would someday bring back to them. Of course, many Karens in Burma have long since become Christians, feeling that the missionaries' Bible is "the lost book," but for the most part, these old legends are now forgotten and are no longer much of a factor in causing people to become Christians. … But as we traveled to the home of the Telakhon chief, our imaginations were stirred by the possibility of a group of 6 or 7,000 people deciding "en masse" to become Christians! However, we found that it will not be that easy! The chief and his closest disciples listened attentively to all we had to say and agreed with us at many points. But they did not feel that the Bible is "the Lost Book," because, they said, that will be a magic book which can be read by all Karens, no matter what the dialect, and regardless of the fact that they may be illiterate!

Furthermore, they could not understand why we made Christ the focal point of our teaching. "The Telakhon believe in one God and have a good moral code—is not that enough?" (We didn't tell them how often we have heard that viewpoint!) We explained that we would know nothing about God except for Christ, and that the world lacks not moral codes but people who are motivated by the love of God, which makes the struggle to live up to a moral code unnecessary. We also described the role of Christ in making salvation possible for all men.

Space does not allow us to describe our conversations in any detail, although sometimes we traveled for two days without seeing anyone. We feel that eventually many of these people will turn to Christ, but we must be prepared to wait anywhere from two to ten years.

Rev. Paul Dodge

May 6, 1963, Winnie to Paul's parents:

Do want to get a line off to you to let you know we are all fine and "back in the work groove again." Brooks is a "9 day old" today and is a grand baby. … We probably will leave here for Bangkok July 2nd, as it is quite a process to leave and we have vacation time coming to us, so feel we need it most as we prepare to go. I've done some sorting and packing but have loads yet to do!

June 27, 1963, Winnie to Paul's parents (from Bangkok):

Well, lots of water has "gone over the dam" since I last wrote. I'll only say I'm glad those days are over! I guess the best way to explain what I mean is by beginning on June 11th. Brooks had a coughing spell about suppertime, and I thought he had swallowed some fuzz. The other 3 boys had severe colds and coughs, but Brooks hadn't had any runny nose, so I was quite surprised when the next morning he had lots of nasal congestion and proceeded to have a severe coughing siege which frightened me. I gave him Penn Strep and sulfa and Benzoin inhalations, as he was very lethargic, cold and cyanotic. That evening he had another attack of coughing, so we brought over the electric suction and oxygen. We used nose drops and had 2 hour watches all night. The next day, Friday, he seemed improved but in the late afternoon he went into a deep sleep with gasping breathing and so I said we had better call for the helicopter, as I was concerned!! Paul had the Border Patrol wire for a helicopter, and we began packing in earnest! We knew SEATO was having maneuvers and, too, the telegram could very well not get through. Saturday Brooks was improved so we wired them not to hurry. (This they never got!) Sunday at 9 a.m. the helicopter arrived and at 10 we left and (as it was a new jet one) we were in Bangkok at 12 noon. Even though Brooks was better we came anyway as Paul still felt punk and Brooks had an umbilical skin tab to be removed and a circumcision to be done.

June 6, 1964, Winnie to her Mom, after furlough year:

Today had a potluck dinner after church; wasn't a bad turnout. I'm back studying written and spoken Pwo Karen for 2 hours each day and also teaching my Thai nurse aides 1 hr. a day. The boys study each day and should be finished this month. They enjoy the competition at Thai school. … It's good not to have the total medical load now that Doug and Helen are back. … Paul's teaching English to the 2 Thai teachers and Tryphena, so he's busy, too.

July 26,1964, Winnie to Paul's parents (from Bangkok):

Went to S.S. and church in p.m., then supper "out" with the Dr. Hurlburts (not going to Sangkla but back to the U.S. Public Health Service in Saigon, Vietnam).

September 14, 1964, Winnie to Paul's parents:

The rain came last night and brought the river up some, which means maybe we can get our diesel gas all the way up! We hope you had a nice 40th anniversary.

Rev. Paul Dodge

September 29, 1964, Winnie to Paul's parents:

Tonight, we had the Thai nurse over for supper. She is the first of the Royal King's family to become a Christian and I guess the pressure is quite great. She is a good nurse and is very sweet and retiring. Our floods have now receded, and this Saturday our Mission Secretary, Cecil Carder, and the Disciples' Secretary will come for a visit. … Paul has the Trail breaker bikes going now, so imagine he will be "on the road" as soon as the rains cease. … We've really enjoyed S. School with the Baptist and Disciples literature. Helen teaches Forrest, Pam, and Dan, and I teach Sherwood, Glen, and Cathy. (Paul's note: the Thai nurse's name was Peaprom, but I forget the "nam sakul" [surname]—one which impressed the mailman when he saw it.)

From Paul's Newsletter # 10:

We have been back in Thailand since July 11 and back on the station since Aug. 8. We made the usual three-day trip in one day, thanks to the fast "jet" boat which our co-worker, Dr. Doug Corpron, brought back with him from furlough last year. We arrived on a Saturday evening and were greeted by the workers and by the ten boarding students who live in the hostel, which was completed just before our furlough. The kindergarten has been open four months and has more than twenty day-students in addition to the boarders.

October 10, 1964, Winnie to her Mother & brother:

> This is overdue but it has been go, go, go! Our company arrived Monday evening and then left Thursday a.m.... Paul went down for a week with our Secretary, Cecil Carder, to get permission to open the school (1st grade) next April, so I'm alone with 3 boys with colds. Sherwood went down, too, to "try out" city schools but won't go until January.

October 27, 1964, Winnie to her mother & brother:

> Saturday worked at the hospital as usual. Sunday had S.S. for older missionary children, and Thai service at 11 a.m. with 60 present. In p.m. Paul counseled with a Thai TB patient (been here 2 ½ months) who has been reading the NT [New Testament] and now the whole Bible, and he accepted Christ! Please pray for Mr. Chum. His lung damage is extensive. ... It is real hot, as October can sometimes be. Our corn is about 6" high, and beans, too. Have already planted a second corn. ... Paul is out making a railroad tie fence at the boarding school today. [These railroad ties (also called "sleepers") were from the bed of the abandoned "Death Railway," a short walk from the Kwai River Christian Mission.]

November 20, 1964, Winnie to her mother & brother:

> Just now Paul is off on a 3-day evangelism trip. He has with him a Dr. Stern (anthropologist from Washington state) who is studying our Karens. They hope to do a little hunting, too. The school should get registration by April, they promise us.

Rev. Paul Dodge

November 29, 1964, Winnie to her mother & brother:

I can't imagine why you haven't received our letters!! I've written nearly every week. However, they [the letters] can only go down when a boat does! Those have been few and far between this fall… We will be going to Bangkok the day after Christmas for Conference. It is at Bangsaen on the ocean (where the Worleys work). Our Thai nurse has a two-week vacation on our return to Sangkhla, sooo—plus the fact that 8 W.H.O. Thai fellows are coming up to work on 2 diseases, Filariasis and Scrub Typhus! Busy, busy!

March 1, 1965, Winnie to Paul's parents:

The 10th of March we plan to leave on the Telacon trip (till the 27th)—Paul, S.P. [Sherwood Perry, oldest son] and Glen and I, so I must begin to get things together. A Doc is coming from Chiengmai to cover for Doug so he can go. [This was Ed McDaniel, Phil's dad. Phil's mom, Charlotte, also came on that trip and taught kindergarten to the younger missionary kids.] There will be seven elephants. … Paul baptized Somboon a week ago yesterday and then went for 2 days to his village this week. Tomorrow he is going to below Thakanun, as on his return from Bangkok the jet boat broke down. So, they are going to fix it and do an evangelistic survey of the area at the same time.

Early History

March 1, 1965, Winnie to her mother & brother:

> The boys all had the mumps while Paul was gone, which is good timing. … We had one of the anthropologists and his interpreter over for Sunday dinner yesterday.

March 25, 1965, Winnie to her mother & brother:

> We got in last night from our "trip to the Telacone." Sherwood & Glen went with us, and Forrest and Brooks stayed with the doctor's wife, Helen. The doctor relieving Doug goes tomorrow, so I'll not get to give you all the details, as it is now 11:30 p.m.! The first day we went by Land Rover over the new mining road to an old camp site where we had to get out and walk, as it had rained the day before and the trucks couldn't go any farther, they said. … Paul and Doug and Dr. Stern (anthropologist) had gone the day before (wanted to climb the biggest mountain and still there out hunting). The elephants arrived and took the boys, OlivePa and boxes, etc., and we hiked four hours into Metherng. The next day was a short one via elephant (picked up 2 more elephants at Metherng) to Thi Lai Pa and there washed clothes, swam and taught the elephant men English. The next day was a beautiful trip through real picturesque jungle areas with yellow, pink, red, violet and white orchids growing wild in the jungle. The elephant boys cut them and put them in their hair or gave them to me. The next day we travelled all day and slept in the jungle with fires. The last day we travelled through Burma and arrived at Ti Mau about 4:30 p.m. They greeted us like "lost brothers." … I have stacks of mail to

read yet, but we have 17 patients (supposed to have only 10), so I haven't had time to read the rest, only yours. Your pkg, is in Kanburi and Paul will get it when he goes to Bangkok April 10 for meetings.

March 29, 1965, Winnie to Paul's grandmother:

We all arrived home safely on the 24th & 25th... It was an excellent trip and we were well received. How we praise God for the baptism of a Telacone man whom Paul met on his 1st visit and gave God's Word to. He read it and believed!!! He's also a leader of 10 families in Burma and now he will lead them, too, to know our precious Savior!!! ... The Chief of the Telacone again refused Christianity but his followers are most interested.

Early History

April 14, 1965, Paul to his Grandma:

I have been in Bangkok several days and am on my way back to Sangkhla. I recall that your birthday is this month, so I'll try to finish this and get it in the mail before I start upriver. I'm always glad to get out of the rush of Bangkok life and get back on the peaceful river. As usual, I'm taking back some fresh fruits and vegetables and medical supplies, and this trip I have to take some bottled gas, too (four 110 lb. bottles) as ours is running out. We brought a Gas stove back with us, you remember, and we really enjoy it as compared to kerosene… Right now, I am sitting in a crowded train, waiting for it to leave the little station. We are at the town of Kanjanaburi, which is our state capital, and is the place where 14,000 Allied prisoners of war are buried. They died putting in the railway which the Japanese built from Thailand to Burma. It used to run by Sangkhla, but now only this lower half is used. That is why we switch to boats or jeeps for the last part of the trip. This time of the year we go as far as Takanun, the county seat, by boat and take the jeep the rest of the way. If all goes well, I should be home by tomorrow night, in time to get ready for a service on Good Friday. There have been 2 baptisms in Sangkhla in the past few months, so we are quite encouraged.

Rev. Paul Dodge

April 21, 1965, Winnie to Paul's parents:

Well, things are busy, busy here! Just now we have a group of 9 young Christians from a village not far from Bangkok who are going to help in evangelism and build a TB unit for us. Our hospital has 14 patients and some very sick ones as well as 3 dope addicts in for rehabilitation!! Doug (our Dr.) goes on a 5-week vacation tomorrow, so yours truly will be in charge. … Everyone here is quite well now. Paul had a bout of amoeba while in Bangkok but okay now. Had a nice Easter… Good Friday we had no special celebration, as Paul wasn't back yet.

May 11, 1965, Winnie to Paul's parents:

Our patient load has dropped to 8 for the first time in 5 months, and it came at "the right time" as my aide has had to go to Burma, as her grandmother is very ill. We are thankful that Olive Pa's daughter, Olive, came home, so I'm training her… Our work camp built the rest home for our T.B. patients, and also our Karen cook has come to know Christ mainly from their ministry, so we are most thankful! … Our 2 school teachers arrived last week, and school will begin on the 17th… They are both nice Christian Thai young men—Phiphat and Duang Dee.

Paul's Christmas newsletter, written in October 1965:

With both Dr. Corpron and a Thai nurse on the station most of the time now, Winnie's work load will be considerably lighter than it has been at times in the past, although teaching Glen and Forrest, in addition to being responsible for some of the administration of our ten-bed hospital, promises to keep her occupied. Paul keeps busy with local teaching and preaching, station maintenance, village evangelism, and business trips, interspersed with language study and office work. We are all in good health and are hopefully looking forward to an expansion of our program in the coming months. We are especially desirous of finding the resources for building and staffing a Christian Witness Center in the heart of our town, and of reaching into the outlying villages with a combination literacy, evangelism, and medical program.

December 8, 1965, Winnie to her mother & brother:

Helen may get a ride down by helicopter today, so I'll hurry and get this off. Everyone is fine here and now our Thai nurse has left us again the days are more than busy. Sherwood will get home about the 20th and we are hoping we will have some time to enjoy him this time. Thanksgiving was mostly entertaining. ... Paul is off via Trailbreaker to visit south of us where there's a Christian family. We were invited to eat with some Burmese men who have fled from Burma for political reasons. ... Had a note from our Telakhon Christian who spoke of poverty and food shortage there.

Rev. Paul Dodge

December 30, 1965, Winnie to her mother:

Arrived home with Helen & brother. Sherwood and the 2 Corpron boys arrived home with Helen on the 21st (Tues.) and were 24 hours late due to motor trouble. On Wed. morning we did surgery (hydrocele) and in the afternoon a hemorrhoidectomy, then in the evening we went to the Christmas pageant put on by our Bible woman in Netate village (10-minute walk). Glen was Zaccheus and Forrest, Joseph (with his coat of many colors), and Sherwood was a wise man. They all performed very well and there was a local dance team to do a folk dance afterward, so it was 10:30 + before we arrived home. The next day we had a sports program in the afternoon put on by the teachers here; then in the evening we had a community program with a creche scene, religious and secular (Thai-USIS) movies and a traditional folk dancing group. I served 56 dancers with cookies and Kool-Aid. The morning of the 24th I made creampuffs…wrapped gifts, and in the afternoon went to the hospital as usual. … Christmas night we had the annual Mission pitch-in dinner here. There were over 50…with us, eating on chairs and on the floor. Paul, dressed as Santa, came and delivered the exchange gifts and bonuses to the delight of all. There were also slides and movies. Sunday after church we had a family dinner (I made Christmas donuts) which 65 of us enjoyed, followed by a short Christmas program and then the baptism of Cathy Corpron and Glen in the river. That evening we had our Christmas Communion service. … Yesterday we slaughtered a cow. There was also a Mission meeting this week, and night before last we had to drill burr holes on a man that had been beaten on the head. He died the same night from so much brain swelling. Come to find out, the man was in love with someone else's sweetheart! Paul and Doug have been working on the generator, as it was leaking oil. There has been a flu bug around but except for Brooks having a cough we have all been quite well. Tomorrow there will be games and soccer at the Court House for the community and then the same on the first, plus a supper and dancing (mostly drinking!!) in the evening. We will attend some, but probably the two families will join for games, etc., in the evening. ... Sherwood goes back to school on Sunday the second. We have enjoyed him so much, but the time has gone much too quickly. Paul must take the car down to Bangkok for registration in 2 weeks, so will see him soon again. His brothers sure do miss him when he goes. ... Paul will be making a trip to Three Baskets Valley (near the Telacone) about the 25th of January to survey it with a Presbyterian agriculturist with the prospect of Christians from Burma inhabiting it and growing wheat there, as it is much higher and cooler there than here. The Christians in Burma are under a lot of (surveillance) and would like to make a move...

PS Telecone trip is in February (3). Hope to go, but nothing certain now.

Rev. Paul Dodge

January 28, 1966, Winnie to her mother & brother:

Just a note to let you know Paul arrived home safely on Monday. We are all fine! Forrest celebrated his birthday today and had 2 of the Karen boys plus the Corpron children in for a party. … This morning I gave 76 shots at the government school for Typhoid/Cholera and this p.m. another 44 here at the Mission school plus 8 others (including Paul!) There is some cholera already this year in Bangkok.

July 8, 1966, Winnie to her Mom:

Arrived back safely (from vacation in Malaysia) after 2 days in Bangkok. … The Corprons go tomorrow on their vacation. Our Thai nurse "Phiphrom" came back to substitute for my vacation and may stay on for 2 more months. This is a help, as one of the aides is going to the beach with Corprons. It's 12:45 a.m. (had to order hospital drugs, etc., tonight, so will get 5 hours' sleep before getting up at 6 to get the engineering Dr. (about a bridge here) fed so he can return with Corprons to Bangkok. It is monsoon season here!

August 15, 1966, Winnie to her Mom (from Bangkok):

Well, our week at International Church Camp was very busy! Paul had the Jr. High Bible study group and a boys' cabin of Juniors. I had a cabin of Jr. High girls and was camp nurse plus "the family" so kept "on the go." They had a very full program and it's well that we have this week to do our year's buying before we go to

Chiengmai for Mission Conference Aug. 23–28. We also must register the boys in school and have dental work, too, so our days will be full.

September 17, 1966, Winnie to her Mom:

The first three boatloads of building supplies have arrived and there are still at least two more to go. Paul has already found a "bug" in the drawings for the roof trusses so it looks as if we will have a "good time" as building construction begins again!! This week we purchased land for the Christian Witness Center and Paul is now ordering the roofing and lumber for a "shell" as that is all that our $2,000 will stretch to do. As more funds can be found we will complete the building. ... Today a Moslem Burmese man who 9 months ago fell out of a coconut tree and broke his spine, paralyzing him from the neck down, told our Christian aide that he wanted to become a Christian!!! Pray for him as he reads his Burmese Bible and people witness to him, that he may truly understand and accept Christ. He now has partial use of all his extremities. Himay is his name.

September 30, 1966, Winnie to her Mom:

The Corprons got back safely. Helen is still very thin but seems pretty well otherwise. ... Paul will be out visiting villages next week. If Forrest is better, I might go with him. I also want to resume my Karen language study this fall. Paul is now studying Mon 2 hours a week.

October 9, 1966, Winnie to her Mom:

We have all had colds but keep "on the go." Two days ago, Paul and I went to Bikli area west of us to the village where Nau Too She, our Bible woman, is now living and teaching. There are no Christians in that village; however, we have 5 Christians in a village a 3 hour walk in from there. She says that there are two young men in that village who are interested in becoming Christians. There we gave DPT shots and stayed overnight, then the next day on the way back stopped at two more villages and gave DPT shots too. They had an epidemic of whooping cough some months ago. This was the last shot of the series. We also heard the gossip that one of the Christians in that village had begun the use of opium. Please pray if it is true that he will be willing to take the cure. We are building a Christian Center because this is what the Thai Christians on the committee feel will be much more successful. Furthermore, some feel that the church building should be built by the Christians here and not by Americans. Well, we have many thoughts on the matter but won't stop now to explain.

Early History

October 20, 1966, Winnie to her Mom:

> The last of the building supplies have arrived; so, clearing of the land, etc., of the Christian Community Center will begin soon. It has also been suggested that since the Somerville Church would like to give $5,000 to it, that this structure be constructed in such a way as to be a church, too. Soooo, we'll see.

December 3, 1966, Winnie to both sets of parents:

> It is most unusual for me to write a duplicate letter, but time is slipping away and I'm afraid that you won't hear at all if I don't write tonight and to both parents. Here we are all fine and the boys left last Sunday at 6:30 a.m. and arrived in Bangkok at 10:30 p.m., so were in time for school at 7:15 Monday. We had a nice Thanksgiving together and my only regret was that Doug was away, so I had to be "Doc" and so my time with them was really very little. Paul goes to Bangkok tomorrow for ExCom meetings… This will be followed by the Church of Christ in Thailand's annual meetings, so it will be the 17th before he will be returning home and we have decided that we will take the boys out a week early from school as there won't be anyone to come up with them later, and would be quite an added expense. … Helen, the doctor's wife, has been in the hospital again while they were down this time; she is having some of her chest symptoms again… We had this 2 ½ lb. preemie baby just before Thanksgiving and it was unable to suck, so I have had to gavage it around the clock every three hours besides being "Doc" so my free time has been nil.

43

Rev. Paul Dodge

December 18, 1966, Winnie to her mother & brother:

Doug did go down on the helicopter on Tues. and Paul and the boys were flown up, along with an obstetrician from Chiengmai who was in Bangkok for meetings and Paul talked into coming for five days. He just returned via boat to Bangkok today. The hospital is still full and lots of malaria just now.

December 30, 1966, Winnie to her Mom & brother:

I'm wondering how you folks spent your day, Christmas? My day started at 4 a.m. when I was called to deliver a baby. Our baby boy arrived at 6 a.m. and was fine. I then returned home to celebrate the Christ Child's birth. We had a nice Christmas … and we were so happy to hear that Helen's surgery revealed nothing except a slightly enlarged liver, and she will be returning the 3rd via helicopter. Doug returned yesterday. We have been very busy up until about 5 days ago, but now it is fairly quiet. … We will be having company about the sixth of Jan. One of our Baptist missionaries from Japan is coming with four Japanese lay people. Our boys will return to Bangkok on the first, as school begins on the third. They are both fine. There is a very great possibility that Glen will go back to the third grade. The strain of trying to keep up shows in his personality at home, so I'm quite sure even though he loves his fourth-grade teacher, and she him, that in the long run it will be best. I fear that Forrest is going to have to do the same unless I can be relieved of all the doctoring and nursing responsibilities. I feel badly about it because it is mostly due to our irregular teaching last year for both of them.

Anecdotes

Raising Beef

One of the most vivid memories of those early years—and I'm sure we must have photos of it—was the butchering of cows. There was no market, and meat was hard to come by, although rarely a little pork would be sold by a peddler. So, we built up a herd which over time reached 20 or so, counting calves, by buying Brahmin cattle from Burma (which was probably illegal) and we would shoot one a month. Our two families would use the largest share of the meat, but as the staff grew in number and we opened the hostel and the school there was quite a demand to meet. A vivid memory is of Winnie sitting on a plastic sheet which was stretched out on the porch floor on which the quarters of beef also lay, the two of us consulting a cookbook which had diagrams of various cuts and apportioning the meat to the various households and institutions. A real mess, but it met a real need.

Hunting

I fancied myself to be quite a hunter, but rarely brought anything home of real significance—although I did bag a Sambar deer (like an elk) and a barking deer (the size of a police dog).

Kerosene-powered refrigerator

We had refrigerators which ran on kerosene. Once a week I would turn it off in order to trim the wick so it would burn clean. They had a very small freezer which could not hold much. Once in a while we would make ice cream in an ice cube tray by mixing powdered milk, sweetened condensed milk and other ingredients. The serving size for each family member was just an appetizer!

Near-drowning

One event which I will probably never forget was my near-drowning experience just downstream from the houses. It had rained heavily all night and I got up early, as usual, and went to make sure that our outboard motorboat was okay. I was shocked to see that the river had risen 9 or 10 feet overnight! Uprooted trees were being swept along in the muddy current and the boat had also been carried away. I spotted it on the other side of the river, about 150 yards downstream. This was our only transport in the rainy season, and I was afraid that it would soon be carried further away or smashed by the debris rushing down behind it. Being a reasonably good swimmer, I decided to strip down to my underwear and swim diagonally with the current, figuring to land where the boat seemed to be hung up. I was able to do it, but when I had almost reached the boat I was caught in a swifter current because the river was pouring into a rice field. I slammed into the roots of the small tree which was between me and the boat. The roots were not strong enough to allow me to climb up on them, but by grabbing them I was able to keep from being pushed against the base of the trunk. The water was pouring over my head, but I could pull myself up enough to get a breath. I knew I couldn't keep that up for long, so I took a deep breath and worked my way down the root system in hopes that there would be room enough under it to be able to get to the downstream side of the tree. Thank God, there was, and I climbed up onto the trunk and waited until a large boat came and took me and the outboard boat (which wouldn't start) back to the landing. I was shivering and had thorns in my arms from the river debris. Breakfast was quite late that morning!

Late Night Midwifery

We were awakened in the middle of the night by a man calling from underneath our bedroom window, "Maw, khrup! Maw, khrup!" (Doctor! Doctor!) (Doug was on furlough then.) The man explained that his wife was in a difficult labor (probably breech) and the village midwives had given up. Could Winnie go and try to help? They lived in the village on the other side of the river, so Winnie would have to cross it in a tippy dug-out which had only a few inches of free-board. (For some reason we did not have the outboard available then.) But she told me to stay with the kids, and taking her medical kit and a flashlight, she went into the darkness with this stranger. Hours later she returned, tired but pleased that she had saved both the baby and the mother. What a woman – like the pioneers of old!

Paying Workers in Gold

In order to saw the lumber for the hospital, hostel, and other buildings, we employed Mon men who created saw pits by digging a trench over which a frame was built. The elephants would roll the logs up a ramp onto the frame; then the men—one above and one below—would cut the logs in two by using a long saw with handles on each end. They would then use a chalk line, using charcoal in a coconut shell, to mark the cuts needed for the various sized boards which they could get out of each half. We would keep track of how many boards of the different sizes and then I would have to calculate that into cubic feet or meters. There were several crews, plus laborers of various sorts, so records had to be kept for each man's amount due (in Thai Baht). They were mostly Mon from Burma, however, so instead of Thai currency they wanted to be paid in gold, which they could take home with them at the end of the job! Not only that, but they wanted the gold in differing forms—some wanted nuggets of a certain weight each, and others wanted chains of varying weights and lengths! That meant that I would have to go to the gold shops in Chinatown, Bangkok, select the gold according to the orders, and then bring it back up-river. That's when I bought a revolver, as a lot of people knew what my errand was! Sometimes the boatman and I, and usually some other passengers, would have to sleep on a raft which served as the home of a family if we didn't make Thakanun before dark. The quiet sound of a dug-out canoe paddle cutting the water would wake me (a light sleeper in the best of conditions) and I would put my hand on the revolver until I knew that the visitor was not to be feared. Should I have relied on trust in God rather than a gun? Perhaps. But I had heard of an OMF [Overseas Missionary Fellowship] missionary in northern Thailand who had been killed for a much lesser reason; so, I felt that self-protection was in order. Right or wrong, it made me braver!

Speaking of boats, at different times we had some great ones which shortened the travel time in the rainy season considerably.

End Notes

1. Dr Cressy was a specialist in the study of the work of the Christian movement in East Asia, having analyzed the strategies of churches in 7 Asian countries. This report was based on a survey made at the request of the Church of Christ in Thailand, printed in 1959 in Thailand.

2. Dr. McGavran, a 3rd generation missionary to India, was the founding Dean and Professor of Mission, Church Growth and South Asian Studies at the School of World Mission at Fuller Theological Seminary. *The Bridges of God: A Study in the Strategy of Missions* was originally published by World Dominion Press in 1955 and republished by Wipf and Stock Publishers, Eugene, OR.

3. It is not clear to me (Paul) how McGavran knew about this group, whether he only was aware of unevangelized Karen in that general area and identified the Telakhon after learning of John Sams' report after his meeting Olivepa in Mae Sod, or if their legend of the Golden Book of Life to be returned by "the White brother" was already known.

4. Russell Brown, Secretary for S.E. Asia, and, as I recall it, Marlin Farnum (the Overseas director for the Baptists, who was skeptical about our desire to have a school but was persuaded before he left).

5. We often overworked the vehicle [Land Rover], overloading it and driving it up steep stream banks which sometimes threatened to overturn it. Crossing deep streams required that we remove the fan belt

and then re-install it on the other side. The aluminum body was terribly hot, so we usually kept the top part of the body off. Other memories of Land Rover travel include the tense crossing of bridges made of thin logs with scary gaps between them. We knew we were in danger of dropping a wheel in when the person guiding us over would get wide-eyed!

6. Paul Dodge to Doug Corpron: Doug, I think that this group must have been Allen Acheson and some friends from International Church [Bangkok].

7. The study of Karen was under the tutelage of Olivepa and Olivemo, who had moved from Mae Sod (where John Sams had met them in 1955, and Carl Capen [ABM Secretary] and Paul Dodge had interviewed them in 1960). Olivemo was a native speaker of Pwo Karen and was the most reliable informant, having easily adapted to the local dialect. They and part of their large family (all of whose names were from Shakespeare plays and began with "O") moved to Sangkhla in November 1961. Soon joining them was Olivepa's sister Mary, who befriended a local lady (Pa Thong Dee) and began teaching children in her house in the nearest village. Her influence was inestimable.

8. Paul's note: I believe that this doctor was Tom Roberts, who served at Overbrook Hospital in Chiang Rai.

9. This group of JUSMAG (Joint U.S. Military Advisory Group) officers were led by Gordon Young, a 3rd or 4th generation MK (missionary kid) who was brought up in a remote part of Burma, spoke Lahu like a native—along with other ethnic languages—and was a renowned hunter. He wrote books about his experiences, one of which is *Tracks of an Intruder*. His father, Harold Young, established the Chiang Mai zoo. Gordon had taught me how to tan animal skins, a hobby which I enjoyed. Locals who had shot any unusual animal or reptile knew that I would be interested in buying the skins for preserving them. One time a hunter brought me the hide of a large Himalayan Sun Bear, and as the Corprons were on furlough I decided to use their bathtub for the tanning process. To my chagrin the chemicals dissolved the enamel coating on the tub, so when the Corprons returned I met them at the boat landing and said, "Before you go into the house, there's something I need to tell you!" A new bathtub arrived after a short while to make up for my misadventure.

10. Esther Greenmun came from the Mae Sariang Christian Hospital to "learn the ropes" at this one, stay and deliver the baby when the time came, and stay on a few weeks more until Winnie was able to take over again.

Chapter 2

A Conversation with Dr. Doug Corpron

Jungle Medicine

Excerpts from a video interview recorded by Carol McDaniel Licht

January 19, 2019, Yakima, Washington

About Douglas O. Corpron:

Dr. Corpron was the founding doctor of the Kwai River Christian Hospital. He saw patients first in the breezeway under his house, then in a small dispensary (converted storage shed), and finally in the new hospital, which he had helped to design. He was also responsible for the acquisition of equipment and for public relations.

Span of service at KRCH: March 1961 through June 1967

Preparation

Phil: You arrived at the site of the future Kwai River Christian Hospital in March 1961, but a lot had to happen before you actually moved in.

Doug: My history there [in Thailand] was for two four-year terms, the first two years of which were spent in language school. I was recruited by the United Christian Missionary Society to go to Thailand to do this job. I had wanted to go back to China. I'm a China missionary's kid. My dad was in Anhui Province for a whole career.

Phil: Your dad was a doctor, too, right?

Doug: My dad was a physician. He is considered by the Anhui Provincial Hospital—a 2,000 bed hospital today—as the founder, and I have been honored by them more than once now as the son of their founder, which has been incredible.

I went [to Thailand] with my wife. By that time, we had 3 kids. We landed in Bangkok and went to work on the language. The decision to go and start a new program among the Karen on the Burma border had been done by two missions: the United Christian Missionary Society, which is Disciples of Christ, my mission sending group, and the American Baptist Mission, which had a long and deep history among the Karen in Burma and were brought in because of that.

John Sams, who was part of the decision-making process as to where to locate, was challenged to try to find a location in which these two boards might consider locating the joint mission. He made many trips along the Thai-Burma border, coming upriver from Kanchanaburi. They did make the decision that there is this one spot which was on the river and they did determine it was going to be navigable during the rainy season, and because of that, they decided that that is where they would establish the mission.

The Beginning

Phil: When you arrived at the site of the future Kwai River Christian Hospital in March of 1961, what was there?

Doug: My wife, Helen, and I had been preparing for a number of months and we had sent food supplies up. Much had already been done, and we were going up to two newly constructed houses. John Sams, being located in Nakhon Pathom, which is halfway between Bangkok and the Kanchanaburi area, had arranged for a building team to go upriver in October. He had also hired people to haul gravel and sand up onto this site prior to the builders getting there. In a matter of a couple of months, they completed two houses. He said he had gone to Bangkok and bought I think it was maybe 70 tons of materials that they put in barges and shipped up along with the builders and they went to work in the middle of the jungle with nothing around them and built two residences. There was another couple—missionaries of the American Baptist Mission Society—Paul and Winifred Dodge. Paul was an evangelist and Winnie was a nurse. And so, Winnie was my main assistant and in charge of the nursing staff and often filled in for me when I was out somewhere, using a treatment guide that I had put together for people to use when I wasn't there.

Paul and I and others in the mission team had been up there several times. I had gone up prior to our moving our families up and offloaded things from a barge: some of our furniture and food supplies. Paul and

Winnie had done the same thing. The workmen, who were big-city Thai, were not very happy being located in mosquito-infested malaria country, and more than one of them had a bout of malaria while they were there, but they moved on ahead. Many of them were living underneath these newly constructed houses, which were typical raised two-story homes to get the houses up where the breezes were.

Phil: So, when you first got there [with your family], there were these two houses: one for the American Baptist evangelist and nurse [Paul and Winnie Dodge and three sons] and one for you and your wife [and by that time four kids], but there was no hospital yet!

Doug: Right.

Phil: But that didn't stop patients from coming to see you.

Doug: Almost immediately the word got around that there was this foreign doctor that had arrived. One of the very first patients happened when we had just arrived. We hadn't even moved all our things upstairs. All of a sudden here came a man who had blown off much of both of his hands. That's an injury that you and I talked about previously that we both saw. The Karen and Mon would make a homemade bomb out of bamboo. They would drill a hole and put gunpowder in there and a fuse, and the thesis was that if they threw that bomb and it exploded in the water it would stun the fish in the river and they would come floating up and they would get quite a lot of fish to eat with one explosion. But the problem is, periodically one of these bombs didn't get thrown soon enough, and it would explode in the hands of the man who was trying to do it, and this man had done that, and he had actually blinded himself at the same time. And he was in bad shape. But here he was, and I was trying to do what I could. I put up boards on top of a couple of barrels, laid him out there, and Winnie was there, and we finished cleaning up his shattered hands, most of which were blown off. We actually gave him a unit of blood that one of us donated (probably me because I'm type "O" and was a universal donor). Unfortunately, he had lost so much blood, that he stayed in shock and he died. And I thought, "This is not a very good beginning for a new doctor in the jungle." But the attitude seemed to be that they were amazed we had even tried to do anything. And that was kind of refreshing and a new look at the attitude of this community.

It was amazing how quickly we were busy and pretty soon I had several hundred patients coming in, and my wife, Helen, said, "We cannot have the underside of my house used as the hospital with my children running around."

Whenever a patient would come, they brought their whole family, and they were the support system. Relatives knew that they had to come and cook and take care of the patient. We needed them. You and I have talked many times about how—when you were making rounds—you never knew quite where your patient was because if a baby was there in a sling underneath the bed and the family was up on the hospital bed, they would have to remind you who the patient was.

Phil: So, your wife didn't allow continuation of hospital activity under the house. Where did you see patients?

Doug: "You have to do something!" [said Helen] So, there was a storage shed we had built about 50 to 100 yards downriver, and we decided we had to turn that into a treatment clinic. We built a little temporary "sala" [a roofed-over open platform with benches] for a waiting area outside this treatment shed where people could wait in the shade and out of the rain. So that's where we had the shift of medicine, and people would come and go there and no longer were staying underneath our house. And that was what we had to work with the first two years.

Early Hires, Construction, House Calls

Doug: We set up a dispensary with a pharmacy in one half of that storage shed. I hired two people besides having the help of Winnie regularly. One, whose name was Sudah, was very valuable because she was Thai-educated. She was a local Pwo Karen and fluent in her native language as well as Thai. And then the other person I hired was a man called Surin. He was a high school graduate and was bright. I trained him to start doing many things: first laboratory work—blood work and looking for malaria parasites and all the other things we tried to do—and eventually we had a little X-ray and he trained to do that. In fact, he did my operative anesthesia: managed the anesthesia machine after we used open drop ether to manage the induction. He [Surin] had the Mon language. He was also fluent in Thai. You and I spent a considerable amount of time in language study. I had spent two years learning the Thai language. But we were never through using interpreters where we worked because we encountered the Mon language, two dialects of the Karen language, and the Burmese language. We were never done working with languages, but it is still true that most of the time the Thai language that you and I had studied was the key to our ability to communicate.

Phil: You were seeing patients in this storage shed. Meantime, the hospital building was going up, correct?

Doug: There were plans. There was an architect missionary who was part of the Presbyterian mission; his name was Taylor Potter. The plans we had for the two houses were drawn up by him. That's how we were able to get the materials together.

Phil: So, now we have American Baptists, Disciples, and Presbyterians all working together.

Doug: One of the refreshing things about—as you know—working in Thailand is that we were working under the auspices and as the coworkers of the Church of Christ in Thailand, and we could forget our labels and work together and plan together. We had help from people like Taylor Potter, who was delighted to help. We already had some materials. And we were determined as quickly as we could to start building not only the hospital, but also a boarding house for students who were staying there and studying in the local school. Also, we had national coworkers and we needed new residences for them. We selected a site which was maybe 200 or 300 yards away from the homes, where we located the hospital. So those buildings all got underway quickly between 1961, when we got there, and the summer of 1962 when we [the Corpron family] left on furlough.

We had an American Baptist missionary, Chet Galaska, who had a device [a hand-operated mechanical press] for making compressed soil blocks. There was a material that was everywhere underfoot which is the residual soil of a rain forest, at least in that area, which they call "laterite." If you take that—it's heavy clay with small gravel pieces— you could moisten it up, and there was a formula where you put in a small percentage of cement with the laterite [about one part cement to about 17 or 20 parts laterite]. You could put this in the hand-operated machine and press out one block at a time. We used these for the construction of our hospital walls.

Phil: Those blocks: you tested them, right?

Doug: We were saying, "What do you mean? The rain's going to come during the rainy season, and we'll have water beating down on these walls, and these blocks are just going to melt away!" Well, we carefully sun-dried them, and we took two or three down and put them in the river and watched them carefully. They sat there and didn't dissolve at all for a number of weeks. So, we were reassured. We made hundreds of these blocks and used them for all of the inside and outside walls of the hospital. We left openings in which we carefully put Thai-made louvered glass windows that you and I lived with for a number of years. And those were the fundamental materials we used in building the hospital.

Phil: By making the blocks locally, you saved a huge amount of money over what it would have cost to purchase cement blocks in the big city and transport them to the construction site!

Doug: And, of course, we were getting busier and busier, you know, and by 1962 we were desperate to get over to the new hospital building. It had a roof on it. Not all the walls had gone up yet, but we were beginning to have clinics over there. We had set up our pharmacy and dispensary. We were doing outpatient medicine in that shell of a building as it was being completed.

Phil: I understand there was one particular patient you cared for: a very influential man in the community. And your good influence with him, or his good influence with you, served you well later on.

Doug: Oh yes, you're thinking of the abbot of the Buddhist temple who became nationally famous. He was Mon. The Mon were probably as large a population in the Sangkhlaburi village area as the Karen, and they were a strong Buddhist community. And the abbot, who became nationally known as Luang Por Uttama, was a young man then. My coworker, Surin, was a Mon, and so they knew each other well. This was after we were established, and we had an X-ray unit and a lab going. The abbot came over with a history of coughing up blood and said he would like me to examine him. X-ray and lab tests proved that he had a small open tuberculosis lesion, and we started him on therapy for a whole year. My assistant, Surin, dutifully went across the river— a substantial walk—regularly to give him his streptomycin shot. He was [also] taking INH. He had a full recovery. That was a significant relationship we established.

One time we had a new police chief in town who decided he might get some bribe money from me if he jailed my assistant Surin. Many people who ran small businesses would take materials from Burma and resell them in Thailand for a profit. There were many things coming from Burma, smuggled across the border all the time. Well, Surin was arrested on the basis of having some of that—his wife was selling a few things. When I got back from a trip and found him in jail, I went over across the river and talked to Luang Por Uttama and said, "We have a problem. Our friend Surin has been put in jail, and I need your help."

He said, "Don't worry about it." And the next day he was out of jail, and a couple weeks later that police chief was gone from the town! And we heard at the clinic that the word in town was, "Just don't mess around with the doctor because he's a friend of Luang Por Uttama."

Those were all issues that gave me reassurance that we had local safety and I felt comfortable traveling around in the villages. Much of my early medical work centered around doing a lot of house calls. I didn't just sit in our clinic waiting. If there was someone in the Mon village or in the main Sangkhlaburi village, I would go over there and do house calls. And I have one picture that shows me coming back from a house call with my doctor bag in one hand and a big fish in the other. I had been paid for that house call!

Surgery, Walking Blood Bank, Sinking OR Table

Phil: You had some very challenging patients early on.

Doug: I might begin first by talking about a man called Jute, who was a young Mon boy. It was the earliest case of major surgery, and it was done in that clinic on that homemade [wooden examining] table. We didn't have proper screening. We had people looking in while we did this.

Phil: Curious relatives?

Doug: That's right. Nurse Winnie Dodge and I sterilized the instruments. We had a pressure cooker sterilizer. The diagnosis was easy because you could see the wave of peristalsis from this enlarged stomach trying to squeeze food past this obstruction, undoubtedly due to the multiple duodenal ulcers he had had. He was gradually starving to death, and I knew that if I didn't do something, he would die. We were going to do what we could do. We used spinal and local because this was kind of high up for a spinal. I made a small incision in his abdomen and found a loop of bowel—probably jejunum—hooked the loop of bowel into his stomach; did a lateral anastomosis; opened it up and closed up. And it worked like magic because he immediately began passing food through his stomach, which he hadn't done for a long time. And pretty soon he started gaining weight—20 or 30 pounds—and got his health back. He actually got involved helping us, eventually working at the hospital. He was kind of like a walking advertisement because everybody in the village knew about Jute dying as it were. And there he was walking around doing well. And that all happened even before we had the hospital going, which was a fun part of his story.

Phil: I think there was another case that you did early on that was rather nerve-wracking. Can you tell us about that?

Doug: Oh! The bur hole case! There again, that was before we had a hospital. I was called to see this young man who was lying unconscious on the floor in a house not far from the mission compound. I had to go up a rickety ladder under the floor of the house and there he was, and I examined him, and I could see that he had a dilated pupil on one side. And his story was that he had fallen. He was a mahout, an elephant driver, who had fallen off his elephant and had struck his head and had been unconscious since that time. He clearly had an intracranial bleed of some kind. And here I was a gung-ho young doc wanting to do things. And I knew that if he had a subdural hematoma, and I could do a bur hole, which is not a very big procedure, it might be lifesaving. And so, we determined to do that. We got the materials together. I did not have a proper medical bur, which importantly has to be round so that once you penetrate through the skull you don't plunge into the brain with your bit. But I had an old-fashioned wood bit and a hand crank, and we sterilized those up. We didn't have to do any anesthesia because this man was unconscious. We went to the house—his little hut—climbed up and set up a Coleman lantern. By that time, it was getting dusk. We made a small incision. Of course, again, we had family standing around. This was rainy season and there was a termite hatch out. I remember termites flying into the wound while trying to do something for this young man: successfully making a bur hole on the proper side, based on his blown pupil and, unfortunately, finding that he did not have a subdural hematoma but had some form of intracranial bleeding or swelling that resulted in his dilated pupil.

Phil: And all of this took place in his house!

Doug: In his house.

Phil: A house call for neurosurgery!

Doug: A half a mile walk from where we were living. And I got to thinking, "Oh my goodness—because he did not recover; in a day or two he died—what must these villagers think of this weird Western doctor using these weird pieces of equipment on the brain of this boy, and he died. 'Look what happened!'"

But the attitude seemed to be more like, "Well, this is one of those outcomes of modern medicine, but it is still better than what we had before!" At least that seems to be the way it was because we certainly had no change in how our busyness kept growing and growing.

Phil: Well, they could see you had done your best to help the patient.

Doug: I hope that's what they thought. That seemed to be right.

Phil: So, tell us now about the man with the bear bite.

Doug: That was after we moved in [to the main hospital building] and got going after 1963. We heard that there was a canoe with a man in a bad way coming up the river. We went down to see what the situation was, and here was a man who it turned out had been in a confrontation with a sun bear. According to his story, the bear got his whole head in its mouth and they were on the riverbank and they rolled down together into the river, and when they hit the water the bear let go. This man had a severely fractured jaw. It was so loose that his tongue would drop back, obstructing his airway when he was sitting up. So, he was kneeling on hands and knees in the dugout canoe as they rowed him up. And, of course, he had lost a tremendous amount of blood.

I determined that he had other injuries. He had multiple lacerations and his face was terribly torn apart and he had this fractured jaw. I was able with some local anesthesia to wire his jaw back together again and did some beginning repair of the major lacerations. We were able to give him a unit or two of blood. I called, and the Thai Army helicopter was willing to take him to town. He ended up actually at the Bangkok Sanitarium [Adventist] Hospital. I'm not sure whether they went straight to Bangkok or to Kanchanaburi. He had multiple surgeries and made a full recovery and I saw him there maybe a year later still holding forth at the Bangkok Sanitarium Hospital. That was pretty amazing.

It does bring up one subject: the issue of giving blood. It had become often enough that one of us on staff would give a unit of blood, but we couldn't keep doing it. We talked before about Luang Por

Uttama with whom we had developed a warm relationship. Surin, my lab tech, suggested the idea of working together with the Luang Paw to determine the blood type of as many young Mon workers that he [Luang Por Uttama] would appoint to come over to the hospital to have their blood typed. That way a walking blood bank would be created, and we did that. We had maybe 30 men. They were all young working men and the Luang Paw just told them that that's what they were going to do. So, they were "volunteers" for a blood bank, and we used that several times, depending on their blood type and their availability. I'm sure you had the same issues with blood supply.

Phil: We didn't have that same cohort of young men in the walking blood bank, but some of the people on the hospital staff, including myself, as well as some of the teachers at the Christian school would occasionally be willing to give blood. Of course, we always tried to get blood for a patient who needed it from the patient's own friends and relatives if we could. That was the first avenue.

Doug: Well, you and I, I think, Phil, were determined to do as high a quality of medicine as we could, given the fact that we were in these isolated situations. I was determined to have X-ray, determined to have as much lab as we could figure, and a good operating system going. We had this "fancy" operating table that you had to live with as well, that as it aged, would no longer hold its hydraulic pump. So, we would prop up the table at the proper height.

Phil: It would slowly sink, and not only that, it would sway a little bit from side to side. The swaying, we never did find a good solution for. The sinking we could, because we cut a piece of wood to prop up the table from underneath, just the right length for each doctor that operated, depending on how tall they were and what type of operation they were doing.

Doug: I'm not sure where I got the operating table: probably a used one from somewhere else.

Phil: Yes, the operating table was definitely a used one. It had a plaque on it from a hospital in the States.

Doug: It's still, I think, important to say that I didn't feel like I had to make apology for the quality of medicine that I practiced, nor did you because we still had the basics in tow. We didn't have a lot of the fancy things. And of course, the world has changed in terms of the world of MRI's and CAT scans these days and all the automated laboratory work.

Phil: So much good can be done with basic equipment, and in the field of public health, with vaccinations and safe water supply and sewage disposal.

Making Contact with the Telakhon

Phil: You took at least one trip deep into the jungle to visit the Telakhon.

Doug: The story of the Telakhon is important, particularly in the decision making [about where to locate the mission work]. They had an ultimate leader called the Phu Jite [or Phu Gyaik]. The Phu Jite who was famous was still alive when I made one of the initial trips. We had a coworker we haven't spoken too much about, but whom you knew well: Olivepa. His daughter Olivia became a very loved and trusted worker of yours through the years. Olivepa was hired by John Sams. He [Olivepa] was British trained—a bright man—who had a long history of the Karen Free State effort in Burma. But he came there [to the Kwai River Christian Mission] charged with helping us work with the Karen and knew about the early thinking of Don McGavran and his motivation to make contact with this group, the Telakhon. He put together with five or six elephants a five day [each way] trip. We went from Sangkhla, camping along the way. I remember them cooking rice in big tubes of bamboo, and that was delicious rice cooked in that way over an open fire. I remember sleeping in a tent along the way, and hearing animals go by at night, wondering who was going by, and going all the way to this Telakhon village. Here was this subgroup who spoke Pwo Karen and Olivepa was able to communicate with them, and we met the Phu Jite. They had regular worship services. They had kind of a combination of Buddhism and animism and a religion of their own, which was quite distinctive. Allan Eubank, who was a missionary of our board, somehow was fascinated with this, and he never let it go. Allan worked in Nakhon Pathom and then in Chiang Mai and he made I don't know how many trips to that area. Usually, after they [the Allan Eubank family] moved to the Chiang Mai area, they would come in from the north. But those first trips [to the Telakhon], where we established our relationships, began in Sangkhlaburi. The young women who were unmarried all wore white. You could tell who was married and who was not. They were a very tight group with a lot of their own customs. They had this tradition that someday the white man with the book of truth was going to return: the white brother who used to be part of the family. That story didn't seem to be too real with the Telakhon at that time. But still they were receptive to having the mission workers come whenever they did.

Phil: Do you recall whether that trip to the Telakhon was one of the occasions when my dad [Dr. Edwin McDaniel] came to cover the hospital while you were away?

Doug: I believe that it was. You know, your father was a very close colleague, and somehow he was the one that was always able and willing. He was a busy man in the Chiang Mai medical world, but he was willing to come. That was a three-day trip for him or more. Whenever I had a need … if I was going to be gone for any length of time [he would fill in]. When I went down to Bangkok for a month because my twins were coming— and that was one delivery with twins that I was not wanting to do in the jungle—we waited a whole month down there. Your father came and took my place for that whole month. His friendship and support were very important. [Editor's note: The twins were born September 23, 1965 in Bangkok.]

Travel in the Wet and the Dry, Jet Boat

Phil: Could you describe a typical trip from Bangkok to the Kwai River Christian Hospital?

Doug: There was a train we could board on the Thonburi side of Bangkok and get to a little town called Wang Pho, which was basically the end of the rail line.

Phil: About how long did that train trip take?

Doug: That would take about 6 or 8 hours [on a train pulled by a wood-burning locomotive]. So that was the first day. And there was a little hotel in Wang Pho where we stayed multiple times with family, with kids, with guests. It was a pretty typical Thai hotel [for those days] with mats that you slept on. There was a restaurant we ate in. From there we could go by hang yaow boat ("long tail" boat). In the heavy rainy season when we moved up after coming back from furlough in 1963, we loaded there [at Wang Pho] with large rice barges going upriver. We took a lot of equipment up. By that time—five kids—that was quite a trip. If it was dry season the hang yaow (long tail) boats did not go well beyond the main stop village of Thakanun. We had gotten acquainted with the Chinese merchant who was up in that village who was very welcoming to us staying there in his home. And we would eat in a little restaurant there. Then if it was really dry season, we had our mission Land Rover: it would meet us, or we had left it there. We would pick it up and drive from there to the mission. Or if there was enough water, we could also have a long tail boat take us right to the mission station. The jeep ride from Thakanun to Sangkhlaburi was really problematic. There was not a [proper] road. We were usually going on roadways that were developed by large logging trucks that traveled from village to village and accessed the river in places, and if there was not a bridge, you went down one side and up the other. If you were luckier, there were two logs across that creek, and you'd have somebody get out of the jeep and get over on the other side and guide you so that you had one wheel on each log. There were a couple of spots like that.

Once we were coming back, and we had the family and we had a stack of eggs—about 10 or 12 big containers of eggs—and kids in the back of the Land Rover. In the tropics you don't keep the top on—it's just too hot to run with it on—and the jeep had no air conditioning. So, the issue of rolling over was a real hazard. We had a driver, and he was going down the gully, and to go up the other side, he had to "goose it." The engine died and he backed into the stream bed really hard and the Jeep flipped over and off flipped the eggs, and off [flipped] the kids! Luckily, no one was hurt—and we saved most of the eggs.

One thing I might talk about is the Rogue River jet boat. I should mention that because that was one of my not very good ideas! But I'm a fly fisherman and I love the Rogue River, which is in southern Oregon. Jet pumps to drive riverboats were just getting going. They are very popular now—all over the West you see them. The jets are greatly improved. But I felt that that was the perfect answer: that the hospital needed to have one of those Rogue River jet boats. They were plywood boats. The one I ordered was 16 or 18 feet long. I think it was 18 feet. It had an inboard engine—a great big inboard engine—with a Berkeley pump that worked beautifully. It was just like the model, but it was a bit smaller than the ones they run down there [on the Rogue River in Oregon] with tourists going upstream for the ride.

A Conversation with Dr. Doug Corpron

Well, I used mission money, and we got that boat, and had it shipped to Bangkok, and got it on the Kwai River, and it worked beautifully. The trouble was, it also used so much gas [gasoline] that I could not keep gas enough to get to the hospital and back. So, I had to store gas in 55-gallon drums along the way based on the distance I could go with that boat before it needed to be refueled. I would leave gas with what I thought was a trusted friend. And then we would use the boat in and around the mission, but if we had a long run, when we got to the drum where we were going to fill the gas tank again, it had turned into water somehow. Somebody had stolen the gasoline! I never could solve the issue of how to keep gas safe to supply this boat, and so we ended up using it less and less and it ended up sitting there.

I just heard from Roy Myers, who was the physician who immediately followed me, whom you know because he has gone back multiple times to help at the Kwai River Christian Hospital. He said, "I was the one who found that boat tied up at the mission and I realized that it was not going to be useful, and I found somebody in the U.S. Army who was delighted to have it, and they took it to Bangkok." He said they were running VIPs around Bangkok and going up the klongs [canals] and stuff with my boat. So that's the saga of the Rogue River jet boat.

Phil: You mentioned earlier about doing operations and taking X-rays. What did you do for electric power?

Doug: Well, our first major generator was a two-cylinder Lister: a British generator. It was an outfit that worked beautifully, and we were able to wire power to the whole mission. We had strict times, as you did: certain times in the day—usually in the evening—when we were able to share electric power with the whole mission. And that was the power we used at the hospital. If we had emergency surgery or the need for an X-ray, we had that power plant we could turn on and use it for our needs.

Phil: Was that a hand-cranked start then?

Doug: It was, and it took a lot of maintenance. You and I were talking about not being trained in medical school to take care of the multiple pieces of equipment needed. One time I counted up 13 pieces of mechanical equipment that I was taking care of!

The diesel fuel had to be kept in 55-gallon barrels. There was often rust in the bottom of the barrels and it would be sucked into the fuel tank. The injectors had microscopic openings and would get plugged up.

On one occasion I had taken down the Lister generator and was cleaning it. Trying to be meticulous, I had laid clean parts out on surgical sheets from the hospital. A visitor asked, "What kind of surgery is this?"

Happily, the instruction books for the Lister were helpful and we could usually figure out what to do.

By contrast, we had a US Wisconsin outboard engine (50 hp) on which we attached a jet pump. It was a great rig for our 16-foot aluminum pram. Wisconsin said, "If you have a carburetor problem, just take it to the nearest dealer"—not much help in the jungle!

Chapter 3

Up the River Kwai and Back in March 1965

By Dr. Edwin McDaniel, April 1965

About the author of this letter:

Best known for his work in family planning in the north of Thailand, "Maw Mac" ("Dr. Mac") was also a long-time friend of the Kwai River Christian Hospital, starting long before son, Dr. Phil McDaniel, had even entered medical school. Besides filling in as a relief doctor (see below), he also helped find nurses, volunteer doctors, and used his connections to procure equipment and supplies.

Dr. Ed McDaniel filled in at the Kwai River Christian Hospital multiple times over three decades. He covered the hospital twice in 1965 for 3–4 weeks each time: once so Dr. Corpron could go visit the Telakhon and once so that Dr. Corpron could be present with his wife and family in Bangkok while awaiting the birth of their twins. Dr. Ed McDaniel covered the hospital briefly once or twice during the two years between Dr. John Freeman's watch and Dr. Phil McDaniel's watch. He also served as relief doctor about 10–15 times during son Phil's watch. Following is a letter and diary of his very first trip to the Kwai River Christian Hospital, which was in March 1965.

McCormick Hospital
Chiang Mai, Thailand
April 23, 1965

Dear Friends,
Those of you who have read the book and/or seen the motion picture "Bridge on the River Kwai", or read "Bamboo Doctor" or "Miracle on the River Kwai", may sometimes have said to yourself, as

I often had, "I wish I could go there someday and see for myself the scene of the infamous 'Death Railway'. I'd like to get even a slight realization of the horrors the Allied prisoners of war went through when compelled to construct the railway that was to connect Siam to Burma and strengthen the Japanese hold on the region and promote their 'Coprosperity Sphere of Asia'!"

As many of you already know, among the several foreign missions cooperating to promote the work of the Church of Christ in Thailand (in effect a "United" church) are the Presbyterians, American Baptists, and the Disciples (United Christian Missionary Society). About five years ago the American Baptists and Disciples, in cooperation with the Church of Christ in Thailand, founded a new mission station at a little village called "Sangkhlaburi" on the upper reaches of the Little Kwai River, on what used to be the most northern part of the "Death Railway", close to the Burma border. This is an area difficult to reach and very needy. The Disciples sent Dr. and Mrs. Corpron to set up a small hospital, and the Baptists sent Rev. and Mrs. Paul Dodge to set up a hostel for Karen children and promote an evangelistic outreach to the Thai, Karen, Mon, and Burmese people in the area. Since Mrs. Dodge is a nurse, and the hospital has no other nurse, "Winnie" Dodge has spent much of her time in hospital nursing.

About three days journey north of Sangkhlaburi (which the Japanese called "Nikki") live several thousand Karen tribespeople, called the "Telakhon Karen". These people have a religious belief that at one time, many thousands of years ago, they had God's Book, which they called the "Golden Book". But, one day, the man in charge of the book laid it on a stump while he burned the stubble off his rice fields. The book caught fire and burned up. But someday, according to this belief, a white man would bring God's word, the "Golden Book" back to them! Mr. Dodge had already visited the Telakhon Karen people twice before, but never had the doctor or nurse gone. Dr. Corpron had never felt he could leave his hospital for the three weeks necessary for the trip.

So, the combination of my having long wanted to visit the River Kwai area, plus Dr. Doug's desire to accompany Mr. Dodge on this year's trip to the Telakhon Karen, served to make Charlotte and me decide to make the long trip to Sangkhlaburi. So, on 1 March we left Carol to continue her schooling in Chiang Mai and went to Bangkok in company with Miss Margaret Strane, the Fraternal Worker [that is, missionary] medical technologist at McCormick Hospital, who was to instruct the new lab boy at the Kwai River Christian Hospital.

Here are some entries from our "diary":

1st day (5 March 1965):
Taxi from guesthouse to railroad station at Thonburi. Train left station at 8:05 AM. Sat third class (the only class!). Took pictures of Chinese vegetable gardens along the railway tracks. Train not too crowded. People happy as most Thais seem to be all the time! Stopped at every little station. Most of the way we traveled over the "Death Railway". About 10,000 [later estimates are much higher] men died mostly of cholera, malaria, starvation, beriberi, and overwork. Prisoners were mostly British; but many Dutch, Australian, Malay, and Indian, too. Also, many Thai and other forced laborers.

2:30 PM train slowly crawled along the top of a creaking trestle built on a shelf of solid rock carved from the side of a cliff by prisoners of war working in blazing sun with no sunglasses to protect the eyes and mostly no shoes to protect their feet from the hot rocks.

Arrived at Wang Po, almost the end of the line, about 3 PM, put up in clean but hot little wooden hotel. After a bath, supper of kow-pat (fried rice) in a moderately clean restaurant across the street, took trial ride in mission jet boat on nearby Kwai Noi River! Quite a thrill.

2nd day:
Up at 5:30 AM because boatmen wanted to make an early start. Breakfast in the same restaurant at 6:30 AM—Ovaltine and fried eggs. Left boat landing at 7:30 AM. A very fast boat and quite a sight to see the 25-foot jet of water come out of the back! The 200 hp engine drives us along at two or three times the speed of the best native hang yao ("long tail") boats but drinks up the gasoline like a thirsty horse drinks water! About 14 5-gallon tins used on the trip. Very cold at first. Put on coat and pun-muang jacket (dark blue homespun farmer shirt). Hot later. Lovely scenery along the way, including many wild birds and a few wild monkeys. Arrived at upper boat landing at "Ta-ka-noon"

about 2:30 PM. Loaded freight and people into a dilapidated old Land Rover and left for Sangkhlaburi, our destination, about 3 PM. First part of road is used by a mining company and is very rocky. Then we turned off onto a dirt road that runs through the bamboo jungle. A nice shady, pretty drive, but all the time had to dodge overhanging bamboo branches because this Land Rover has no top or windshield! Got stuck in mud holes and high spots in the road several times. Fun to see the driver "winch out" of these places! Our driver is a very capable chap. Crossed through the riverbed several times! Water is very shallow at this time of year; and the riverbed very rocky. Water rises about 16 feet in the rainy season. Finally arrived at the little town of Sangkhlaburi well after dark. Surprised to see wooden houses and city electricity. Arrived at the hospital on the other side of the river at about 8 PM. Hospital has its own electric generator. Missionary houses are of wood, but well-built and lighted. After a welcome shower-bath and good supper, to bed.

3rd day:

Got cold during the night. It goes down to 58° F sometimes, even at this hot season. Used two blankets. After breakfast, Dr. Corpron, the Disciples doctor in charge here, showed me around the small 10 bed hospital built about two years ago. Plenty of TB and malaria here. There is also a heroin addict "taking the cure".

4th day:

Dr. Corpron, Dodges, and several other people left by Land Rover about 9 AM for their trip to the Telakhon Karen area. They will find elephants waiting for them about a half day drive up ahead and go most of the journey on elephant back. Now that Winnie Dodge is gone, my only helpers in the hospital are Miss Margaret Strane, who has come to teach the lab/X-ray-technician, the "Mon" young man named "Surin," who is the lab technician and speaks and writes Mon, Burmese, and a little Thai and English. (His wife has hemoglobin E-F disease, has a hemoglobin of only 6.5 and is almost full term). He has a big, golden-teeth smile and seems very willing to work. "Sudah" is a newly married Thai girl who has trained as a nurse aide and also works as pharmacist, cashier, records clerk, and OR assistant. She speaks good Thai and seems to be a willing and capable worker. She also speaks Mon [and

Karen] and is often my interpreter. "Jute" is a young Mon man who was rescued from death by Dr. Corpron doing a gastroenterostomy a couple of years ago after the patient was brought in nearly dead of starvation from a stomach obstruction. He talks good Thai and is my Mon interpreter. I often have to call him from his work in the surgery supplies room to help me talk to the Mon patients. Tryphena is an attractive Karen Christian woman, here to get some basic medical training. She is a hard worker and a great help. She knows a little English and is useful as my interpreter for the Karen patients. Five languages are spoken here: Thai, Karen, Mon, Burmese, and English. If the patient doesn't speak Thai or English (and most of them don't), I have to use an interpreter, which slows down the work some. Usually there are not many outpatients I am told; but today, for some reason, there are 27 and I am kept busy almost all day long. But a swim in the nearby river in the late afternoon makes me feel fresh again, and a good supper at Mrs. Corpron's house restores strength. The afternoon and evening have been very hot.

By this time, you may well be tired of reading. So, we will close this letter and continue our "diary" in the near future. Next time: What the Telakhon Karen said when presented with God's Word. Did they accept it as their long-lost Golden Book? We also hope to tell you about our Thai baby daughter.

Thank you all for your prayers. May God bless you each one.

Most sincerely,

Edwin B. McDaniel, MD

[The diary continues as what appears to be a rough draft for days 5–21. Whether this was ever sent out as a letter, I do not know. –Editor]

Up the River Kwai and Back

Days 5-19: About 10 OPD [outpatient department] patients every day. Inpatients overflowing the 10 beds most of the time. Had 17 inpatients one day. Lots of malaria, much of which seems to be of the special chloroquine-resistant strain. We are having to use quinine on these. Also, lots of hookworm, bad anemias, scrub typhus, and beriberi here. The pretty Burmese woman with leprosy who lives three days walk from here, looks better now after a week's treatment and went home today with her husband, baby, and a six-month supply of DDS, vitamins, etc. She is very grateful.

We also get patients with wounds caused by cutting hands and feet with harvest or jungle knives. Most of them don't come in until many days later, and then, only because the bleeding won't stop!

Fortunately, no major surgery so far. Really appreciate a trained OR crew when put out here where there isn't one! Even getting the proper drapes is quite a job! Did a debridement of a foot wound and an incision and exploration of a huge scrotum, both under low spinal.

The woman with hemoglobin E-F disease delivered in bed a few days ago. She was brought in at the last minute. Baby is full-term and looks nice. Fortunately, there was no postpartum hemorrhage. She had 500 mL of blood a couple of days before delivery, which raised her hemoglobin from 6.5 to 9.0. She will have to have repeated transfusions all her life, as there is no cure for disease, which is something like thalassemia.

Getting a lot of letters written and some good reading done in OB. Only one mail delivery, and we have been here almost 3 weeks! Took a Land Rover trip about one hour north of here a couple of days ago, to see the remains of one of the three bridges over the River Kwai. After the war, the tracks on this part of the "Death Railway" were torn up and taken away. A lot of the hospital paths and roads are built with "sleepers" from the railway bed, many of them with the spikes still in them. There's not much left to be seen of the railway bridge except for a few old piles, a few pieces of track underwater and the dry roadbed on the land. It reminded us of a terrible chapter in the Japanese war.

Dr. Edwin McDaniel

Yesterday went in the small mission outboard jet boat on an ambulance call about one hour and 20 minutes downriver. The water was very shallow, and we hit big rocks several times, but it was a fast, pleasant trip with beautiful scenery and birds all around us. Most of the people in the village had malaria! Brought back a baby with advanced pneumonia and malnutrition and a man with a huge scrotum, so painful he couldn't walk. Arrived back at the boat-landing just before dark.

Day 18: Charlotte, who has been teaching kindergarten to the smaller missionary children all this time, got a nasty wasp sting this afternoon which caused a huge, red, painful inflammation of one thigh. A short time later she had chilly feelings and a little fever. Put her on antihistamines.

Day 19: Work as usual. Charlotte feeling better but leg still a bit red. The travelers to the Telakhon Karen were due back today but didn't arrive.

Day 20: Dr. Corpron and his party got back at 2 AM this morning! They had a good trip. Turned over all the hospital cases to him. What a relief! I hadn't done general practice for the last 12 years—only OB.

It has been a very interesting experience. Miss Strane, Charlotte, and I left by Land Rover on the return trip. By now some rain had fallen, and the mud holes in the road through the bamboo forest were deeper than before and "winching out" was more frequent and more difficult than on the trip in. At one point, when the winch failed, it appeared that we would be stuck on the road all day! But we got out and finally reached the river at Takanoon at 3 PM, too late to start the trip downriver. A merchant in Takanoon offered us the use of a large room above his store, for sleeping. Since there is no hotel, we accepted with thanks. There was a squat toilet in a well-built outhouse with a door that could be pulled shut down the street at the warehouse about one half block away. After a pour-bath in the open area in back of the store and supper of boiled rice and meat soup at the restaurant across the street, went to bed in the hot room above the store. A man of the house slept in one corner. Charlotte feeling chilly, hot, and aching, but uncomplaining.

Last day: Up at 5:30 AM. Breakfast in restaurant across the street at 6:30 AM, boiled rice and chicken soup again. Charlotte feeling fine today. Loaded stuff in mission jet boat and off downriver by 7:30 AM. Again, cold but warmed up quickly. Raised canvas of boat about 10 AM. Stepped ashore to photograph jet boat racing by a pretty waterfall and under the railroad trestle of the Death Railway. Rode jet boat until 4 PM with a stop at Wang Po to take on 10 more peeps of gasoline [each peep holds about 5 US gallons – Editor]. Arrived at Kanchanaburi, collected the mail, photographed the war cemetery where Allied prisoners are buried, ate supper and drove into Bangkok. Got lost, but finally arrived at the guesthouse at 2 AM.

Sunday, 28 March: Charlotte down with a shaking chill, and fever to 105.6°F. Falciparum malaria parasites found on blood smear. Evidently her prophylactic Daraprim taken all during her stay in Sangkhla was ineffective. Put her on the quinine brought from Sangkhlaburi for just such an emergency.

Wednesday, 31 March: Arrived safely back in Chiang Mai. No more malaria. Thankful for an interesting trip and safe return home.

Chapter 4

The Myers at Kwai River Christian Hospital and Mission, Thailand, 1967–1970

By Dr. Roy Myers, June 2019

About Roy and Gillian Myers

The Myers (both doctors) moved to the hospital in June 1967, taking over from Dr. Doug Corpron. "Dr. Roy" was the second director of the Kwai River Christian Hospital. He did general medicine, surgery, and obstetrics. Gill did some general medicine, pediatrics, and public health. After the Dodges left, she took over the hospital treasury job as well.

Span of service: June 1967 to July 1970 plus multiple volunteer stints years later in retirement.

While we were in Medical School in Johannesburg, South Africa, Dr. Robert Nelson, the Field Secretary for the United Christian Missionary Society USA, suggested we could get married as students. We happily accepted this suggestion and were married in June 1962. The plan was to go to India once we had completed all our medical education and received our medical licenses. We went to the Missionary Orientation Program in Stony Point, New York in January 1966. Tamar, our oldest child, was delivered in June of 1966. At that time, we got news of a change in our ultimate destination. We were to go to Thailand! Dr Corpron and his family were to return to the States and a replacement was urgently needed at KRCH. The only things we knew about Thailand were the movies "The Bridge on the River Kwai" and "Anna and the King of Siam". We had a lot of catch-up reading to do.

We arrived in Bangkok and were started immediately in the Thai language school in September of 1966. Our luggage only arrived in December with all our medical books, and we were expected to write the Thai Medical exam for our Thai licenses in January. We were told not to worry as it was expected that we would fail as most doctors did and then rewrite later. This did not sit too well with us, but we had no option. Much to our joy and the surprise of others we passed on the first attempt. We only had a total of 7 months of Thai language before moving to the "Jungle Hospital".

During our Bangkok stay we took the opportunity to visit the UNICEF headquarters. We were able to persuade them that they had NO work in the hospital area. They were surprised and immediately checked up only to discover that they did not. They readily agreed to support us even though we were not a government organization. They provided us with 5 tons of materials yearly. We received powdered milk, vitamins, cod liver oil and vaccinations which were the backbone of our village outreach program.

We made our first up-river trip before the Corprons left. It was in the dry season and quite an experience for ex-city people. It started early in the morning with a 4-hour car trip to Kanchanaburi, where there is a cemetery to the many British, Australian and Allied forces soldiers who died while constructing the Death Railway from Bangkok to Burma in the Second World War. Then an hour rail trip to the boat landing site at Wang Pho. The rail line literally hugged the cliff with the river flowing alongside through the mountain passes and over numerous concrete bridges. We had a colorful group of fellow travelers ranging from local farmers and their products, chickens, vegetables, military persons, and locals. The long-tail boats are only wide enough for two people per seat, with 10 rows of seats, and the propeller is on a 10-foot-long shaft which made it possible to jump rapids. The boat ride was fascinating but after 6 hours of engine roar and hard seats, began to lose its appeal. To spice up the trip we fortunately passed by a 6-foot king cobra crossing the river ahead of us swimming upright in the water. We were also treated to an engine breakdown. Our driver had to make a jungle walk to a nearby village to get a new engine while we all sat waiting for his return an hour later. We ultimately arrived at Takanun (Tongpapum). Tamar tolerated the trip well till the next part by jungle road, or rather track or path. Paul Dodge, the pastor, met us here with the mission Land Rover. We had our evening meal and then set off in the dark. The 60-kilometer trip took 6 hours of bumps, twists and turns, and having to get out and walk when we crossed dry riverbeds, but the vehicle went down and up hills to do this. Getting out to walk was a precaution in case of an accident. The "road" was created by the lumber trucks hauling teak logs from the forests. This first trip of these city-born-and-bred people with a 9-month baby was a real wake up. What had we gotten ourselves into? On arriving at the mission, we were greeted by Doug and Helen [Corpron], who urged us to take a sponge bath and check ourselves in the mirror. We were brown from head to toes from all the dust kicked up off the road. Yes, a real dirt road. This trip really gave us a taste of what was to come. We were introduced to the staff of the hospital, hostel, school and church. After a short visit we returned to Bangkok and language school having had an unforgettable experience which has lasted a lifetime.

We returned to the hospital in mid-1967. Our furniture, food and toilet supply for a year was on its way in a barge, as the river water level was still high enough to reach the hospital. A new phase in our lives had started. We were now working with Winnie and Paul Dodge. She was the chief nurse and had been holding the hospital open till we arrived. He was the hospital administrator, which suited us as we became familiar with the type of patients we would be working with and what life would be like living in splendid isolation. We met with the Thai preacher and learned what his outreach would be and soon found out it was not directed towards the patients nor the Karens and locals. This was a problem for us. We were into nondiscrimination. We met the Thai teachers who were having emotional difficulties living in such isolation. The obvious solution was to help local people and students to feel that teaching was a good calling.

The hospital was staffed with Winnie and local Karen people and Ebra Sanba. She was a Karen from Burma who was a registered nurse who had recently arrived at the urging of Olivepa Thadin, the Karen elder leader in the area. He had represented the Karen people in London at the negotiations to create a United Burma with all of the hill tribes and the Burmese. At that time the Burmese military took power of Burma and arrested or killed the hill tribe leaders and subjugated all. Olivepa came to Thailand as a political refugee and then settled in the Sangkhlaburi area on the mission and he and Olivemo became the hostel parents. Olive, his eldest daughter, was a hospital aide with Tryphena, Saella, and Benita. Surin was the lab technician and also did all the X-rays and anesthesia by open mask ether. Other hospital people were Jit and Lincoln as gardeners and Rebecca as the admission clerk. There were other workers whose names elude me now. Harmiet [also spelled Hla Myint] was our general maintenance man with help from Aphee.

We also had a group of resistance leaders against the Burmese Army who had escaped to our area and were living adjacent to the mission. They all spoke excellent English and we had wonderful discussions about life and the sadness of war, loss of nationhood, and what persecution was like. Despite this loss, they continued to struggle for recognition and freedom as a person, as a people, as a nation. At times it was hard to remember we were so isolated and yet so involved with life and struggle. We were totally accepted into the Karen family.

Towards the end of our first year the Dodges went on furlough to the States and did not return to KRCH. We decided to repaint and clean the hospital. There were betel nut stains on the floor and walls which really required hard scrubbing to clean up. We had to try to re-educate the patients and families to spit into spittoons. We also had a blockage of the toilet system due to an overload of ascaris worms [roundworms] passed by patients. This got us onto a prophylactic treatment of all patients against the worms. Leading our digging crew and wearing rubber boots we were successful. I felt it important to show by example.

Gillian became our new hospital treasurer and we discovered how poor the hospital was. Belt tightening was the order of the day. The records were not good; receipts of transactions were poor. The village chief and others tried to double charge us for goods and work. When Gill showed him his signature of received payments, he tried to deny it and then told us that "Acharn Dodge" paid him and we were stingy and causing him to "lose face".

Without the connections Doug [Corpron] had in the States, we had to find new ways to support the hospital. On our second trip back to Bangkok for a missionary meeting we went to the Thai Public Health Department with our concerns for TB and malaria in our area. As a result, we became part of their field programs. For each case we diagnosed of malaria or TB we had to send them a blood smear or sputum sample. If our diagnosis was correct, they provided the medication free. Surin, our lab technician, was 99% correct.

Clarence and Lucille Welch, retired hog farmers from Missouri, who were working in the Nakorn Pathom area, were sent up to help us with maintenance and to teach a different method of pig farming. Instead of free roaming, pigs were penned and rapidly fattened and marketed quicker. Gill, Clarence, and Gareth, a local Karen, spent many evening hours playing guitar together. In later years we learned that Gareth was the head of the music program at the Christian College in Chiang Mai. We were sad to see them [the Welches] go on furlough, but they returned as the managers of Bangkok Christian Guest House. They had been great fun and most helpful to us and the Mission.

Ester Greenman, a Baptist nurse, replaced the Dodges at the hospital. She was also joined by Emilie Ballard, who had worked with the Burmese Karen Christians for many years as an evangelist.

On one of our early visits to Bangkok we met a Disciples army chaplain based in Bangkok. He was interested in our work, so we invited him to visit. He took us up and was so impressed that he used the mission as an R&R retreat for soldiers. Over a period of a year over 100 soldiers came to stay in our house and the hostel. We had many intense discussions on religion, life, and the war in Vietnam. They came in groups and stayed for four to five days, bringing their own K rations, which Gill combined into edible food. Daily bread came out of the oven at about 2pm and they lined up like ants to devour slices. The army was also very supportive, giving the hospital blankets, food treats, blood for our patients (not really allowed) and medications about to go out of date but still very usable. Bangkok-based army doctors also visited, providing much companionship and discussion on medical and surgical issues. Through them we were able to dispose of a large fuel-hungry Rogue River-style jet boat. This had been donated through the Corpron contacts when he ran the mission. No one knew how to drive it and it cost much more than a regular boat to run. The military were going to use it for a village outreach program but ultimately took it to Bangkok and used it to entertain visitors and ranking officers. It was a weight off our backs. It had been stuck on the pylons on the stairway from the rising and falling of the water level during the rainy season on many occasions. To lift the boat off the post was quite difficult. Fortunately, there was no damage to the boat.

With our working with the Thai Public Health Department we met members of the Liverpool Tropical Medical School from England. They were advisors to a Thai medical school. On their visits to check on our work and treatment of malaria and outcomes, they were able to keep us updated on treatments. The retiring head of the Liverpool program, Dr. Elliot, had been a prisoner of war in the mission area under the Japanese during WWII. He gave us a copy of his diary of his experiences. We were able to show him old upturned boxcars and bridge and railway remains. We remained friends with his successor Dr. Dion Bell for many years. A copy of the diary is now at the Australian Death Railway Museum on the road from Kanchanaburi to Sangkhlaburi [at Hellfire Pass]. The museum is in memory of all the Allied and particularly the Australian POW's who died while building the Death Railway line [from Nong Pladuk in Thailand to Thanbyuzayat in Burma] in order to connect the railway systems of Singapore, Malaya and Thailand with the railway system of Burma during the Japanese occupation.

Amongst the many visitors to "Hotel Myers", as there were no hotels in the area, was Dr. Mashall, an Egyptian Public Health physician from the World Health Organization, who came up to KRCH for mosquito control operations in the area. He had Peace Corp staff spraying homes in the villages to kill mosquitos. We had him spray mission houses, the school, the hostel, the church, and hospital. We hoped to set an example for the locals. The work was done in cycles with return visits.

With the 5 tons of UNICEF contributions, we were able to do village visits by Land Rover in the dry seasons and by aluminum boat in the rainy season. The milk powder and vaccinations were a great attraction for the villagers. We made use of local schools and the village leaders' homes to distribute the materials and teach public health. I had a cultural lesson with my first local anesthesia operation. Thinking how important privacy was, I found the most isolated location in the home to do the procedure. Midway through I had the sensation of "watching eyes" and turning around, saw a large audience watching. After that, I did all procedures in full view of the crowd—real live theater—a teaching moment.

River travel was often easier than travel by road until we had a breakdown with engine trouble. We had to pontoon our way downriver until it got dark. Aphee, our boatman, found a large riverside house where we stopped for the night. Ebra, Aphee, and I bought a chicken, which Aphee killed and stripped the feathers and skin like removing a glove. It was then cooked over an open fire. The owner gave us spices and rice which we ate in the firelight. We slept on the bamboo floor and next morning pontooned our way home.

Land Rover trips were very different but also with many unexpected events. We had to cross rivers with the water lapping at the doors. Crossing bridges made of logs, we often had to move the logs to accommodate the track width of the Land Rover, which was narrower than that of the lumber trucks. At times we had to make new roads because of fallen trees. Our worst experience was sliding off the logs at the crossing and getting stuck in the mud. This occurred on a trip to Bangkok for the surgery to Niki's neck [second daughter]. She was born with a tumor in the neck. We were unable to lever the vehicle back onto the road. We needed an elephant! After an hour we heard the dragging chains coming towards us. The mahout [elephant driver] felt we should push rather than pull, but after buckling the back of the vehicle we pulled. I was in the driver's seat with the engine on, the elephant leant forward and then took off pulling the vehicle easily out of the mud. What strength in those legs!

We had thought Niki would be born in Bangkok, but after a trip towards the end of Gill's pregnancy when we made the trip with a delivery set as a precaution, no baby. We returned to KRCH and Niki arrived in our hospital. She was the third missionary child born on the Kwai River Christian Mission compound [Dan Corpron was born in 1961 in the Corpron house and Brooks Dodge was born in 1963 in the Dodge house.] It was a wonderful and scary experience. I completed the delivery, and Ebra, my assistant, did the suctioning of the airway with a resultant loud cry. She cleaned and wrapped Niki and gave her back to a very happy Gill. Ebra's relationship with Niki still remains very strong. Ebra is like her second mother. After an hour in the hospital we wheeled Gill back to the house, the delivery completed.

The next trip was also an adventure. Niki had a rapidly growing blood vessel tumor in her neck. We went to the SDA [Seventh Day Adventist] Hospital [in Bangkok] and the tumor was excised under general anaesthesia. She had to stay in hospital a few days, so Tamar and I went ahead on home, taking a truck ride for the last 60 kilometers. The road was not in a good condition and the driver was going a little fast. Going around a bend in the road, the truck veered off into a tree. I saw the accident coming and with Tamar on my lap, feet braced on the dashboard and holding her tightly we hit the tree, which stopped the truck solidly. We were uninjured but a little shaken up. The truck was dented but still functioning; so, we completed the trip home. A week after the operation, through contacts, Gill and Niki got a Border Police helicopter ride back to the mission station. Gill had to feed Niki in the Commandant's office and then followed a long and tortuous flight. The pilot was doing his first trip upriver and had to follow the river closely. The consolation was the fantastic view she had of the terrain: jungle trees and tall bamboo growths, villages and rice paddies and the river. They landed at the border patrol site, and Gill walked home, carrying Niki [who also had bilateral casts on her legs to start correcting her club feet]. This was the time of no phones in the jungle.

The hospital was busy with lots of sick malaria patients and general surgery patients. They arrived by many forms of transport from walking, ox carts, dugout canoes, regular long tailed boats, and being carried in a longyi, a circular skirt-like male clothing, supported by a bamboo pole with a person on each end and the patient lying in the loop. Some of these patients had been carried for days through the jungle. Patients had injuries from mine blasts, cuts from hatchets, tree falls, or infections, pneumonias, and heart problems. Many of the patients paid their bills with rice instead of money. Paul Dodge had overseen the building of a rice barn so the rice could be stored and later shipped and sold down river. We heard of how the rice merchants would sell rice at a high price after the harvest season was over and indenture the farmers to them by buying rice on the field when the farmers had no money to buy next harvest season's rice. This was a vicious cycle. We changed things by not sending the rice down river but holding it till the rice prices rose and then under-selling the rice merchants. This allowed the farmers to sell their own rice at fair market prices. This did not make the merchants happy, and soon there were threats against our lives. Our Mission chiefs in Bangkok then decided to move us to Chiang Mai to work in the McCormick Hospital surgery department under Dr. Harold Hanson till things quietened down. I was delighted as I was doing operations with guidance that I had to do at KRCH. Ten days into this I came down with severe jaundice requiring hospitalization myself. Laboratory tests revealed viral hepatitis. I remained very yellow for 6 weeks and underwent a liver biopsy which showed healing liver cells. Within a week I was back to normal and back at work. Gillian also worked while in Chiang Mai at the McKean

Leprosy Hospital. The children were left with a nannie. We soon got word that it was safe to return to KRCH. In our absence there was an outbreak of typhoid. Ebra [Sanba], Emilie [Ballard], and Esther [Greenman] were holding the hospital open and working. There had been many sick and some dead patients. The headman and other leaders asked the Mission to bring us back. We were happy to return and had a most productive and fulfilling year. I did a lot of surgery and Gill was very active with the Public Health program and the children. Economically, the hospital was on a sound footing and our thriftiness had paid off.

Our experiences had helped us in our future decisions on returning to South Africa. Gill went into Pediatrics and Public Health and I went into General Surgery. We had developed very strong and deep relationships with the large Karen family in the area making us feel part of their extended family.

We both completed our specialty training and also moved our whole family to the States, settling in Maryland. Gill completed her residency in Public Health and Preventive Medicine at the University of Maryland and also did her master's degree at The Johns Hopkins Medical School. She then went into the Anne Arundel County Health Department from which she was recruited to be the first Medical Director of the Maryland State Program of HIV Aids at a very trying time. Aids was newly discovered, greatly feared, and very scary to the public, who now needed to be educated about this disease. Later she joined the Prince Georges County Health Department until her retirement. I did a Fellowship in the R Adams Cowley Shock Trauma Center, part of the University of Maryland Medical Center, and stayed on till my retirement.

The Myers at KRCH/KRCM

In our retirement we went back to the new [Huay Malai] KRCH for about 2 months a year till 2015. We have remained in close contact with Ebra and other Karen family members. We both look back most fondly on our days at the KRCH. The experiences greatly enriched our lives, making us open to new people, ideas, and points of view. We learned to listen and try to understand others and accept different lifestyles and philosophies. The hardships made us more appreciative of the good things in life and how to share with others. It has made us who we are today.

Roy, Gillian, Tamar and Niki Myers

Chapter 5

Recruited for the Kwai River Christian Hospital

By Ebra Sanba, April 2019

About the author of this chapter:

Ebra is the longest-serving nurse (32 years) at the Kwai River Christian Hospital to date. She speaks five languages and possesses a wide range of nursing and midwifery skills. She was a key person in keeping the hospital open.

Span of service at KRCH: 1967-1999

    I never heard about the Kwai River Christian Hospital wanting a Karen nurse from Burma. Before I came to work at KRCH, I was working in Maymyo B. M. H. (Burma Military Hospital). As usual, every year, we have a month annual leave. I was going home to Bassein to visit my mother and stay with her for a while. I rode on the train from Maymyo to Rangoon and my brother met me at the station. We went to stay at my friend's house for a night and were going to go to Bassein the next morning. We arrived at my friend's house at 2 PM. Then at 5 PM two ladies came to visit me. I was very happy to see them. One was my cousin's sister. I thought that my cousin's sister wanted to send things for her mother. We had had no contact from each other for many years, and I was surprised to see her. Then both of them started to talk about KRCH. They said that there is a mission hospital near the Thai-Burma border. There is a missionary doctor and nurse working in the hospital. The doctor wanted a Karen nurse from Burma to come and work in KRCH. Thai nurses came and worked for one week, went back to Bangkok, and never returned. They do not want to work in a rural area. The missionary doctor, Dr. Corpron, asked Olivepa to look for a

Recruited

Karen nurse from Burma. The two ladies said many things about the hospital. I listen to them, and at last I told them I cannot go because I am on leave and will have to go back after my leave. The most important thing now is to go home and see my mother. They said I can come back after one year. I said I cannot go. I strongly refused. Then I said if I don't report back to work there will be a big problem for my family. We talked for a long time, then the house owner asked the two ladies, "How long are you both staying here? There is a rule that if we have guests staying at our house, we have to report to the headman (names, where from, and length of stay)." The two ladies said we are going early in the morning.

Then my brother asked me, "Are you willing to go with them?"

I said, "No. I don't want to go. I am not ready to go. I have a job and have to report back to work after my leave."

Then my brother said that the house owner is very worried and nervous. He said, "If you won't go, they will not leave the house."

Last of all I had to agree to go with them. I told my brother to take things I brought for my mother and family. I know my mother will ask him about me.

So, early in the morning we left for the train to take us to Moulmein. Then we went to the riverbank and stepped on a boat.

At 3 PM we arrived at the place where the guide was to take us. We started walking. I am a village girl, but most of the time I stayed in the city. I was not prepared for this journey. It will be a long, difficult, and dangerous journey. At that time Burma is in a very bad situation between the Karen and Burmese. Because we were still in Burmese territory there would be danger even in Karen villages. We always avoid going in the village. We walked outside the village. We walked the whole day start from early morning till dark. We always reach a hut in the field and sleep for the night. In the early morning the two ladies got up cook rice and fish paste with chili, packed in banana leaves and started the journey. We are in the Karen territory. On the way we passed many Karen soldiers, but they did not ask any question. We walked every day for almost 3 weeks. Then the guide told us we are getting near the border. This is the last big Karen village. We went outside the village. There is a house with an old man staying with three grandchildren: two male and one female. He is a cousin of Olivepa, staying out of the village. The Karen soldiers always pass their house, and sometimes rest there. We stayed there longer, almost a week. Then I asked why are we taking so long this time. We were longer there because a message came that we are not allowed to pass that area because they thought I was a Burmese spy coming from Burma. With a heavy heart I was very worried for my family back home. "I am not a Burmese spy. What am I going to do now? If I cannot go forward, how can I go back? The Burmese will say I am a Karen spy!" But after a day, a message came that we could continue our journey.

There was a group of the men going out to work in the forest. We can go with them, so the next morning three elephants with five men came to get us. One lady rode on each elephant. The men walked. We arrived at their place at almost dark. It was raining. We passed swift streams and rivers, but we three ladies were on the elephants. There were three bamboo houses. It's a big forest with big logs ready for the elephants to pull them down to the river. Then early in the morning, the ladies cooked and packed and we started our journey again on foot. It goes on every day. Then we reached the river. We crossed on a bamboo raft to the other side. We walked and saw the three pagodas at Three Pagodas Pass. We sat down and ate rice. The guide said one pagoda is on the middle; that is the borderline; the other is on Thai side, and the other is on Burma side. We still had to walk. Then we continue on to cross the Thai border. We met 2 Thai border policemen. They asked us where are we going. The guide said in Thai, "KRCH". So, they let us pass.

The guide arrived first at Olivepa's house. Then half an hour later we arrived. Olive ran down to meet us. We shook hands. She asked me, "Are you the Karen nurse Dr. Corpron asked my father to look for?"

I told her, "Maybe."

Then she said, "Dr. Corpron left just this morning. You came late!" I was so tired I did not say anything.

Then she said, "Tomorrow is Sunday. We will go to church."

The next day we went to church. The church service was held in the mission school hall. Paul Dodge led the service. After church, we shook hands but did not say much.

Then Olive said, "Do you want to see around the hospital, mission school, and hostel before you go back to Burma?"

"Yes", I said.

Recruited

We went to the hospital. Everything was so quiet. Sunday is a quiet day. Then we came back to Olive's house. I was very worried thinking, "How am I going back? News will spread that I went to Thailand."

Then one lady told me not to worry. "You can come with me. I am going back to Moulmein next week." I was still very worried. The Burmese will check me and ask many questions.

Next day was Monday. Olive dressed up and went to work. She is a nurse aide in KRCH. About an hour later, she came home and said, "Come to the hospital. The new doctor wants to see you."

So, I went.

Dr. Roy Myers was there. He asked me, "Do you speak Karen?"

"Yes."

"Burmese?"

"Yes."

"Thai?"

"No."

"English?"

"A little."

"Do you know Dr. Corpron?"

"No."

"We are doing our ward rounds. Come with us." So, we did our ward rounds with Esther Greenman and Winnie Dodge. [Both these ladies were nurses with the American Baptist Mission.]

After rounds, Dr. Roy said I must come to work tomorrow.

"Move to the hostel this evening." So, I moved to the mission hostel. [This was the Christian boarding house for elementary school students.]

I shared a room with a nurse aide from KRCH. As soon as I moved in, the nurse aide gave me a mat. She took out a big quilt. She said, "This is for you. Dr. Corpron's wife left this quilt. She said to give it to the new nurse that is coming from Burma." I was very thankful because I have nothing. I could not bring anything.

The next day I went to work in KRCH. That was 4th July 1967. I worked with many missionary doctors and nurses and volunteer doctors.

Dr. Corpron asked Olivepa to look for a Karen nurse from Burma. I came but never had the opportunity to work with him. The first doctors I worked with were Dr. Roy and Dr. Gill Myers. They were very good to me. They helped me in everything I need. They help me all the time even until now.

Then I worked with Dr. John Freeman.

Dr. Phil [McDaniel] was my last doctor I worked with.

I came to work in KRCH on 4th July 1967. Retired 23rd June 1999. That is how I came to work in KRCH. I came on foot from Burma to Thailand.

Chapter 6

Village Health and Friendship Bridge

By Dr. John Freeman, January 2010

About the author:

John and wife, Nancy (RN), reopened the hospital after it had been closed almost four years for lack of a doctor. He expanded the village health program and set up a school health program. With the help of local craftsmen and village leaders, he undertook the construction of a bridge over the Ranti River (a tributary of the River Khwae [Kwai]), using materials from the abandoned Death Railway. You can find out much more about the Freemans' time at KRCH from John's book, Jungle Episodes.

Span of service at KRCH: March 1974 to May 1977

[This chapter was copied from "Ministry to the least."]

On our first visit to the hospital [in 1974] we were struck by the remoteness of the place as well as the difficulty of transportation. On the other hand, the Kwai River is the most beautiful river that I have ever traveled on. It was at that time a place of beauty on the jungle trails and the rivers.

At the time of our work, there was a serious concern about the possibility of a communist takeover of Thailand. The U. S. had just pulled out of Vietnam and communist rebels were operating just up the road from the Kwai River Christian Hospital. So, with that in mind, we worked to reopen the hospital with as simple an approach as possible in the likelihood that all missionaries would have to leave.

The village health program seemed the way to go as it had the potential of preventing many more illnesses and deaths than a small hospital could take care of. At that time, when a person got sick enough to go to the hospital, he was usually too sick to get there. So, with the help of Olivia [Thadin/Saiduangchai] and Josie [Falla], the village health program took root and lasted about 25 years and prevented thousands of children's deaths. With all the village health work, Olivia still had time to keep up her veterinary practice that centered mainly on castrating pigs. The hospital work was made a joy by having Ebra [Sanba] who could handle anything in the hospital. Of course, all the others who worked in our little hospital at that time made the medical practice a happy time. The nurses even had a little sense of humor as at the end of clinic one day they informed me that there was still one more patient. The waiting room was empty except for a dog and some chickens. Josie motioned that the patient was outside; so, I went to look and found only an elephant. He had a rash that covered his whole belly. All the salve in the hospital would not cover that.

We did, though, have a full-service hospital. There were a few times when embalming was performed. We stocked medicines for animals and as I mentioned, Olivia had her sideline business.

One thing that Nancy and I remember is that we had to produce most of our food. Nancy soon had a flock of chickens and I had a hutch full of rabbits. Then there was the pig always in the pen. The goats lived under the rabbits in their little house. We soon had a garden going that produced most of the vegetables that we needed.

The varmints were always lurking somewhere, but they were there to add interest. The first year while [daughter] Jonlyn was still crawling, we killed about 40 or 50 scorpions on the floor of our house. Of course, there was the occasional "takap" (centipede), which was a frightening sight. A cobra lived around the pumphouse, but I never had a stick when meeting him, so we decided to live and let live.

When there was a little slack time, we could find entertainment, such as the time I helped Nai Chert and the Mon carpenter build a bridge across the river [Ranti]. That was an interesting little venture.

All the wonderful people there made it a very pleasant place to spend three years. I would do it again without thinking about it and our children remember the life on the Kwai with great fondness.

John and Nancy Freeman

Chapter 7

Midwife, Lady Health Visitor,
Mobile Clinic Coordinator

By Olivia Saiduangchai, April 2019

About the author of this chapter:

Olive, Oliver, Olivia, Ophelia, Orlando, Oscar, and Oswald were all sons and daughters of Olivepa and Olivemo. "Olivepa" means "Olive's father" and "Olivemo" means "Olive's mother," both names derived from "Olive," their firstborn. Olivia headed up the mobile clinic program from 1975-84 (until the hospital was moved from Lainam to Huay Malai), bringing healthcare to remote villages on a regular schedule. Even after the move to Huay Malai, she continued to oversee an "under-5's" program as well as family planning and prenatal care at the hospital. Villagers from six nearby villages came regularly for these preventive services.

Span of service at KRCH: 1975–2005

Training and work in Burma

I did my training as a healthcare provider in Burma as a midwife and Lady Health Visitor. I finished my midwifery training in Burma on the 3rd April 1962 at the Dufferin Women's Hospital, Rangoon. After I finished my bond as a midwife, I applied for Lady Health Visitor School in Rangoon. I finished my Lady Health Training on the 31st August 1966 and served the government for four years for my bond.

The Rural Health Centre was staffed as follows:
1. Health Assistant: 1
2. Lady Health Visitor: 1
3. Midwives: 5
4. Malaria Assistant: 1
5. Leprosy Technician: 1
6. Smallpox Vaccinator: 1
7. Gardener: 1

The main duties of a Lady Health Visitor are as follows:
1. In charge of the Mother and Child Health Clinic
2. In charge of midwives
3. Survey and collecting of family folders
4. Health Education
5. Home Visiting
6. Join Rural Health Centre Mobile Clinic Team
7. Meet with midwives once a month
8. Attend a Health District meeting once a month and send reports

My training included the following:
1. Field work at the Leprosy Clinic
2. Field work at the TB Clinic
3. Field work at the Mental Hospital
4. Field work at the Venereal Disease Clinic
5. Field work at the Contagious Disease Hospital (CDH)

My main duty was to follow up on patients by visiting them at home and finding out if they had any problems. During the training, we attended lectures and, at the same time, did home visiting. In a big city like Rangoon it's crowded. It's not easy to find the right address. Sometimes I felt sorry for the car driver. Most of the patients are poor and change their job often with new address. Occasionally, the whole day we can visit and follow up only one. But as a team, we did our best and worked together well.

Moving to Thailand

I heard about the Kwai River Christian Mission and the Kwai River Christian Hospital from my parents [Olivepa and Olivemo].

Midwife, Lady Health Visitor, Mobile Clinic Coordinator

My parents asked me to come home and live with them [at the Kwai River Christian Mission]. They didn't want me to stay in Burma. At that time, I was working in the Health Department, Burma. As soon as I knew my parents wanted me to come home, I put in my resignation [after finishing all my bond with the government]. I had to wait for a year until I could resign because they could not find anyone to replace me. I prayed to God saying, "If I can come home, I will be happy to do whatever job is available." I came home in April 1970.

There is a difference working with the government compared to working with the mission. Working with the government means we must do our duty the best that we can. But with the mission, we endeavor not only to help people's health, but also to attend to their other needs (example, when we see they need food, clothes, etc., we cannot overlook it). As Christians we need to show people our love and care and pray for them.

Wash Girl, Evangelist, and Village Health Program Coordinator

At the time I came home, the Kwai River Christian Hospital was closed [for lack of a doctor].

The first job I got from the mission was at the hostel as a wash girl because the wash girl was sick. I worked for two months with no salary.

The second job was as the evangelist to Kwe Kya Toe Village to replace Kru Sai Kham who was going to work at another village. I also accompanied missionary Emilie Ballard on her village trips. The salary was about 500 baht per month. [The exchange rate at that time was 20 baht per US dollar; so, this salary would have been about US$25 per month.] I know that God used me and let me work with the mission. I thank God for that.

After a few months the Kwai River Christian Hospital reopened as a clinic. I helped Ebra [nurse from Burma] and Josie [nurse from Australia] who were taking care of the patients. We did everything that was needed for the patients (washing, cleaning, cooking).

As soon as Dr. John Freeman came, he found out about the difficulties of communication and transportation in the area. To bring patients to the KRCH was difficult. Sometimes patients came to the hospital when they were very sick and it's too late to help them. So, it's better we reach them before they get very sick. Dr. John decided to start a mobile clinic. As I had been working with the Public Health Department in Burma at a Rural Health Centre, going out to the villages and spending a few days was no problem for me. I like to travel, meet people, and make new friends. It's a joy for me.

Chapter 8

Memories from My Early Years in Thailand

By Nurse Jan Vertigan/Yawan, August 2019

About the author of this chapter:

Jan came to Thailand as a missionary nurse with the Australian Baptist Missionary Society (later called Global Interaction) in May of 1977. She and a small staff held the Kwai River Christian Hospital together during a challenging time. Dr. Bina Sawyer was nominally the director of the Kwai River Christian Hospital during the time between Dr. John Freeman's leaving (May 1977) and Dr. Phil McDaniel taking over (April 1979). Dr. Sawyer made occasional short working visits during this period but lived most of the time in Maesariang in the north of Thailand, where she worked at Maesariang Christian Hospital. Dr. Keith Dahlberg, also of Maesariang Christian Hospital, and Dr. Ed McDaniel, based at McCormick Hospital in Chiang Mai, each made at least one working visit during this time period, but most of this time, the KRCH was without a doctor physically present. Travel between Maesariang or Chiang Mai and the Kwai River Christian Hospital took 2-3 days one way in those days.

Span of service at KRCH: May 1977 to February 1994

First Ten Days in Thailand

Having made a commitment to God to be involved in cross cultural mission overseas, there came decisions of when, where, and what mission.

Many decisions later, I was arriving in Thailand on 30th May 1977 just 2 weeks after the Freeman family had left Thailand to return to the USA. Dr. John Freeman had been the sole physician at the Kwai River Christian Hospital for the previous three years. I was met at the airport by Jan Stretton (fellow missionary nurse assigned to KRCH) and Ray Burman (evangelist missionary recently moved to Sangkhlaburi with his wife, Shirley). We made it back to the Bangkok Christian Guest House just before the midnight curfew (ban on being out on the street).

The next morning Jan and I were immersed in the bustle and aromas of Chinatown searching for parts for the water pump and buying hospital supplies. There were medicines to purchase and other hospital business to attend to.

We made a trip to Manorom Christian Hospital to meet with Alan and Charlise Davis, Leprosy Mission staff, who advised regarding KRCH patients with leprosy.

I was being sent by Australian Baptist Missionary Society to move straight to work at Kwai River Christian Hospital rather than starting my missionary time at language school. The previous Australian nurse, Josie Falla, had returned to Australia, and Dr. John Freeman's departure was leaving Jan Stretton as the only expatriate staff member at KRCH, and the mission didn't want her alone, especially as the responsibility was big. Also, it was still a period of communist insurgency.

Ten days after arrival, we set off in a little old truck packed full of hospital supplies—through Chinatown and past early morning tai chi enthusiasts—on to Kanchanaburi. Past that city we started to get into beautiful mountain country that, in many ways, reminded me of Tasmania's west coast mountains, an area where Jan and I had first met and worked together. I'm so glad Jan was sitting in the middle. I was next to her in the "window seat." However, there was no actual window. In fact, there was no actual door! She was dropping off to sleep and leaning onto me. If she had been in the "window seat" she might have leaned right out of the truck!

We drove to the boat landing at Bak Saeng, Sai Yok Noi. This was the first year of using this site as previously it meant a train trip from Kanchanaburi to Wang Po station and hauling supplies down steep steps to the landing. I noted one of the raft houses with a young boy caring for a pig in a pen on the raft. Aware of my minimal language we smiled at each other and I was aware that, for most of the world, a smile is the international language.

Finding two Sangkhla brothers, with their boats, was a relief (as of 2019 S'ngop still had raft houses, restaurant, and local boat tours in Sangkhla). The river trip was on a pristine clear day—I have described it as being able to see every leaf on every tree—the views were breathtaking, yet also highlighted the remoteness. There were stops along the way at floating raft houses: shops with toilets out over the river where the resident fish knew when the facilities were in use!

The river was low, as the rains had only just started. We crammed into the smaller boat, with all the supplies, and headed up-river for Tha Khanun (now Thong Pha Phum). From there on we had to avoid rocks and negotiate rapids. After around 10 hours from departure, we arrived at Sangkhlaburi town with the then new Mon bridge glistening in the sunset glow.

The stunning views and the peaceful scenes all set me praising God for the beautiful place He had led me to come and work.

We came around into the Ranti River and to the boat-landing below the "doctor's" house. With no resident doctor and none in sight, this house was now to become the new "maidens' mansion" with up to 4 single ladies in residence.

Having settled in and eaten, we anticipated a quiet evening sleep and a first view of the hospital in the morning. Then, in the darkness of evening, Nanu, the male nurse aide, was downstairs calling "Jan, Jan"—"a patient"—but was he saying "shock" or "shot"? We needed to go to find out.

A baby was crying incessantly with little strength in his arms and legs. The mother was blaming the DPT vaccination given recently. The possibilities could be many—polio? viral? malaria? meningitis? [but no stiff neck]. No telephone, no radio links; the next nearest hospital back in Kanchanaburi we had passed through at daybreak.

So then, time to turn to the textbooks on the shelves. We found an entry regarding pertussis vaccine encephalopathy (later papers discount this complication). The article ended with the words, "any child with these symptoms should always be managed in a major hospital with all facilities for resuscitation!" And there we were in this little jungle hospital with no doctor—we were "it".

Now the challenges that God had brought me to had become obvious just hours after my arrival.

But I knew that God would be with me through all the challenges as well as in the joys.

Jan Vertigan/Yawan

Hospital without a Doctor

At the time of my arrival in Thailand, there were no indications when another resident doctor would arrive to take up the hospital work.

The professional staff consisted of Jan Stretton (nurse on site since 1974), Ebra (nurse at KRCH since 1967), Olivia (midwife/public health who had joined the KRCH staff 1974) and now Jan Vertigan (nurse). We worked with a team of locally trained nurse aides, lab and other staff. Jan and I were missionaries with the Australian Baptist Missionary Society.

Arrangements had been made for some doctors to visit occasionally but there was no regular schedule. There was no telephone or radio contact, so the best way to make contact with others was to re-trace the trip I had made, back to Kanchanaburi city: 8–10 hours by boat then find a vehicle to continue the trip.

There was an "anamai" [government health station] in the local township for simple treatments. We could request their assistance in radio-calling for a border police helicopter to medivac out very serious cases that we could see may benefit from treatment in the city [Kanchanaburi, the provincial capital], but they were hesitant to take any who were not citizens and many locals didn't want to leave the area anyway.

We knew that Jan Stretton was to return to Australia in December for her first 1-year furlough. Hence, a pressing need for me to learn as much as possible before she left. This was another reason why I had been sent straight to KRCH, by-passing language school for the time being.

Oranut, a language teacher from Chiang Mai had given me a few basic lessons in Australia where she had been visiting. Oranut arrived in Sangkhlaburi a month later to assist several missionaries and also run Thai classes for interested local Karens. So, I was able to communicate at a basic level by the time Jan and Oranut left in December.

The only local person who had a reasonably good grasp of English and was also fluent in Thai was Chatri, Jit's older brother, who did all the lab, X-ray, and dental work at KRCH. But he, too, left in December to return to Chiang Rai with his wife (whom he'd met while doing lab training with Margaret Strane at Overbrook Hospital) and their baby son. [Years later, Chatri would become Jan's brother-in-law when Jan married Jit.]

With no doctor, no fellow Aussie nurse, and no hospital manager, a lot of administrative and medical work was heading my way.

Loes de Vos had previously served with ABMS [Australian Baptist Missionary Society] in Papua New Guinea and arrived to join the KRCH staff in August 1977. [She remained as the pharmacist and later added work with the Candlelight Project for children with disabilities until 1999].

By the end of 1977, the hospital would need to be re-registered for the following year which required 2 nurses and one doctor. This meant it was essential for me to do the registration exams (thankfully, in English). These I completed by late 1977. As Ebra and Olivia were not able to register, Emilie Ballard was to be the second nurse. She had trained and been a USA army nurse during WWII. She had worked for many years in Burma until all missionaries had to leave. She then moved to Thailand and although not planning to do hospital work, she did register as a nurse. [Emilie celebrated her 100th birthday on July 22nd, 2019]. But a doctor was still required, and Dr. Keith Dahlberg had returned to work at the MaeSariang Christian Hospital, so they were willing for Dr. Bina Sawyer to take official responsibility for KRCH. However, Bina would continue working at MaeSariang and make occasional visits or arrange for other doctors to come. These visits happened, on average, about every 2-4 months for 1-3 days each visit. The only long visit was from Dr. Ed McDaniel who came with his Thai daughter and stayed around 10 days.

During 1978 we received great news that Dr. Phil McDaniel had been accepted as the new full-time missionary doctor for KRCH.

In July 1978 Ray & Shirley Burman, fellow Australian Baptist missionaries had been in Thailand 2 years but in Sangkhla just over 1 year, now working in outreach among Pwo Karen. One Saturday they were travelling down river for meetings and escorting a mission visitor. Shirley wouldn't have seen the imminent boat collision and was killed instantly. The only way to confirm the news, brought by other boat drivers on the Sunday, was for a group of local leaders to accompany me to the Kanchanaburi hospital the next day.

The following month Phil, Melba, and Linette McDaniel arrived, and, following TBMF conference, they then travelled with Loes and myself in what became a most dramatic trip. Heavy rains had flooded the river. One failed attempt to reach the boat landing by road—requiring a return to Kanchanaburi overnight—then meeting the boats at a closer destination, saw us on the swollen river for a slow trip. At Tha Khanun I assured the family that, although timing meant we would reach Sangkhla in the dark, all boats carried a spotlight to show the way. However, as darkness fell our boat had no such luxury!! Our driver seemed to sense the way well until we headed into some bushes and a disturbed snake was attempting to join our boat. We made a hurried retreat!

It was great to welcome them and Phil as the doctor, but their time then was short lived as the family returned to Bangkok to take up language study. Phil had arrived in Thailand at around 9 months old with his missionary parents and had a good grasp of conversational Thai. But he needed more than childhood language and then to focus on reading and writing. The family returned to Sangkhla in April 1979 for Phil to take up the role of full-time doctor in residence.

During the almost 2 years since I had arrived and without a full-time doctor, there were many times when I knew the care that we were called to give to patients was far beyond my own training and experience. I was reminded of words that had been shared with me by a fellow nurse, "God calls us to be faithful and not necessarily successful".

A few cases:

A boy arrived so oedematous that he was like a taut balloon about to pop. Diagnosis: nephrotic syndrome.

Soon after, we had a visit from some returned prisoners-of-war [Allied POW's during WWII] and family members. One man was a doctor. After chatting, I asked if he knew much about nephrotic syndrome (hoping for some advice). He responded: "Oh, hardly ever see it these days." Then he immediately said that the group needed to leave. I commented that our doctors were here, now, as I pointed to the medical textbooks in the bookcase!

By the time the boy went home he looked normal again and on high dose prednisolone and instructions to have high protein/low salt diet. Not long after, he returned with recurring oedema. He was taking the medicines—so what had been his diet? Well, of course, the local cure-all diet: rice and salt! He had been pleading to return to the hospital where he had been given eggs, fish and meat to eat.

It was because of the care of this boy (grandson of the headman) and a couple of others from Yakadee [also called Wiakadee] village, that Olivia made plans to return to the village to follow up on a previous failed attempt to commence an under-5 clinic there. I was able to accompany her on this trip by boat, then by oxcart. This was the start of many years of clinic visits to Yakadee and nearby villages.

After staff devotions one morning, Ebra went to a waiting family, then called me to see "this baby with tetanus."

The only cases I had ever seen were in my training hospital when two patients were brought to the operation room to have tracheostomies as part of their management. This 3-day old baby had been born in her home village and brought with parents to KRCH by a relative who was a boat driver. The umbilical cord had been cut at birth in a traditional way—with freshly cut, sharp bamboo. Bamboo should be relatively clean; however, the machete used to cut the bamboo would have been the one used for all kinds of garden and other work.

Our old textbooks advised the use of phenobarbital which gave great results to control her spasms. Later, turning to a more recent textbook, it said do not use phenobarb; the drug of choice was diazepam. However, the results were poor, so back to the initial treatment with good results.

Jan Stretton and I had to be away for the annual TBMF [Thailand Baptist Missionary Fellowship] mission conference and wondered if baby WahSawPaw would be there on our return. Ebra's first greeting was, "Do you want to see your tetanus baby?" She did well and returned home to a normal life.

A lady presented with liver pain. Her history and her X-ray, compared to the textbook, were classic for amoebic liver abscess. Medication wasn't resulting in any significant improvement. The family wanted to take her home and "feed the spirits." I explained that the patient's condition was due to the "fii" (abscess) not the "pii"(spirits). Finally, they agreed to stay a little longer, so time was critical. The same older textbook described, in detail, the method of aspirating an amoebic liver abscess. I was extremely nervous, having been taught the dangers associated with liver biopsies. After reading and re-reading and much prayer, I sought to follow instructions regarding the point to aspirate: back came 450 ml of pus the colour of chocolate milk, just like the text book described. After aspirations on 3 occasions and medication she went home well.

A couple of years later one of our fellow Australian Baptist missionaries came, with our missionary doctor from Bangladesh, with the same diagnosis, for treatment at Bangkok Nursing Home (then the Bangkok hospital with the best reputation for treating foreign workers throughout Asia). Apparently, the decision to aspirate was made and then cancelled. Tragically, he died of a ruptured amoebic liver abscess on Christmas day with his wife and twin infant daughters still in Bangladesh.

I thank God for the good result in our lady's case.

Some other memorable cases:

- A baby with a pyothorax [pus in chest cavity] that needed to be drained
- The man who had been attacked by a tiger that he had shot when it was attacking his cattle. It caught up with the shooter and mauled him before it died. We managed to medivac him out but at the expense of 2 other patients who were scheduled to fly out by the helicopter. One man died (probably late stage cancer) and the other man went home (partial paralysis after a fall from a coconut tree).
- Our lab technician, Chatri, had been delirious, with cerebral malaria. In his confused state, he tried to get to the river with a risk of drowning! While under treatment, he had 11 family members sleeping in his hospital room overnight. He recovered well.
- And many more ....

I made many mistakes in my language attempts (and still do sometimes). One night I wanted to learn the Thai word for the moon, so I asked my 2 nurse aides, "What is the word for that "fai nai fah" ("light in the sky")? Through their laughter I learnt the word "phra-jan". But my phrase "fai nai fah" became a standing joke to remind me that

I had a lot to learn! It reminded me that, in language learning, it is better to learn to laugh at ourselves, along with others.

We were remote, and living far from familiarity, but we did have local friends. The remoteness was highlighted one Friday that I was off duty. I was listening to FEBC [Far East Broadcasting Company] Christian radio when I realized the story was of Jesus carrying his cross. I realized that this was probably Good Friday, but with only Thai calendars and no other missionaries there at the time, I had no way of confirming this. The local church had made no mention of this as far as I had understood. I became aware that I wasn't only separated by distance but also separated from church life that was so familiar.

Almost 2 years after my arrival Phil and Melba McDaniel had completed their language study and moved, with Linette, to take up residence in Sangkhlaburi, with Phil now the resident doctor at Kwai River Christian Hospital.

Jan Stretton had been on 1-year home assignment and 3 months of refresher language study and returned at the same time as the McDaniels.

I was then able to attend the Union Language School, fired up with the desire to really come to grips with language learning. Having had responsibility for both the medical and administrative work of the hospital, I was acutely aware of the need for improving my ability to communicate.

During my time in Bangkok I lived at the Student Christian Centre along with Thai University students—yet another challenge to communicate, but a good training ground.

As I record these memories about events that occurred 40 plus years ago, it feels as though they happened the day before yesterday. I continue missionary work in Sangkhlaburi, now working with disabled folk in the community. I married Jit (Thumrong) Yawan 8 years after arriving in Thailand.

There are many more stories—of life, of work, of relocation, of family. Maybe, one day, these will make it into a book!

A Night of High Drama!

Setting

Lois Visscher had been a missionary doctor with Presbyterian Church (USA) and had spent 36 years in India. She had also spent a couple of years in Sudan (never wanted to see fresh dates again—every dessert!) and done some relief stints in Vietnam. She then was a volunteer in a Cambodian refugee camp. Phil McDaniel was due for home assignment in 1982, so Ed McDaniel (Phil's dad) made contact with Lois (both Ed McDaniel and Lois Visscher had been PCUSA missionaries). She agreed to relieve.

Lois didn't speak Thai but studied and passed the Thai medical registration exam (in English).

She was a dedicated doctor. She had many "old school" ideas that mostly worked well. She was a strong character of Dutch heritage and was sometimes rather abrupt with people.

Phil, Melba, and Linette returned to Thailand from their year-long home assignment in June of 1983. Melba was 6 months pregnant at the time. She and Linette stayed in Bangkok awaiting the birth. Phil returned to KRCH for two months and then went back to Bangkok to do some further language study while awaiting the birth. This left Lois again as the sole doctor at the hospital.

Relocation [from the original hospital site to Huay Malai] was in progress, and the wet season was on in full. The muddy roads were virtually impassable.

That Night of High Drama

Thursday, September 8, 1983 I was quite tired as I had been up much of the night on call but had promised to make a special birthday cake which took me most of the day (no time to catch up on sleep!). Baby "Arm" was a year old and his birthday coincided with that of his dad, Khru (teacher) Weerasak, headmaster of the United Christian School. The cake—Pooh Bear with a red balloon, made of several cakes joined together, had taken me all day to prepare and was ready to be shared at the party.

The celebrations would be in the form of a worship service in the school assembly hall, an evening meal, and then videos on a small TV screen for a couple of hundred people. The invitation was open, so Dr. Lois went along, too. However, she tired after a while and went home before the party was over in the hopes of enjoying a little peace and quiet.

I was on call at the hospital, so after the worship service, I went to give some injections and check on the patients. When I returned, videos were playing but they had saved me a meal. I sat and ate in the teachers' staff room. It happened that Ophelia (translator for Compassion International) and Jit (relocation foreman) were sitting, chatting there, too. After a few minutes Khru Boonchom burst through the door of the staff room and blurted out, "Dr. Lois has been stabbed!" (His niece, who lived next door, had heard Lois calling for help.) As we three jumped up and followed along the pathway, I asked if the doctor was still alive. "Yes!" As we ran, I instructed Jit to head to the hospital to collect the stretcher.

Bursting into her upstairs unit, there was Lois, conscious, thrusting her arm out saying, "Take me to the hospital and start an IV!" I told her that Jit would bring the stretcher, to which she replied, "Don't wait. Take me on this!" Though injured, she had had the foresight to spread her bedspread on the floor and lie on top: a method for quick transport.

By this time, a bit of a crowd had arrived on scene: enough to carry the makeshift stretcher to the hospital. Everyone from the party had fled home.

Lois had suffered a number of stab wounds to her neck and abdomen. She was having some breathing difficulties. We took an X-ray with our little WWII portable machine. While I was trying to figure out the result, Lois asked to see the films herself, but her reading wasn't much help either.

She told me that if she died to please tell her "son" in India what had happened. This was a young man she had sponsored. She dictated the address. Her brother would be notified by the mission.

Blood loss would be inevitable. Donors lined up to be checked. I was the first donor and there were 3 more.

I realized there was not much we could do locally—she needed major hospital care. But it was nighttime. We had no 4-wheel drive vehicle, no telephone or radio communication, and no way to get another doctor there.

I requested Khru Weerasak and Jit to head out by motorcycle to hunt for a 4-wheel drive vehicle. They returned with the news that the Electricity Generating Authority of Thailand (which was working on a hydroelectric project) had their vehicle, but it had just arrived damaged; it was effectively only 2-wheel drive, which could not make the trip.

Had a 4-wheel drive vehicle been available, she probably would have died on the trip out.

So, I set about to suture the 2 neck wounds—not large, but deep. (Later, I noted that her carotid arteries pulsed right under both these scars. One carotid laceration would have caused death!) One on her sternum was minimal but there was one central wound of unknown severity just below her ribs.

Some police turned up and asked what they could do to help. I responded that they could go out to try to find who did this. Their reply: "But it's night-time; what can we do?"

"Well, it would help if you could start organizing a helicopter medivac out for the morning. We'd like to get to Bangkok Christian Hospital (BCH)."

Through the night we monitored vital signs, gave blood, and kept her comfortable.

All patients and relatives were keen to hurry away, so by the next day the hospital was almost empty.

Morning news: contact had been made with Bangkok Christian Hospital, which was now awaiting the transfer.

A helicopter would arrive. When it finally did, it made a few flyovers.

The Nai Amphur (district mayor) arrived—he'd only just heard the news. When the helicopter headed to the new (relocation) town site, he headed off by car to stress the urgency. It soon arrived. The Nai Amphur stepped out and apologetically explained that the pilots had thought this was like many of their calls, just to take some mildly ill person from the government clinic.

In preparation to fly out with Lois, I returned to her house to collect some of her clothes and necessities.

I noted cigarette ash on the verandah table. Perhaps someone had been passing time while waiting for Lois to return from the party. Inside Lois's apartment, I saw valuables lying around, but with nothing apparently missing. There was a large pool of blood on the bathroom floor where Lois had dropped and pretended to be dead. As best I could determine, no knives were missing from the drawers.

A single flip-flop sandal had dropped inside the fence, perhaps left behind during a hurried getaway.

Preparations were in place to transfer Lois to the helicopter. We needed people to carry charts and X-rays/oxygen/IV and 4 stretcher bearers. But when the time arrived, one stretcher bearer had gone home after night duty. I tried to call a young man sitting with a friend on seats in the foyer, but a nurse aide insisted she could do the job.

So, we all moved in convoy to the school soccer field (the usual landing pad) to wait.

A policeman approached to see if Lois would be able to identify a couple of young men they pointed out in the crowd—a lady had seen them acting suspiciously the night before. Lois hadn't seen them when they attacked from behind. Moreover, the electric lighting at the time of the attack had been dimmer than candlelight. So, she couldn't help.

As I looked in the direction of the young men, I realized they were the very ones I had tried to call to carry the stretcher!

We flew over the beautiful scenery of the Kwai River valley but had little time to admire the view. I had no idea how far this trip would take us and how I would organize ongoing transport. The pilots apologized for the need to stop to refuel at the border police station in Kanchanaburi. I realized then that they would be taking us all the way to Bangkok. This was a great relief. It was also a relief to know we would not be running out of fuel in mid-air! We landed on the roof of the Police Hospital in Bangkok and were met by Dr. Bannasit, director of Bangkok Christian Hospital. He, himself, had previously relieved Lois for a stint.

We were rushed by ambulance from the Police Hospital to Bangkok Christian Hospital. Bob Coats (mission leader) met us there.

Shortly after, Phil McDaniel walked in. Bob asked after the baby. Nathan had been born two days earlier and all this was news to us: news we'd been awaiting.

Doctor exams, plans for emergency surgery, then off to the operating room.

I could finally take a break!!

I realized a friend was visiting from Nepal so an unexpected chance to catch up for dinner.

As we walked past the hospital gate the surgeon met us and explained that they had found Lois's knife wound was a penetrating injury that passed only millimeters between both heart and spleen, through her stomach and sliced her diaphragm. Any of these could have killed her!

Dinner completed, I went on to the mission prayer meeting. I crept in during prayer. Then the house phone rang. The hostess returned with news from Phil that now baby Nathan's second lung had collapsed, and he had another chest tube. I had been thinking that the earlier news of this precious baby meant all was fine.

Home to the Bangkok Christian Guest House to finally sleep—I had now been up for a very dramatic 40 hours.

Suddenly, tension relieved, I could let go and sobbed and sobbed.

However, we had seen God's goodness in so many ways.

Lois improved somewhat but later decided to fly back to the US to recuperate, accompanied on the flight by Winnie Dodge (the first nurse at KRCH; now missionary in Bangkok).

Nathan was able to be cared for in the neonatal ICU of a university hospital. He did well and came home to Sangkhla healthy.

Dr. Eli Cong from Maesariang Christian Hospital was able to cover the Kwai River Christian Hospital until Phil McDaniel and family were ready to return to the work.

No one was ever charged for the attack, but there was speculation that the young men had been hired to attack.

Why? Unknown! There were many people in the area from outside the community with all the relocation work. Maybe someone was upset at something Dr. Lois had done or not done.

Lois claimed from an early stage and continued to say, that she had forgiven those who had done this to her.

Lois did, later, return to continue work in Thailand: She did some more work in a refugee camp and spent some time at Manorom Christian Hospital (OMF—Overseas Missionary Fellowship). Finally, she was granted her wish to return to work at Kwai River Christian Hospital until she felt she was getting a bit shaky during surgery. Then, in her early 70's, it was time to retire.

What an amazing life of service to her Lord and to the poor in so many places.

Editor's note: I visited Lois in the Bangkok Christian Hospital several times. Whenever I asked to pray with her, she reminded me to pray for her attackers as well. —Phil McDaniel

Chapter 9

About the Big Buy

By Pharmacist Loes de Vos, July 2019

About the author of this chapter:

Loes de Vos from Perth, Western Australia, served as pharmacist and purchasing agent at the Kwai River Christian Hospital from 1977 to 1999. Keeping the pharmacy stocked with what was needed without buying too far ahead, required careful planning. Some diseases were relatively seasonal, causing a fluctuation in the demand for certain medicines. In the 60's and 70's, a large shipment could be sent upriver by barge in the rainy season or by truck over jungle tracks in the dry season. Transport of supplies by barge was no longer an option after construction of the dam across the River Kwai Noi commenced in the early 1980's. Fortunately, a good road skirting around the reservoir was part of the hydroelectric project. When this was finally completed, shipments by truck became feasible year-round.

When I arrived in Thailand in August 1977, I started off my time by going to TBMF [Thailand Baptist Missionary Fellowship] Annual Conference. This gave me a good introduction to who all was working with TBMF.

After Conference, Jan Stretton and I set out to do what was then an annual buy of supplies for KRCH.

That first buying trip was really quite small as we didn't have such a large number of patients. We bought what was needed and then found a truck to drive us (Jan Stretton and myself) to Kanchanaburi, where we left our goods with the "Barge Lady" who ran the barge service up the Kwae Noi river when the water level was high enough. Jan and I then found a hotel for a night and the next day left for Sangkhlaburi first by taxi for about an hour to Saiyok Noi. From there by boat which that day took us 12 hours.

The Barge arrived a month or more later when the water was high enough. The Barge when it arrived had more than just the hospital supplies Jan and I had bought. There were supplies of all kinds on board. Things which I can think of are:

- Diesel fuel for the hospital generator and for the water pump
- Gas (LPG) in steel bottles [cylinders] for our houses for cooking and the hospital autoclave
- Kerosene for refrigerators in houses and hospital [Yes, they did run on kerosene.]
- Oxygen cylinders for the hospital. I remember the oxygen tanks being of an interesting variety of sizes.
- A year's supply of toilet paper and laundry soap
- Equipment and building supplies

Soon after starting work in the pharmacy, I realized that we needed to get supplies in more frequently because our storage conditions were far from ideal, and so some things would not survive for 12 plus months on our shelves.

I went down river in February 1978 and as part of that trip did a bit of a top-up buy. This then grew into the "Big Buy" which I did twice a year.

For a Big Buy trip, I would basically stock-take the pharmacy and write up the shopping lists from that. I would then get everyone else to give me their shopping lists.

In Bangkok I would book myself into a double room at the BCGH [Bangkok Christian Guest House]. After taking out the second bed I would get to work. Ringing drug companies and other suppliers was the first thing and organizing them to deliver to the guest house all on the same day. From there I would start packing the supplies into my room. Things which came ready packed in boxes were the easiest. Boxes of laundry detergent (for hospital and household use) and boxes of toilet paper were packed from floor to ceiling. Smaller orders were repacked into boxes for which I wrote up packing lists so I knew where to look for things when I returned to KRCH with all the goods.

It usually took two or more rounds of phoning suppliers to get everything needed.

There were also quite a few things which I had to hunt down in person and this took up quite a bit of time. The fact that the whole of

Bangkok is a bit like one huge department store was helpful. I could cover quite a few things in one trip. This was particularly so with Chinatown. One gets to know where the "plastic bag street" is, and the cloth merchants' area, and the little shop that would make stainless steel goods to specifications. Plastic bins, buckets, and boxes were also found together in this area.

Then there were the companies I needed to go to in order to place orders and collect the goods myself. This included the Government Pharmaceutical Organization (GPO) which made a huge range of simple medicines at good prices.

Another address I visited frequently was the company which supplied medical equipment [such as surgical instruments and laboratory equipment]. I often went to them with samples of what we needed so I could buy an exact match.

When all the buying was done, and I had packed all the boxes into my room there was usually only enough room for my bed and a little path to the bathroom. The rest of the room was floor to ceiling boxes.

The next thing was, we needed a truck to get it to the hospital. I can't remember ever having to organize this myself. There was always someone else who knew how to do this. Eventually, the hospital and mission (KRCH and KRCM) had a truck we could use. The last few trips I made I packed quite a lot into the hospital pickup truck and drove that up to Sangkhlaburi.

I don't know if the whole Big Buy thing came to an end when I left. More and more things were available either in Sangkhlaburi or Kanchanaburi. Also, there were trucking businesses who would deliver from Kanchanaburi and even from Bangkok, though we had quite a job convincing some Bangkok companies how far away we really were. I remember one company rep who decided we really couldn't be that far away and set out to deliver our order himself. I think he expected a couple of hours drive. About 6 hours later he arrived at our door. We then had to send him back 17 Km to town to find the hotel.

Chapter 10

Adaptation and Perseverance

By Phil McDaniel

About the author of this chapter/editor of this book:

Phil was the fifth director of KRCH (after Dr. Bina Sawyer). He is grateful for all his friends and colleagues who contributed memories to include in this book.

Span of service at KRCH: April 1979 to June 2002 and subsequently 11 volunteer stints of 2-4 weeks each.

Background

The Kwai River Christian Hospital was carved out of the jungle in the early 1960s. I did not set foot in the hospital until September 1978 and then, only for a brief visit by way of orientation before starting Thai language school in Bangkok. Finding doctors and nurses to staff the hospital had been a vexing problem from the very beginning. This was due in large part to the remoteness of the outpost and the challenges of transportation and supply. Doctors Doug Corpron, Roy Myers, John Freeman, and (briefly) Bina Sawyer all preceded me as directors of the KRCH. Each of us had to function as general practice jungle doctor, maintenance man, and chief administrator. We were also involved in staffing, public relations, and equipment acquisition.

In this chapter I'll be trying to paint a picture of how things were on my watch (1979–2002).

Growling and Grunting in the Jungle at Night

I first learned about the Kwai River Christian Hospital in March of 1965. My dad, who was a missionary doctor in Chiang Mai in northern Thailand, volunteered to cover the Kwai River Christian Hospital for Dr. Doug Corpron so that he could participate in a trek deep into the jungle to visit the Talako ethnic group. My mom, Charlotte McDaniel, and a laboratory technologist, Margaret Strane, accompanied my dad on this trip. (See chapter 3 for my dad's "diary" of that trip.) They were at the KRCH for about four weeks. I was a junior in high school back in the States at the time. My dad made a tape/slide show [and here I am talking about cassette tape and Kodachrome slides!] to tell about his experience. On the tape one can hear the snapping of his "cricket," indicating when to advance to the next slide. Alas, I have not been able to locate the slides! However, having later become familiar with the area, I am able to reconstruct some of the images in my head. My dad described in one of his letters from that time how they could hear the sound of wild animals in the surrounding jungle at night. The Sangkhlaburi area was hyperendemic for malaria and hookworm. Dad describes cases of severe anemia due to malaria and/or hookworm. Just a few days after leaving Sangkhlaburi, my mom came down with high fever, shaking chills, plus headache and body aches. Malaria smear done in Bangkok on the way back to Chiang Mai was positive for Plasmodium falciparum malaria parasites. This brought the misery of malaria close to home! With early diagnosis and treatment, she made a good recovery.

Call

My "call" to serve in Thailand as a missionary doctor did not consist of a voice or a vision, but rather the inspiration of role models. My grandfather had run a mission hospital in Nakhon Si Thammarat in southern Siam (Thailand) and established a "leper home" (leprosarium) in the same area. My father served as the only doctor at Overbrook Hospital in Chiang Rai, Thailand for about 4 years and then headed the department of obstetrics and gynecology at McCormick Hospital in Chiang Mai and was a pioneer in family planning in northern Thailand. Although my grandfather died before I was born, his legacy lived on in the stories my dad told about him. My dad was a model of service to others inside and outside the hospital.

Our house in Chiang Mai was just across the street from McCormick hospital. I became familiar with the hospital, running errands for my dad. He had installed the first telephone system and the first public address system at McCormick Hospital. He had also greatly upgraded the water system. Having installed these things, people expected him to fix them when they malfunctioned. He would call and ask me to bring over a multimeter, a wrench, an extension cord, a fan, or a flashlight.

Dad arranged for me to observe operations from time to time. The ones I remember specifically are a C-section, a cleft lip repair, and reduction of a dislocated hip.

When it came time for me to go to high school [9th through 12th grades], I chose to go to Stony Brook School in Long Island, New York. My dad had attended this school. My brother, Ed, was about to begin his senior year there. Attendance at daily morning chapel was compulsory. The masters (teachers) at the school took turns giving the chapel talk. In my senior year, Mr. Karl Soderstrom gave a particularly memorable talk based on Jesus' parable of the sheep and the goats. This reads in part, "Truly I tell you, whatever you did for one of the least of these brothers and sisters of mine, you did for me." (Matthew 25: 40, New International Version of the Bible). From that time on, I made up my mind to try to prepare to be a missionary doctor.

Preparation

I attended Wheaton College and then the University of Illinois College of Medicine. After that I did an internship and residency in internal medicine. Knowing that I might end up in a remote place where I was required to do some surgery, I spent one year in Mason City, Iowa in a surgical "preceptorship" which allowed me to get quite a bit of experience in general surgery and orthopedic surgery in just one year. Following that year of surgical training, my wife, Melba, my daughter, Linette, and I went out to Thailand under the auspices of International Ministries of the American Baptist Churches. Melba and I began Thai language study in Bangkok. I remembered some Thai from growing up in Chiang Mai. However, the dialect I grew up speaking was the northern Thai dialect. In language school we learned to speak, read, and write the Bangkok dialect, the official language of the Kingdom.

The medical and surgical training I received in the USA was a good start, but I felt a little weak in the area of obstetrics. I knew that at the Kwai River Christian Hospital I would have to do C-sections and breech deliveries. My dad was head of the department of obstetrics and gynecology at McCormick Hospital in Chiang Mai. He arranged to have me spend a month in Chiang Mai working with him and his colleagues in order to gain some experience in OB.

According to my log of procedures from my month in Chiang Mai I did the following:

- Normal spontaneous vaginal delivery: 6
- Breech deliveries: 3
- C-sections as assistant: 4
- C-sections as operator: 6
- Tubal ligations: 10

While I was getting experience in obstetrics and picking up some Thai medical terminology, Melba was making gains in Thai studies with a tutor.

During that month in Chiang Mai, a public health team from McCormick Hospital comprised of student nurses and their instructors plus a volunteer dentist made a trip to a remote village in the hills to provide vaccinations and some rudimentary medical and dental services to hill tribe people. I went along as an observer.

The dentist stayed quite busy extracting decayed teeth. There was no electricity; so, his operating light consisted of a flashlight held by a volunteer. One afternoon I took my turn as flashlight holder. After he had pulled a couple more teeth, he turned around and said, "Aren't you going to be going to that hospital on the River Khwae? You may have to extract some teeth there. Why don't you let me hold the flashlight and you extract the teeth? I can help you."

So, my preparation for work at the Kwai River Christian Hospital consisted of three years of training in internal medicine, one year of surgery, six months of Thai language study, a month of obstetrics, and an afternoon of pulling teeth!

What the Patients Thought of the New Doctor

"You're an intern, aren't you?"

That's a question I was asked by a fellow passenger in a pickup truck serving as a taxi. I was still pretty new at the Kwai River Christian Hospital. Apparently, I looked quite young. Being asked whether I was an intern was rather deflating after all the time and effort I had spent preparing to be the doctor in a hospital where I would be the patients' last best hope. As time went on, patients gained confidence in me to the point of expecting TOO much.

"Doctor can't you operate? Please just try! If I die, I won't blame you!"

That request was from a patient with end stage heart failure due to chronic, untreated hypertension. He had total body edema. His lungs were waterlogged, and he was very short of breath. I felt compassion for him, but his problem was not one that could be treated surgically! We did the best we could to treat his condition with medications, but his case was hopeless, and he died in a few days. I'm not sure I ever convinced him that surgery was not the answer to his problem.

A young lady with one of the most beautiful faces I have ever seen asked me to operate on her face to correct what she perceived to be some asymmetry. I told her that her face was already pretty and that I could not improve on perfection!

Patients with large cancerous growths sometimes came seeking treatment. It was heartbreaking to have to tell them that their growth was unresectable. In most cases these tumors were beyond cure or palliation even in a big city hospital. Referral would have been futile.

What the New Doctor Thought of the Patients

I assumed the post of hospital director in 1979. At that point the hospital was a 10-bed hospital with just a few inpatients at any given time. Outpatient numbers had been meager. The hospital had been limping along the previous two years with only occasional visits by Dr. Bina Sawyer, Dr. Keith Dahlberg, or Dr. Ed McDaniel (my dad), all busy missionary doctors serving in the north of Thailand.

The spectrum of diseases which I saw when I began my work at the Kwai River Christian Hospital was rather different from the spectrum of diseases I had been seeing in Chicago, Illinois and Mason City, Iowa. I had to adjust my "index of suspicion" for various conditions. For example, a patient presenting to the Kwai River Christian Hospital with high fever "has malaria until proven otherwise," in contrast to a patient presenting to a hospital in Chicago, where malaria would have been one of the last considerations. Pulmonary tuberculosis was very common at the KRCH, including very advanced and sometimes multi-drug-resistant cases. We also saw TB of the spine, meninges, kidneys, joints, and other extra-pulmonary sites. Psychiatric illness was common. Diseases we thankfully saw only rarely were tetanus and rabies. Toothache was very common, sometimes associated with tooth abscess. Of course, coughs, colds, sore throats, belly aches, headaches, and dizziness, which are common the world around, were common there as well.

Patients sometimes came to the hospital with a fracture due to falling out of a house. The houses in that area were typically built on stilts to keep the living area high and dry. The space under the house was often high enough for a man to stand up straight. Most of the living area upstairs had walls consisting of woven bamboo. However, there was often a porch area where cooking and washing was done. This was often open on one side. If an occupant of the house became inebriated or was prone to sleepwalking, he or she might walk off the porch and fall to the ground.

Men sometimes broke bones or fractured their spines when they fell out of trees from which they were harvesting coconuts or betel nut.

Patients had numerous options for treatment. They could go to a general store, the kind that sells fishing nets, flashlights, rope, and cooking oil and ask the owner for a packet of medicine to treat a cold, a fever, diarrhea or whatever it was that was bothering the patient. Medicine obtained this way was quick and cheap, but not well targeted as to the cause of the ailment. A typical packet would contain five or six pills of various shapes and colors, none of them labeled, but with a fair chance that one of them might help the patient feel a little better. For many patients, this was the first line of treatment. There were some shops on the Thai-Burma border where one could get injections for various ailments and even IV fluid, infused right there in the shop.

Patients could go to a government "anamai" (midwifery/first-aid station) for prenatal care, vaccinations, and minor ailments. In the 1960's and 1970's, there was only one station for the entire district of Sangkhlaburi, as I recall. Staffing of this government health station was somewhat irregular.

Traditional midwives were available for home deliveries. They used techniques on difficult deliveries which were sometimes quite forceful, such as aggressively massaging the uterus or applying foot pressure on the uterine fundus. They also had various techniques for terminating early unwanted pregnancies. Sometimes these methods damaged internal organs.

Shamans were consulted often, especially for psychiatric illness, seizures, and conditions that were otherwise mysterious.

There was a traditional bone setter in the community. He did his work without the aid of X-rays. He used bamboo splints. I thought it was hair-raising—or at least overly optimistic—how early he let his patients begin using their broken extremity again. Surprisingly, the bones often healed, albeit sometimes a bit crooked or shortened. Other times the bones did not heal. That's when the patient came to me. Did patients ever abandon my treatment and go see the traditional bone setter? I suspect so. They didn't like how long I kept them in a cast or in traction.

Aggressive pinching and rubbing of the skin, especially over the clavicles, was used to diminish nausea.

Cupping and massage were frequent modes of therapy.

A patient could get treatment at one of the local Buddhist temples. This treatment might consist of application of holy oil or holy water. The monk/healer would sometimes blow on the affected area. "Tattooing" of a red medicine just beneath the surface of the skin over the area where the patient was having symptoms was yet another treatment available in some temples.

In those days patients often went to an "injection doctor", especially for fevers. Unfortunately, the "injection doctors" did not always use sterile technique (more on that below). A patient presenting to an injection doctor with fever might be given a shot of "Novalgin" or "Bonpyrin" (both are brands of dipyrone). They lower fever and decrease pain. This medication has been banned in the USA since 1977 because of toxicity. Another favorite of injection doctors was quinine. This is very painful when given intramuscularly (the route that injection doctors used) and can cause local tissue damage. If the patient actually did have malaria, the injection might help temporarily, but even two or three injections would not be enough to reliably treat malaria. If the patient did not have malaria, quinine injections exposed the patient to pain, expense, and risk of infections.

"Can't you give me a shot?" During my first two or three years at the Kwai River Christian Hospital, it was not uncommon after discussing his diagnosis and treatment with a patient, to have him turn around and ask for an injection. The patient felt shortchanged if he had to leave without a shot. We did not, however, give shots on demand

and tried our best to explain to the patient that oral medication was often as good or better than a shot. IV fluid was often regarded with the same exaggerated confidence as shots. In fact, sometimes when the receptionist asked a patient what he had come to see the doctor for ("chief complaint"), he would reply, "I've come to get IV fluid." It was felt to be good for many ailments, especially tiredness and lack of energy!

Fountains of pus: injection doctors apparently did not always use sterile technique. In my first five or ten years at the Kwai River Christian Hospital it was not unusual to have a patient come in with a huge buttock abscess at the site of an injection that he had gotten from an injection doctor a week or two previously. These injection abscesses were sometimes very large and accompanied by fever. Diagnosis was usually quite straightforward, and we undertook treatment right away. In my surgical preceptorship I had been taught, "never let the sun set on an abscess." Most abscesses were opened easily under local anesthesia. Sometimes the pus inside was under so much pressure that when the tip of the scalpel blade dropped into the abscess cavity, the contents squirted up in a small fountain. The pus was typically a light brown color and quite malodorous. If the patient came early on in the abscess formation, drainage usually resulted in rapid recovery. If the patient delayed a week or two, there could be considerable amounts of dead fat and muscle in the walls of the abscess. This required surgical removal and subsequent painful dressing changes.

"The Burmese are coming!" That's "the Burmese" as in "the Burmese army". This news signaled the beginning of another dry season offensive of the Burma army against the rebel Mon and Karen groups.

In Burma (Myanmar) there had been a decades-long conflict between separatist groups such as the Mon, Karen, Chin, Kachin, Shan and Arakan and the central Burmese army. These conflicts had been going on ever since approximately the end of World War II. The two separatist groups just west of the Thai-Burma border from us were the Mon and the Karen groups.

The Mon army and the Karen army each laid land mines against the central Burmese army. The Burmese army laid land mines against the Mon and Karen. Mon and Karen soldiers would sometimes step on Burmese landmines and occasionally, by accident, on their own.

Injured Mon and Karen soldiers would be brought across the border to the Kwai River Christian Hospital since they would not be welcome at any Burmese hospital!

Unfortunately, civilians occasionally stepped on landmines laid by Mon or Karen or Burmese soldiers. They also came to the Kwai River Christian Hospital for treatment.

During these dry season offensives, Karen and Mon soldiers with gunshot wounds from the battlefield on the Burma side would also be sent to the Kwai River Christian Hospital. These were often messy, but the landmine injuries were worse. A patient who had stepped on a land mine typically arrived with one foot completely blown off and the other, damaged by shrapnel and burns. On the side missing a foot, there would be mud and jungle vegetation blasted up into the spaces between the muscle groups.

The patient had to first be stabilized. This sometimes required giving a transfusion to replace some of the blood loss. Following this would be administration of some type of anesthesia so that the worst of the mud and sand and vegetation could be irrigated out from between the muscle planes. This preliminary wash was sometimes done outside of the operating room so as to keep the operating room relatively uncontaminated. Occasionally, the rinse was done in a grassy area behind the hospital using a garden hose. We were confident that the water in the hose was much cleaner than the jungle mud in the leg stump. One of my surgery mentors often said, "The solution to pollution is dilution." After irrigating out most of the mud and jungle debris, we took the patient to the operating room for his [or, in the case of civilians, sometimes "her"] amputation.

Landmine injuries often arrived in the middle of the night. This was particularly draining. Each case triggered the multi-step process of stabilizing the patient, giving anesthesia, doing the preliminary wash, then the surgical prep, and then the amputation itself. All this required much more time and effort than, say, an appendectomy, but what made it especially annoying was the fact that it was an injury which had been inflicted on the patient by another human being who was himself at risk of suffering a similar injury.

It all seemed so senseless. As selfish as this may sound, I sometimes felt a victim of the conflict myself whenever I had to get up in the middle of the night all bleary-eyed and peddle down to the hospital to try to help another victim of a war with no winners. I would think to myself that this could have been avoided if the warring factions would just be reasonable and negotiate rather than fight. The weapons used in these conflicts came from China, Italy, Germany, the Soviet Union, and the USA. I felt as though the governments of these countries could have exercised better control over what happened to the weapons manufactured within their borders if they had been so motivated.

The battlefield was not the only place from which gunshot wounds came. Village disputes sometimes resulted in someone punctuating his wishes with a bullet. The disputes were typically over one of three things: money, a woman, or timber. The weapons used in village disputes were often of ancient vintage. Some were muzzle-loading firearms that used homemade black gunpowder for the charge, rags or coconut husk for the packing, and miscellaneous scraps of metal for shot. If the patient was fired on at close range, some of the packing was apt to enter the wound along with the shot. This made for a nasty wound that was prone to infection.

Hunters who didn't have the means to upgrade to something more modern, had to use these old muskets to bring down game. They discovered that the soft metal that toothpaste tubes were made of in those days could be used to make crude shot for these muskets. The Kwai River Christian Hospital had a toothpaste exchange program to improve dental hygiene among the school kids. We gave free tubes of toothpaste to the schoolkids but only if they brought in the empties. The exchange rate was 1:1. The idea was that the "empty" showed that the student had actually used the toothpaste in the previously dispensed tube. Some local hunters got wind of this exchange program and asked that we save the empties for them. We made them agree to use the shot they made from these empty tubes only on the animals they hunted, not people!

In my first few years at the Kwai River Christian Hospital I noticed that relatives sometimes brought patients to the hospital after they had already been to a practitioner of herbal medicine or a temple healer. The same phenomenon sometimes happened in reverse: The patient would come to the Kwai River Christian Hospital first and if there was no improvement in three or four days, the relatives would take the patient to another type of practitioner. The trial period for treatment at the Kwai River Christian Hospital appeared to be shorter for psychiatric illnesses than for, say, fever or cough. The feeling seemed to be that a patient having, say, hallucinations or panic attacks was being tormented by evil spirits and that these could be more successfully treated by a shaman (familiar with how local spirits behave) than by a doctor from America.

We rarely did autopsies at the hospital. We were busy taking care of patients who were still breathing. Moreover, we didn't really have a proper room for performing autopsies. Nevertheless, once in a while I asked for permission from relatives to do an autopsy on a case where I felt it was particularly important to find out, if possible, the cause of death. On rare occasions the relatives themselves would request an autopsy. This happened mainly when the relatives felt that the patient had died in a mysterious manner. If the autopsy revealed gallstones, kidney stones, or bladder stones, this was taken as evidence for sorcery. The relatives would typically request the stones, apparently so that they could confront the alleged sorcerer.

There is a type of benign tumor called a dermoid cyst, which typically occurs in the ovaries. This is an embryonic cell tumor which may contain skin, hair, bones, teeth, and cartilage, all in one tumor. Most of the women from whom we removed dermoid cysts were otherwise healthy. Although the patient and her relatives were typically astonished by the contents of these tumors, they were generally willing to take the doctor's word that the tumors were not the result of sorcery.

Mothers often described diarrhea in their babies in an onomatopoeic way: "prap-prap-prap" for frequent small amounts and "jooooot" for more voluminous stool.

Headache pain might be described as "woop, woop, woop" or "jeeeet", with accompanying hand gestures for emphasis.

Colors were sometimes a challenge. The first time a patient told me that he had "red" urine, I began a line of questioning to differentiate the various causes of blood in the urine. I soon learned that "red" urine typically meant nothing more than dark, concentrated urine. When a patient has a respiratory arrest, we say in English that he turns "blue". In Thai they use a word that usually translates to "green" in English. In Mon they use a word that translates to "black" or "dark". The fact that there is not always a one-to-one correspondence between words for colors in one language and words for the same colors in another language can sometimes be problematic. My patients got around this by using what might be called "village colors". For example, a certain shade of red was "pig blood color" and a certain shade of green was "horse poop color".

Constipation is a common problem pretty much the world around. Patients with small hard stools are apt to complain that their feces are like goat pellets. One day a patient came in complaining of hard dry stool. Trying to be helpful, I said, "Like goat pellets, right?"

He replied, "Not goat pellets, doctor! Ball bearings!"

Those who have worked at the Kwai River Christian Hospital or in any other multicultural setting know that patients express their misery in various ways. These variations sometimes seem to follow cultural lines. Some suffer in silence; others have a more demonstrative style of suffering, as though they want to make their misery known to everyone in the hospital. When they are in pain they moan pitifully; when they are nauseated, they retch dramatically.

Grief was expressed not only along cultural lines but also gender lines. When a Mon child died in the hospital, the Mom was apt to wail loudly, slap herself on the chest; run out of the room and then back in again; jump up in the air and then collapse on the floor. The dad, on the other hand, would be silent and shed no tears. Stoically, he would start to make arrangements for the burial.

Deaths in the hospital were usually from cerebral malaria, tuberculosis, meningitis or some other serious infection that had been left until too late. Stroke, heart failure and kidney failure were among the more common non-infectious causes of death. Although in Thai culture the preferred way of dealing with the dead is cremation, the dead who died in the hospital were usually buried in a graveyard at the edge of the mission compound (at the Lainam site) or a few hundred yards from the mission compound (at the Chonglu/Huay Malai site). The need for disposal of the dead in this manner arose from the following beliefs as I recall:

• A death in the hospital was considered unnatural. Taking the body home for burial rites would risk the home becoming haunted by the unhappy spirit.

• Home was sometimes a long way away, making transport time-consuming and expensive.

• Pickup truck drivers were often reluctant to transport a dead body for fear that their vehicle would become haunted, or that potential passengers, at least, would think it had become haunted and refuse to ride in that truck again.

• There was a need for haste as we had no refrigerated morgue.

• Carrying the body to the nearest Buddhist temple for cremation would mean passing houses where the inhabitants were fearful of mischief that might be done by the unhappy spirit of the deceased. However, carrying the dead body in the other direction—to the graveyard on the edge of the mission compound—was OK because it involved passing only houses of Christian families, who did not feel so threatened by unhappy ghosts.

"Patients don't have time to get sick during rice harvest season." That's what I was told by way of explanation for why inpatient and outpatient numbers both dropped during rice harvest season. Other times of year that numbers temporarily slumped were the beginning of Buddhist lent and the end of Buddhist lent [khao phansaa and awk phansaa]. During these times, the patients who did come often arrived in quite serious condition as family had been too busy to bring the patient until absolutely necessary.

The Way things were on my Watch (1979 to 2002)

Referrals

Although we were able to take care of a wide variety of medical and surgical problems at the Kwai River Christian Hospital, some patients arrived needing specialty care that was beyond our ability to provide. Some required radiation or chemotherapy or special surgery. Judging when to try to send complicated patients "downriver" to the hospital in the provincial capital required consideration of several factors:

• Would a referral to the provincial hospital actually result in a better outcome? It would be unkind to insist that a patient go to the provincial hospital if there was no reasonable hope of cure or palliation.

• Did the patient have the right papers to travel? Many inhabitants of Sangkhlaburi district at that time did not have Thai citizenship. Some were economic refugees or political refugees from the Burma side. Some of these refugees had a refugee card which allowed them to reside legally in Thailand. These refugee cards were color-coded to distinguish one type of refugee permit from another. The rights and privileges, including the right to travel, differed from one type of refugee card to another. Patients who did not have some type of card that permitted travel had to do some paperwork to get a temporary travel permit based on their medical needs.

• Was there a relative or friend who could accompany the patient and translate? Patients needed at least one friend or relative to go with them. This often involved some paperwork as well.

• Did the patient have sufficient funds? Although the patient's healthcare was often provided at little or no cost at the provincial hospital, there were many other expenses faced by the patient and his or her attendant.

• Was there someone to look after the house while the patient was gone? Because there was no way to lock up a village-style house, someone had to be found to live in the patient's house so as to keep the house and belongings safe while the patient was gone.

• Was the patient willing to go? Sometimes patients just did not want to go through the stress and expense of transferring to the provincial hospital. They would say, "We will get our treatment here. If we recover, we recover here; if we die, we die here!" Other times the patient would decide to go home, probably to seek traditional remedies. At least this way, they could die in familiar surroundings.

Emergency medical evacuation

The whump, whump, whump sound getting louder and louder announced the approach of the helicopter that had been requested to airlift a patient to the provincial hospital. The Thai border police were stationed not far from the hospital and were willing to radio to their provincial headquarters about 220 km (138 miles) away by winding road to request a helicopter to airlift difficult emergency patients to the provincial hospital. We tried to use this service sparingly so that we would not wear out our welcome with the border police. Typically, it took an hour or two between the time we requested a helicopter and the time the helicopter actually arrived from the provincial capital. The border police generally wanted some assurance that the patient would survive the trip and required that someone on the hospital staff accompany the patient. While we were waiting for the helicopter, we would try to stabilize the patient and do some preliminary wound care (in cases of trauma). Occasionally, while waiting for the helicopter, the patient would improve to the point that they probably could have stayed on at the Kwai River Christian Hospital rather than being airlifted. However, once the helicopter arrived, we couldn't very well send it back empty! After dropping off the patient at the provincial hospital, the helicopter would return to its base in the same city, leaving the employee of the Kwai River Christian Hospital to fend for himself or herself. The staff member would typically return to the hospital the next day by public transportation, but not before doing a little shopping in the city! As far as I can remember, the border police never turned down a request for emergency medical evacuation. Moreover, the need for a permit to travel seemed to get waived in these emergency cases. I am grateful to the authorities for their humanitarian attitude on both counts.

Guiding principles

- "First do no harm!" This word of caution has been taught to medical students for centuries. The intent of this exhortation is to warn doctors away from using treatments that might do more harm than good.
- "What is the best treatment we can give this patient?" It was usually not too difficult to find out the "treatment of choice" by consulting our reference texts. However, we had to take into account the equipment and medicines we actually had on hand and the expertise (or lack thereof) of the practitioners on site. Fracture treatment was an area in which we majored in "closed methods" even when the textbook treatment of choice might have called for plates and screws, a pin or a rod to achieve "anatomical reduction" (that is, perfect alignment). Dr. Norman Hoover, one of my orthopedic mentors, had worked in Vietnam during the war. He noted that many fractures can be treated closed, using a cast or traction instead of plates and screws. In primitive situations, open surgery and placement of hardware may increase the risk of infection and may not be "the treatment of choice".

Dr. Phil McDaniel

Equipment and supplies: some new, most not

Operating room table: this was an item of used equipment procured for the hospital by Dr. Doug Corpron in the early 1960's. It was completely mechanical. A foot pedal raised and lowered it and various cranks changed the slant of certain segments of the table or the tilt of the table as a whole. It had various attachments for special types of surgery. The table was fairly sturdy for many years but began to get a little wobbly in the 1980's. Not only that, it began sinking during operations. On one of my dad's visits to the hospital, he had the gardener cut wooden stakes—various lengths for various operations and operators—that could be used to brace the table against sinking. Eventually, an NGO in Holland donated money to buy a new operating table.

X-ray machines: When I first started at the Kwai River Christian Hospital in 1979, the hospital was using a stationary X-ray machine manufactured by Siemens. I believe this was the original X-ray machine installed by Dr. Corpron in the 1960's. In the 1980's it began to malfunction. We replaced it with a used X-ray machine from a mission hospital that was downsizing. After a few years, that X-ray machine also malfunctioned, and we finally replaced it with a new one in the 1990s. Because it was difficult or impossible to get some patients from their hospital bed to the X-ray room, we obtained a portable US Army surplus X-ray machine. Although not very powerful, it served very well as a portable unit and also as a backup to the stationary unit. Although the X-ray equipment at the Kwai River Christian Hospital was very basic, it was the only X-ray equipment for miles around during the 1960s, through the early 1980s. Patients would be referred for X-rays from refugee camps and from makeshift hospitals along the Thai-Burma border. X-ray technology at the Kwai River Christian Hospital was used primarily as an aid to diagnosis of pneumonia, TB, heart failure, broken bones, and to search for foreign bodies such as bullets and shrapnel. Some patients felt that X-rays were a form of treatment, so were keen to be X-rayed.

Autoclaves: when I first started work at the Kwai River Christian Hospital in 1979, there was already in place a hospital autoclave which ran off of bottled gas. Unfortunately, this autoclave had developed a small crack in its shell which prevented us from getting the contents of the autoclave up to the prescribed pressure. We replaced it with an autoclave which resembled a large kitchen pressure cooker. For the heat source, we bought the widely available and inexpensive gas burner-on-a-stand used by sidewalk vendors to heat the woks in which they made fried bananas and other snacks. This was "appropriate technology". Alas, even appropriate technology requires some attention to detail. One day while I was in the outpatient department examining a patient, I heard a terrific bang coming from central supply (the room where the instruments are sterilized). Investigation revealed that the man operating the sterilizer that day not only had failed to release all the pressure in the autoclave before loosening the nuts that held the lid on, he had unscrewed the nuts all on one side but none on the other. This led to a mighty halving of the lid such that half was blown off and the other half was still bolted in place. Fortunately, no one was hurt.

Laboratory equipment: Up until the mid-1980's we did not have electric power during the daytime unless we started up a generator. It was prohibitively expensive to run a generator all day. We could only afford to start it for X-rays or for surgery. The laboratory tests we could perform in the 60's, 70's and early 80's were mostly limited to ones we could do without the aid of electricity.

We could check a patient's hemoglobin using Sahli's acid hematin method, a color-comparison technique which required no electricity at all.

A microscope which required no electricity was used to look for malaria parasites, count white blood cells, look for signs of infection in the urine, and search for parasites in stool. An adjustable mirror under the microscope stage caught light coming through the window and reflected it up to the specimen!

The centrifuge used to spin down urine was hand cranked.

When we discovered that our Sahli method of estimating hemoglobin concentration (see above) was giving results that were not very reproducible, we decided to switch to a microhematocrit technique for following anemia. This required an electric powered centrifuge that could spin at a rate of about 12,000 rpm. Rather than have the maintenance man, the watchman, or me start up a generator every time we had to run a hematocrit, we rigged up a truck battery and an inverter to run the centrifuge.

Dr. Phil McDaniel

The Kwai River Christian Hospital had no EKG machine until the 1980's and no ultrasound until the 1990's.

Being hospital director in those days meant troubleshooting water pumps, generators, intercoms, and electric wiring as well as medical equipment such as autoclaves, operating room light, and X-ray equipment.

There was always a three-way tension between compensating the staff adequately, keeping patient fees affordable, and maintaining buildings and equipment. Thankfully, there were often churches or individuals who asked if there was any specific need with which they could help. There nearly always was! Their donations allowed us to purchase equipment outside the regular budget.

Once I received a letter from a church in West Virginia asking if I would be interested in the equipment from an army surplus field medical unit. As I recall, one of the members of that church ran a secondhand store. The opportunity had come up for him to purchase this army surplus medical unit (not the type of merchandise he normally would have been buying). The church agreed to pay for it if I decided we wanted it. I did not know exactly what was in the unit, but I had to decide on short notice whether to accept it or not. We took it, and this turned out to be a good decision. My guess is that the equipment was of Korean War vintage, but it could have been even as old as World War II. In any case, it was perfectly preserved: a great collection of surgical instruments, plus splints, equipment for traction, and a few items we couldn't identify! There were no cots, tents, operating room lights, or anesthesia machines. So, it was not a complete M.A.S.H. unit, but the equipment was a welcome addition to our own. I do not recall whether our first portable X-ray unit came with that field medical unit or not. It may well have. It had a tag on it indicating that it had been checked and packed in 1944.

Harold and Harriet Hanson, missionary surgeon and missionary pediatrician, respectively, were working at McCormick Hospital in Chiang Mai when I was growing up. This was the same hospital where my dad worked. When the Hansons later moved back to the USA, they were distressed by the amount of medical equipment that was discarded by hospitals in the USA. They dedicated hundreds of hours of their lives collecting still-useful equipment from US hospitals and shipping it to Africa in containers. The Kwai River Christian Hospital was not a big enough operation to accept a full container of medical goods and equipment. However, the Hansons did ship out smaller quantities of equipment and supplies to the KRCH on several occasions. Harold was able to get a 50% discount for us on a brand-new Padgett drum dermatome (a gadget to harvest skin grafts), which proved very useful for patients with bad burns.

Dr. Koga, who came as a volunteer from Japan twice to do some eye surgery and teach me how to do some eye surgery, sent ahead many brand-new eye instruments as well as a cryoextractor apparatus. He said that this equipment was donated by the Japan Overseas Christian Medical Cooperative Services (JOCS), but I suspect that a large proportion of the cost of purchase and shipment was borne by him.

Medical students and residents coming to the KRCH for a rotation often brought useful supplies such as suture material, sterile gloves, and urethral catheters.

Retired doctors who came out to the Kwai River Christian Hospital as volunteers often trolled the offices of their former colleagues for free sample medications left by drug reps. These included antibiotics, antifungals, and antihypertensive meds.

Christian hospitals in Thailand occasionally donated old hospital beds and side tables as well as sheets, surgical drapes, patient gowns, and surgical gowns. It is not unusual on rounds to see sheets on the patients' beds stenciled with "Bangkok Christian Hospital" or "McCormick Hospital" or "Overbrook Hospital".

AFRIMS

Since the 1980s, the Kwai River Christian Hospital has cooperated with the Armed Forces Research Institute of Medical Sciences (AFRIMS) on several projects related to tropical diseases. AFRIMS began as the SEATO [Southeast Asia Treaty Organization] laboratory to help combat a cholera outbreak. It was renamed AFRIMS in 1977. AFRIMS is a research center run jointly by the medical arm of the US army and the medical arm of the Thai army. KRCH contact was with the US component. Doctors connected with AFRIMS went out of their way to help the staff and patients of the Kwai River Christian Hospital. Not only did they share freely of their expertise on difficult medical cases, but they also found ways to get certain tests done in Bangkok or the USA that we were not be able to perform at KRCH. They also managed to acquire several important pieces of equipment for the Kwai River Christian Hospital. These included water storage tanks, a laboratory incubator, an apparatus to detect G6PD deficiency, and a heavy-duty suction machine that was able to supply piped in suction to the entire hospital. AFRIMS also secured funds for the AFRIMS-KRCH Clinical Center and a large (125 kVA) back-up generator. AFRIMS and KRCH collaborated on a malaria prevention study, a malaria treatment study, influenza surveillance, a fever study and a diarrhea study, all of which yielded information about the diseases occurring in our geographic area: information of interest to both KRCH and AFRIMS.

The Government Pharmaceutical Organization

The Government Pharmaceutical Organization of Thailand (GPO) is a state-run enterprise which manufactures pharmaceutical products in Thailand and sells them at reasonable prices. Having this organization in operation helps to keep the prices of essential medications affordable to the health care system. I did not appreciate the role of the Government Pharmaceutical Organization of Thailand for preventing price gouging until I made a medical mission trip to El Salvador (which has nothing comparable to Thailand's GPO) in 2007. On that trip I discovered that medication costs in El Salvador were roughly comparable to the costs of those same medications in the USA (and much higher than for those same medications in Thailand). For the average Salvadoran, this makes medicine difficult to afford. In Thailand the GPO manufactures essential medications and sells them at very reasonable prices. This motivates the private sector to keep prices reasonable in order to stay competitive. All this was a big boon to the Kwai River Christian Hospital in its effort to keep cost of care affordable to patients.

Support from the Ministry of Public Health

Although the Thai government did not directly subsidize the work of the hospital financially, the Provincial Office of the Ministry of Public Health provided the Kwai River Christian Hospital with family-planning supplies and with vaccines, provided that we recorded statistics and submitted records on how these were being used. More recently, TB medications and even some HIV meds have been supplied by the Ministry of Public Health so long as protocols are followed and reports submitted.

Injuries inflicted by elephants, bears, water buffalos, or wild boars

In June 1982, shortly before we departed for the States on our first home assignment, I wrote the following in a newsletter:

In the past three years we have had no less than five elephant-related injuries. These have ranged from dislocation of the jaw to severe compound fracture of the tibia and fibula. In addition, we had a patient mauled by a bear and several gored by water buffalos or bulls.

Other animal inflicted injuries included a man who had been gored by a wild ox and developed a collapsed lung. An occasional patient came to the hospital with a wild boar bite. The swelling and pain always seemed to me to be way out of proportion to the size of the bite. (The bacterial flora in a wild boar's mouth must be particularly nasty!)

Snakebites

In the catchment area of the Kwai River Christian Hospital we had cobras, king cobras, Malayan pit vipers, green pit vipers, Russell's vipers, and banded kraits. These snake species all had Thai names as well as Burmese, Mon, and Karen names. Some of the poisonous snakes had non-poisonous look-alikes. All of this caused confusion when we were trying to determine which species of snake had bitten the patient. If the patient's friends had managed to kill the snake and bring it in, we could usually make a fairly firm ID. Most of the time, the patient had not even gotten a good look at the snake, let alone been able to retrieve it. If careful inspection of the bite site revealed clear fang marks, we could infer that the bite had been inflicted by a venomous snake. We stocked antivenin for each type of poisonous snake in the area. These antivenins were made from horse serum and carried a small risk of inducing a reaction. So, if several hours had already elapsed since the patient had been bitten, and the patient was stable, we often just gave supportive care and the patient usually did fine. This conservative approach was especially preferred if the identity of the snake species was unclear and the patient's only symptom was anxiety.

In order to get around the problem of many names for the same species of snake, I bought a poster in Bangkok that depicted the poisonous snakes of Thailand. I hung this up in the outpatient department so that a patient could point to the snake on the poster that most closely resembled the one that had bitten him. This allowed us to better anticipate what the patient's course would be and which antivenin (if any) to give.

It turned out that one of our nurses was deathly afraid of snakes. Even a picture of a snake caused her to panic. We had to turn the poster so that most of the time the blank side faced out and the snake side faced in.

Relocation

In 1984, the Kwai River Christian Mission, including the Kwai River Christian Hospital, had to move to higher ground because the dam that was built as part of the Khao Laem Hydroelectric Project was due to flood out the old location. In all, about 25 buildings were involved. The Electricity Generating Authority of Thailand compensated the villagers, businesses, Buddhist temples, and the Kwai River Christian Mission according to the nature and number of buildings on the old compounds and the number of fruit trees and pineapple plants on each compound. The Electricity Generating Authority of Thailand also assigned relocation sites. These sites were not necessarily of the same size as the original. Since the Kwai River Christian Mission occupied two sites prior to relocation, it was granted two sites to which to relocate: one in the "new" [relocation] town of Sangkhlaburi and one in Huay Malai, about 16 km (10 miles) further west. In calculating the compensation value of buildings on the original compounds, the Electricity Generating Authority of Thailand made the assumption that buildings constructed of wood could be largely salvaged and therefore were assigned a lower value than comparable sized buildings constructed of brick or concrete. Much of the effort of relocating the Kwai River Christian Mission consisted of dismantling the wooden buildings on the mission compound, loading the lumber onto a truck and transporting the materials to the new sites. This necessitated many, many trips. There were trees on the old mission compound that were due to be flooded out by the reservoir filling up. These were cut down and sawn into lumber in two-man saw pits.

In a newsletter dated April 1984, I wrote the following:

> Everyone is pitching in. The teachers have all built little bamboo huts at the old site where they are living while their wooden houses are being put up at the new place. The six missionaries still at the old site have all moved together into the last intact missionary residence, a duplex originally designed for two single nurses.

Hundreds of decisions relating to the layout of the buildings, water supply, sewage, and electric power had to be made. Various government permits and certificates had to be obtained. The Rev. Ben Dickerson and his wife Doris, long-time missionaries to the Karen people in northern Thailand, were reassigned to the Kwai River Christian Mission. Ben was put in charge of relocation. An account of every twist and turn related to relocation is beyond the scope of this book, but I must say that there is a certain camaraderie among those of us—whether missionaries or nationals—who went through the ordeal of relocation together.

In a newsletter from November 1984 I enthused:

> One of the first patients to be admitted to the "new" (Huay Malai) hospital was old "Uncle" Pong. He came into the half-finished hospital looking like he had been pursued by the Grim Reaper for some time already and was about to be harvested! He was skinny, disheveled, and looking very tired. Fortunately, he had a treatable condition: lung abscess. I saw the man a few days ago. It was

amazing! He looked strong and steady on his feet and could even smile! At first, I didn't recognize him! In just three months he had gained 9 kg (20 pounds). In many ways he is symbolic of the miraculous events of this past year.

Recruiting and training new nurse's aides

Nurse's aides trained by the RNs were a vital part of the hospital staff. They took vital signs, passed meds, did dressing changes and translated. They all spoke at least two languages. Some spoke four or five. At one point, Jan Stretton, missionary nurse from Australia, had the responsibility of training newly recruited nurse's aides. Beside teaching them basic nursing skills and the importance of sterile technique, she told them this over and over: "The most important person in the hospital is the patient." However, when they took the final exam no one got the question about the most important person in the hospital right. Some said, "the doctor"; some, "the head nurse"; some, "the pharmacist". So much for efforts to nurture a culture of compassionate, patient-centered care.

Problems recruiting and retaining nurses

Finding nurses for the Kwai River Christian Hospital has been a challenge ever since it was founded. Thai nurses have generally not wanted to work in such a remote place. For the first two decades of its existence, the hospital relied on missionary nurses plus Ebra and Olivia.

When my mother died in 1976, my dad set up a scholarship fund in honor of my mother at McCormick School of Nursing for students willing to go work at one of the rural hospitals associated with the Church of Christ in Thailand upon graduation. The nursing students who accepted a Charlotte McDaniel scholarship had an obligation to work at a rural hospital one year for each year she had received scholarship. Most of the scholarship students ended up coming to the Kwai River Christian Hospital to fulfill their bond. Even with this scholarship, it was barely possible to keep the required number of nurses at the Kwai River Christian Hospital to stay licensed. Other scholarships are now available for nursing students attending the nursing school at Mission University (Seventh-day Adventist) and Christian University (associated with the Church of Christ in Thailand). Scholarships have also supported a medical student and a laboratory technologist. An orthopedic surgeon who had done a volunteer stint at KRCH sponsored a promising young lady from the time she was in grade school all the way through pharmacy school.

Volunteers and medical students

Over the years, doctors, nurses, pharmacists, dentists, a prosthodontist, electricians, plumbers, bookkeepers, a carpenter and even a painter have given of their time and talents at the Kwai River Christian Hospital. These volunteers came from Australia, the USA, Japan, Singapore, and from within Thailand. They paid their own travel expenses and even paid for their own room and board while at the same time donating their energy and expertise. Their example was an inspiration to all of us.

Medical students on elective rotations came from the USA, Canada, Australia, England, Scotland, Ireland, New Zealand, and Malaysia to learn something about tropical medicine and public health. Medical students were a mixed blessing when it came to their contribution to workflow. At the start of their rotation they required some orientation and quite a bit of supervision. After they began to learn the hospital routines, which typically took a few days, they would become a help in both the outpatient department and the inpatient department. From the medical students' standpoint, this rotation was an opportunity to learn about diseases that they typically would not see in their home country. It was also an opportunity for them to see how medicine and surgery could be done in a remote setting without highly sophisticated equipment.

Cataract surgery

On November 16, 1981 Melba wrote:

> One of Phil's goals for the hospital ever since he has been here has
>
> been to persuade an ophthalmologist to come for a few weeks and

137

do cataract surgery. Most of the patients in this area with cataracts had no hope of having them removed. They had to suffer year after year with blindness that was potentially curable! Bangkok, where cataract surgery can be done, is an 8 to 12-hour journey away. Most of the cataract patients, too poor to travel to Bangkok, are refugees from Burma. They are forbidden to leave the immediate area. Speaking no Thai, they would be hopelessly bewildered, frustrated, and homesick in the big city. We asked the Japan Overseas Christian Medical Cooperative Services [JOCS] if they would be willing to send an ophthalmologist here for a few weeks. The results far exceeded our hopes. Not only was a doctor found that was willing to come, but Japan Overseas Christian Medical Cooperative Services donated and shipped to Bangkok all the eye surgery instruments needed for the operations (including a several thousand dollar cryoextractor), and the doctor stressed that his desire was to train Phil how to do cataract surgery on his own so that patients could continue to be helped long after he himself had returned to Japan.

So, in the eight working days that Dr. Akira Koga was here, he and Phil performed 2–4 eye surgery procedures a day. The first cataract extractions Dr. Koga did himself or assisted Phil on, but the final five were done by Phil on his own with Dr. Koga merely observing and advising.

Dr. Koga came again in November 1985 for a second visit. This was after the Kwai River Christian Hospital had been relocated to Huay Malai. Dr. Koga coached me on 25 eye surgeries during the 10 days he was at KRCH on that second visit.

Shortly after Dr. Koga's second visit, intracapsular cataract extraction (where the lens capsule is removed along with the cataract) became more-or-less obsolete. Around that same time our cryo-extractor began malfunctioning. The probe just didn't get cold enough to perform the cryo-extraction procedure efficiently. This, even after sending it for repair.

Dr. Lois Visscher strongly recommended that I contact Dr. Veeraphan, whose work was sponsored in part by the Christian Mission to the Blind based in Germany. Dr. Veeraphan, a Thai doctor, had done training in eye surgery in Israel. He traveled with a nurse, a nurse's aide, and a driver/helper to several locations in Thailand on a regular schedule, doing eye surgery, mainly extracapsular cataract extraction with intraocular lens placement. We would announce the date of his next visit and save up patients for his return.

After many years of making 3-4 visits per year to KRCH with his mobile team, Dr. Veeraphan retired from this routine, and another Thai team began making periodic visits to the Kwai River Christian Hospital.

Prostheses

Villagers with a history of below knee amputation after stepping on a land mine had often never been fitted with a proper prosthesis. Some had devised makeshift prostheses using leather and wood. Others used bamboo which they split on one end and wove into a basket. This created a one-piece basket-and-shaft, serving as socket and pylon. A few patients actually had prostheses that had been made professionally, but they were probably in the minority. One challenge in making prosthetics for patients who have had an amputation done following a landmine injury is that the stumps are not always ideally shaped. The blast of a landmine typically leaves a ragged, jagged mess. The surgeon has to fashion the best stump he can with the tissue that is available.

This means that the stump is often not "textbook perfect" in shape, creating a challenge for the prosthetist.

Regardless of when or where the patient had their amputation done, I felt that they should have an opportunity to be fitted with a proper prosthesis. All manner of things have been declared to be "a human right." It seems to me that a good prosthesis ought to be a human right for any amputee.

There were two main roadblocks in the way of providing local amputees with prostheses. One was the expense. Another was the fact that prosthesis clinics all seemed to want the patient to travel to their location not just once, but several times, to complete the process of measuring the stump, making a mold, fitting the prosthesis, and training the patient how to use it. Making multiple trips to the provincial capital or to Bangkok was not practical for many of the amputees in our area. This was in part due to the time and expense of making multiple trips and also to the fact that many of the amputees did not have proper papers for travel.

I finally made contact with a company that agreed to send one of their prosthetists to the Kwai River Christian Hospital to take measurements and make molds, provided that we could get at least 12 (as I recall) patients together at the hospital at one time so that the tech would be able to do the initial evaluation on all these patients on his first trip. We were able to identify the required number of amputees and get a commitment from them to follow through with the process when the time came. Most of the patients on our list came at the appointed time. The rest we tried to round up before the tech had to return to Bangkok. The plaster-of-Paris molds and patient measurements were shipped off by the branch company in Bangkok to the parent company in Taiwan for manufacture of the prostheses. When the branch in Bangkok had received the completed prostheses from Taiwan, we set up a time for the amputees to return for fitting of their prostheses by the same technician who had taken their measurements in the first place. Minor adjustments were made as required. Patients practiced putting on and taking off their prostheses and practiced walking in them. As we had no physical therapy department at that time, gait training was done outdoors on parallel bars constructed of bamboo cut from a thicket on the hospital compound. The bamboo was free. The prostheses were not! As I recall, they cost the hospital on the order of US$1,000 each.

This was a very large sum to ask from the average villager. We had the patients each pay a token amount: I think it was something like 10% of the total cost and covered the rest with charity funds.

The above efforts got us up to date on lower limb prostheses for the amputees we were aware of at that time. Later, more landmine injuries occurred, resulting in more below the knee amputations. Also, among the refugees moving into nearby refugee camps there were some amputees. All these "new" amputees generated a need for more prostheses.

A group of podiatrists from Washington State turned up at the Kwai River Christian Hospital on fairly short notice proposing to fit some of the local amputees with high-tech prostheses called the Seattle Foot. This would be at no cost to the amputees. I believe it was a Rotary project. In any case, their initial objective had been to set up a prosthetics clinic in Laos or Cambodia, where they could supply prostheses to victims of landmines in those countries. The Seattle foot system was an intriguing setup that allowed the creation of high quality, lightweight sockets based on measurements and plaster of Paris molds taken by the visiting podiatrists. A few months later, the finished sockets were delivered to the Kwai River Christian Hospital by a Rotary representative. All that remained was to cut nylon pylons to the proper length, bolting one end to the socket and the other end to a foot of the right size. This modular design made for easy assembly and maintenance. These sockets were made of such a material that a little reshaping could be done, if necessary, after heating up the area of concern with a hair dryer. Having some spare feet in a box allowed us to replace feet as they wore out. The Rotarians even brought out some of Seattle Foot's ATF's. Have you never heard of an ATF? Neither had I. It stands for "All Terrain Foot". It consists of a large "rubber" plug that can be used in rough terrain such as a flooded rice field, where feet of any kind tend to get enveloped by the mud, making the next step difficult. The theory behind the ATF was that because of its shape, it would be less likely to "get stuck" in the mud. Also, it would spare some wear-and-tear on the more elegant prosthetic foot that it had temporarily replaced. Whether due to vanity or to the inconvenience of swapping feet every time they went out into the rice fields, I think most people who received a Seattle Foot prosthesis elected to keep the more fashionable foot attached to the prosthesis regardless of terrain. In any case, the Seattle foot took care of another cohort of amputees.

In the early 2000s an NGO called Handicap International (now called "Humanity and Inclusion") used space at the Kwai River Christian Hospital as a workshop for making prostheses for amputees in nearby refugee camps. Later, a prosthesis workshop was set up on the Kwai River Christian Hospital campus with funds from a program under royal patronage. This program sponsors the production of low-cost prostheses made from inexpensive materials readily available in Thailand. There were some challenges with recruiting and retaining personnel for training in this program. Around the same time, demand for prostheses declined, and finally, much of the remaining equipment and supplies were ruined when a big flood came along. Now amputees have to be referred to the provincial capital. At the time of this writing, these prostheses are free to all, regardless of citizenship, due to a program honoring the mother of King Bhumibol.

Dentures

Phil Horton, a retired dentist from Iowa, came out to the Kwai River Christian Hospital at least seven times to do volunteer dental work. He did fillings and also extracted teeth that were beyond repair. He wrote to me from the USA sometime before one of his visits asking if there was anyone on the staff of the Kwai River Christian Hospital that I thought could be trained to make dentures. He indicated that he had a friend who was a prosthodontist and was willing to come out to the Kwai River Christian Hospital with Phil Horton. He was willing to donate the equipment for making dentures but wanted to be sure that there was somebody at the Kwai River Christian Hospital who could be trained to continue making dentures after he left. Making dentures requires a mind that can visualize things three dimensionally and can understand the concept of molds and counter molds and how various materials behave at various temperatures. As I pondered who on the staff had the best skill set for learning how to make dentures, the answer seemed to lie with Moung Oo, one of our gardeners/maintenance men. This man had an uncanny ability to create spare parts for broken equipment using scrap materials. He spoke Burmese and Thai. This allowed him to communicate with most of the patients. He also spoke a little English, which made it possible to communicate with the dentist and the prosthodontist.

Moung Oo learned quickly and was able to continue making dentures long after the prosthodontist had left. Although the hardware for the impressions and molds was gifted to the Kwai River Christian Hospital by the prosthodontist, the teeth that went into the dentures, as well as the material for making impressions and creating the denture plate itself had to be purchased in Bangkok to replace the original stock as it got used up. The materials had to be purchased in one of two or three shops in Bangkok. The teeth were quite expensive. So, again, we subsidized the cost with charity funds. (The people who needed dentures the most were not only toothless but also penniless, relatively speaking.) I was surprised on a trip to one of these stores, that the teeth they were selling were made in Scotland. When one thinks of Scotland, the first thing that comes to mind is not false teeth! Angus MacNeill, missionary colleague from Scotland, told me, "Ah, they are probably sheep's teeth!"

Mobile Clinic Program

From the early days of the Kwai River Christian Hospital (1960's) efforts were made toward health education, vaccinations, and nutritional supplementation in the communities around KRCH (see chapters 1-3).

The Village Health Program (also known as the "public health program" or the "mobile clinic") was begun by nurse Josie Falla and Dr. John Freeman in the 1970's. It flourished under the leadership of midwife and lady health visitor Olivia Thadin (later Saiduangchai). It continued as a mobile program (by boat, by oxcart, by pick-up truck, and on foot) through 1984, by which time the Khao Laem Dam had been completed and the reservoir had filled, flooding out many of the villages the mobile clinic had served. The good news was that the Electricity Generating Authority of Thailand built a public health clinic in each of the relocation settlements except for the ones immediately adjacent to the KRCH, as the hospital continued to serve the purpose of a public health clinic for close-by villages. The core services which comprised the village health program included:

- An "under-5" program
- A school health program
- Prenatal care
- Family planning
- TB treatment follow-up

Around the year 2000, an "Over-60's" program was developed to encourage fitness and good nutrition in the elderly and to screen them for diabetes, hypertension, and glaucoma.

Olivia Saiduangchai was the main force behind the village health program almost from early days. She continued in that role until her retirement in the 2000's. Her training in public health and midwifery plus her charm and perseverance and her fluency in Pwo Karen, Sgaw Karen, Burmese, Thai, and English, made her a winsome leader and a trusted source of information on health in the community.

Two striking achievements of the village health program were the reduction in the incidence of measles and the reduction in the incidence of neonatal tetanus. The first was due to measles vaccination in the under-5 population as well as in the elementary school population. In my first few years at the Kwai River Christian Hospital, there would typically be a measles epidemic every year or two. After just two or three years of the measles vaccination program, the incidence of measles was cut to just a few cases per year.

Typically, 2–3 cases per year of neonatal tetanus were seen at the Kwai River Christian Hospital in the 60's and 70's. To the best of my recollection there were only 2 or 3, total, from about 1984 on. Neonatal tetanus is caused by unhygienic management of the umbilical stump after home deliveries. This sometimes included application of cow dung. In the prenatal program of the village health project, pregnant women were routinely immunized with tetanus toxoid. The antibodies they developed were transferred passively through the placenta to the fetus, thus protecting the baby against tetanus for the first several months of life.

Postpartum kits were available for women who were planning to deliver at home or who had already just delivered at home. These consisted of a sterile cord tie, a sterile blade, and some ergometrine tablets plus vitamins and iron. These kits were intended to minimize postpartum bleeding in the mother and neonatal tetanus in the infant.

These kits were known locally as the medicine one takes so that one need not "lie by the fire". This was a reference to the tradition that new mothers should lie next to a charcoal fire for a week after delivery, eating a diet of only rice and salt. This practice unfortunately could result in dehydration, malnutrition, and deconditioning.

Anamais (government health stations) increased in number, staffing, and services starting around the time of the building of the dam. They more and more took over the public health needs in the district of Sangkhlaburi.

Water projects

Following relocation of the Kwai River Christian Hospital from its original site to the Huay Malai area in 1984, the village headman for the new location asked if the hospital could find the funds for installation of a gravity fed water project for the village of Yakadee, which was about 3 miles north of the Kwai River Christian Hospital's new location. At first this appeared to be a daunting task. However, with funds from the Baptist Union of Sweden, three volunteers from Australia, and a large workforce of able-bodied villagers gathered by the village headman, the project was accomplished. Over the next 15 years or so, five more gravity fed village water projects were installed under the umbrella of the Kwai River Christian Hospital Village Health Program.

Latrine project

They teach us in public health courses that the improvement in life expectancy in Europe over the last two or three centuries has been due not so much to vaccines and antibiotics as to improvements in water supply, sewage management, and garbage disposal. Having already helped several villages install gravity fed water systems, it seemed appropriate to further enhance the health of the villagers by instituting a latrine project. My idea was to provide participating households with the concrete rings, cement, squat plate, vent pipe, and expertise. The household's responsibility was to dig the pit and to build the shelter over the squat plate. We started with 10 households. The monetary value of the starter kit (concrete rings, cement, squat plate and vent pipe) was about 1,000 baht (equivalent to about US$30). The household was to set up the latrine with the help of this loan-in-kind and then pay back the "loan" at the rate of 100 baht per month for 10 months. This way there could be as many as 10 latrines being built at any one time. Olivia sensed a problem before we even began. She predicted that it would be difficult to collect on these "loans" and she declared that she was not going to be the bill collector. As I recall, little or nothing was ever paid back, and the "revolving" latrine fund made only one revolution before it stalled. Perhaps the villagers knew that the village health program would never repossess their latrines!

I think it is fair to say that over time it became a bit of a status symbol to have an outhouse, and they started springing up here and there without any direct involvement of the KRCH.

Services to refugees

For many years the Kwai River Christian Hospital has served refugees. These have mostly been from one of two refugee camps: Halawkhanee, a Mon refugee camp just inside Burma set up by MSF (Doctors without Borders) and Ton Yang (also spelled "Don Yang"), a Karen refugee camp on the Thai side of the border originally organized by the American Refugee Committee (ARC) and later sponsored by the International Rescue Committee (IRC). There was also a refugee settlement not far from the "Japanese Well". Besides these refugee settlements there were refugees scattered throughout the catchment area of the KRCH. Halawkhanee and Ton Yang camps each had a small hospital that could take care of basic medical and obstetrical needs. Patients requiring surgery, X-rays, or management of obstetrical complications were referred to the Kwai River Christian Hospital, and the sponsoring NGO covered the bill. Refugees with eye problems were permitted to come to the Kwai River Christian Hospital when there was a visiting ophthalmologist. Many of them received cataract surgery plus the placement of an intraocular lens: a service they would likely not have access to if they were still living in their home village back in Burma. At times, refugees were able to get lower limb prostheses through the KRCH. Refugees referred to the KRCH for further evaluation or care were required to have a form filled out by the refugee camp medical officer or his/her designee. This allowed the patient to get through the border police checkpoint. For our part, we had to record

on the same form a diagnosis, and indicate treatment given, and ongoing treatment recommended, so that the patient could get through the checkpoint on the return trip.

Safe House

In the 1990s there were frequent deportations of undocumented immigrants back to their respective countries. A large number of Mon, Karen, and Burmese were sent by the truckload from the immigration detention center in Bangkok to the Burma border about 15 miles beyond the Kwai River Christian Hospital. We could see these freight trucks full of deportees (standing room only) go rumbling past in front of the hospital. Among the undocumented people being deported, there were sometimes people with significant medical problems. They were often brought back to the hospital from the border by the border police and dropped off for medical evaluation and treatment. These patients had a wide variety of problems, some of which could be treated fairly rapidly and some of which required longer-term treatment. Either way, when the patients were well enough to be discharged from the hospital, they were often not well enough yet to make the trek back into Burma. A halfway house dubbed the "Safe House" was sponsored by a refugee relief organization for patients to stay in while they recuperated or continued treatment for their chronic condition. Although the patients at the Safe House were still technically illegal immigrants and, from that standpoint, were liable to arrest and deportation, the Thai authorities kindly allowed the Safe House residents to stay as long as required in order to be treated. Over time, the proportion of patients in the Safe House who had chronic mental health conditions increased. Some of these patients do not know what their former address in Burma was nor how to get there. For many years support for the Safe House and its residents came from the Burma Border Consortium. Since then various other arrangements have been made for administration and support of this ministry to an undocumented and fragile population.

Dr. Phil McDaniel

Potpourri

Autopsy in the graveyard

One afternoon in the early 1980s, a pickup truck trailing a cloud of dust came racing to the entrance of the hospital. An apparently lifeless man was carried into the outpatient department by his friends. He had reportedly been breathing up until about 3 minutes previously. This was a young man, probably in his 20's, who had been in what seemed like good health most of his life. He had deteriorated rapidly in the preceding few days with vague complaints of abdominal fullness and abdominal pain. He arrived moribund and our efforts at resuscitation were not successful. His friends requested an autopsy. This was a fairly unusual request, but his friends were particularly anxious to know the cause of death. I think they may have suspected foul play as their friend had been well until quite recently. I too was curious as to why such a young man should deteriorate and die in such a short time. We had no morgue and had no space set aside for autopsies. I considered doing the autopsy in the operating room. This would have been convenient from the standpoint of lighting and equipment, but I decided against it because we could not be sure that the patient had not died of some overwhelming infection by germs that might contaminate the operating room. I also considered the area just in front of the operating room where stood the two big sinks at which we scrubbed our hands prior to operations. The lighting was bad, and the space was cramped. So, this space was deemed unsuitable. I next considered the staff bathroom, which included a small unused shower area. It would have been a tight fit, but I thought that the trolley on which the cadaver lay might just fit diagonally. This option was vetoed by the staff, who feared that if we did the autopsy there, the bathroom would forever after be haunted. Someone suggested that we could do the autopsy in the graveyard. The grave could be dug beforehand. When the autopsy was finished, the cadaver could be lowered into the earth. Fortunately for me, we had two visiting medical students doing a tropical medicine rotation at the KRCH. They had just completed an elective rotation in forensic pathology. They were keen to do the autopsy and I happily allowed them to do the procedure while I took pictures. The deceased turned out to have widespread cancer of the liver and had died from massive

148

internal bleeding. The medical students took necropsies (biopsies), sewed up the cadaver and let the patient's friends (who had been standing around watching the autopsy) lower him into the grave.

Who's poor and who's not?

I learned early on that I was not a good judge of who really needed help from our charity funds and who did not. We tried to take care of all comers. We kept our fees very low, but even at that, there were some patients who truly could not pay their bills. We had several charity accounts, mostly funded by donations from abroad, some funded by local donations. The relatives of a patient would sometimes come to me and plead for a reduction in their hospital bill. I generally believed their story and complied with their request. Several times I was gently chided later for being "taken in." Ebra or Olivia would say something like, "Oh, that man is not poor! He has buffalos and fields. He could have paid his bill in full."

Then there were poor families who would not make any complaint. They would go sell their last buffalo to get money to pay their bill.

So, I quickly learned that it was better to consult nurses "in the know" before granting any patient charity funds. Eventually we formed a charity committee.

The DOG Fund

We had several charity accounts, some with stipulations as to who qualified to receive help. There was a charity account funded by the Baptist Union of Sweden; one specifically for children, started with seed money from a princess; and there was a general charity account. These charity accounts allowed us to help patients who otherwise would have had great difficulty paying even a modest hospital bill.

The charity accounts were helpful, but a problem arose with regard to accounting for donated goods. Visiting medical students and doctors often brought with them donated goods such as urinary catheters, latex gloves, chest tubes, and medications. Clearly, the intent of these donations was to reduce the cost of care for patients. If the item which a patient required was available as donated goods, then the patient would not be charged for that item. However, a volunteer pharmacist visiting from Australia pointed out that under this system, whether a patient benefited or not from donated goods depended largely on luck and timing. For example, a patient might arrive in the morning requiring a certain item. If we had a donated one in stock, he would get it free except for a small handling and storage fee. On the other hand, if another patient arrived the same afternoon requiring the same item, but there were no donated ones left, he would have to pay the regular price.

The pharmacist suggested that we set up a Donated Overseas Goods account. He said we could call it the DOG fund. As donated goods came in, the pharmacist would estimate roughly how much it would have cost to order those items from Bangkok, and that amount of money would be credited to the DOG fund. The donated items would then be rotated through our inventory and priced the same as though they had been purchased from Bangkok. The DOG fund became a virtual charity account that could be used to help any patient in need regardless of whether the supplies and medicines used to treat him/her had actually been donated or not.

Adoptions from the hospital

We did not run an orphanage at the hospital. There would have been very little need for one. In that culture children are highly valued and even if both parents died, the child would generally be looked after by grandparents or by the family of an aunt or uncle.

I can think of only two babies that were turned over to the hospital for care. One was born prematurely to a single mother who already had six or seven children. The mother left the baby in the care of the hospital while she returned home to her other responsibilities. The baby was not expected to live, but with intensive nursing care in an incubator she began to gain weight and achieve some of her developmental milestones. It was cumbersome for the nurses on night duty to take care of this infant in addition to the regular inpatients. Eventually, Ebra, Olivia, Jan Stretton, Chris Gage (volunteer nurse), Loes de Vos (the pharmacist), and Melba agreed that they would look after the baby in their homes at night in rotation. Eventually, the baby became strong enough to be placed in the care of an adoption agency in Bangkok called the Holt Foundation. She was adopted by a couple in the United States and kept in contact with some of those who looked after her at the Kwai River Christian Hospital. I arranged to meet up with her and her adopted mother in Bangkok in February of 2008, and we traveled up to the Kwai River Christian Hospital where a very nice "meet your birth family" celebration had been arranged by nurse Lea Lindero.

The only other baby I can remember being left at the hospital was a premature female baby of a Mon lady who already had 6 children. The lady's husband had gone on a trip 5 or 6 months previously and never come back. A day or two after giving birth, the baby's mother informed us that she had to go back to the refugee camp to get some belongings if she were to stay around and help care for her very premature little girl. We expected her to return in a day or two, but she did not. Days merged into weeks and weeks into months. The baby gained weight and strength and was ready to go home, but there was still no mother in sight. This was a conundrum for the hospital. We were not staffed or equipped to raise an orphan. We sent inquiries to the leaders in the main Mon refugee camp and also to several other Mon settlements explaining the situation and asking whether they could find this baby's mother for us. The Mon leaders reported that they were unable to locate the mother of the premature baby. We then asked whether we had their permission to put the baby up for adoption, and if so, could they find a reliable family to adopt the baby. It turned out there was a childless Mon couple very interested in adopting the baby. He had a steady job and Thai citizenship. It was felt that this would allow the baby to eventually obtain Thai citizenship with all the benefits that accrue to that legal status. With the knowledge and consent of the Mon leaders, we set a date on which the Mon couple could come claim the baby, provided the biological mother had not returned before that date. The prospective new parents began setting up their house to accommodate the new baby. They bought bedding and baby clothes and mosquito netting.

Lo and behold, just a few days before the deadline for the biological mother to claim her baby, she showed up! "Where's my baby?" Most of us felt that the baby's future would be much brighter with the couple who wanted to adopt her than with the biological mother, who was poor and single and already had six kids. However, she was not willing to give up her baby even after speaking with the prospective adoptive parents. She said that during her trip to get the belongings at the refugee camp, the Thai authorities did a snap roundup of undocumented aliens. Since she was outside of the refugee camp at the time, she was at risk of arrest and deportation. She explained that she had fled into the jungle and had been in hiding there almost the whole time since her departure from the hospital. The baby was turned over to the biological mother. The Mon couple were very disappointed. We do not know how the little girl fared after that.

Phil's skull

When I was about to enter medical school, Dr. Jack Miner, the father of Andy Miner, my best friend in college, gave me a human skull. While this may seem like an odd gift, it was actually a very valuable and very useful one for someone getting ready to study human anatomy. The skull had been given to Dr. Miner by the widow of a deceased physician friend of his. Dr. Miner, who was an obstetrician, apparently thought I could make better use of the skull in anatomy class than he could in his obstetrical practice.

When my family traveled out to Thailand in 1978 to begin our first term as missionaries in Thailand, we were required to itemize all the goods in our freight and indicate whether they were new or used. We also had to put a value on each item. The skull was clearly used, both by the original owner and by subsequent medical people who studied the piece. As for putting a value on the skull, I was at a bit of a loss. I didn't know what skulls were going for in those days or whether they could even be bought. Obviously, the skull had been priceless to the original owner. I don't remember what I put for a value in the end. I do know that the skull proved very useful, particularly for explaining various X-ray views of the head and in learning and teaching the technique of inferior alveolar nerve block for dental procedures.

So, I have two skulls: one on the end of my neck and one in a box on a shelf in Thailand labeled "Phil's Skull". I do not plan to ever bring that one back to the USA. There would be way too many questions in customs!

Elephant injuries

Elephants can be very dangerous when they are unhappy. They are big and powerful and have numerous means by which they can injure a human being.

The tusks can be used to skewer a man. The elephant's trunk can be used to draw the unfortunate victim over its tusks.

The trunk can also be used to squeeze the victim and crush his chest wall, or it can be used to toss the victim up in the air and let him crash to the ground.

The mouth can be used to bite the face of a victim while the trunk holds him in place.

An elephant's massive forehead can be used to compress a victim's body against a rigid object.

An elephant may use one of its feet to trample a victim.

By rolling over a victim, the elephant can utilize its immense weight to break bones in the arms and legs as well as injure the victim's chest and abdomen.

Bull elephants periodically undergo a phase called "musth" during which they become irritable and aggressive.

In my 23 years at the Kwai River Christian Hospital I saw victims of nearly every one of the above types of elephant injury. One may well ask how a person could survive any of the above assaults. In some cases, there was an element of luck, such as when an elephant trying to use its forehead to crush a man's torso pushed him up against a bamboo thicket. Luckily, this thicket had just enough "give" in it to allow the man to sink back into the thicket far enough to avoid being fatally crushed. He got away with a few broken ribs.

Once an elephant tried to skewer his mahout on its tusks, but they had been recently sawed off, and were too short for a successful skewering. At times a victim managed to escape thanks to the extraordinary courage of a friend who rushed in at great risk to himself to extricate the victim.

"A Japanese dog bit him."

Kawasaki, Suzuki, Honda, Yamaha: as motorcycles proliferated, so did motorcycle injuries. Some drivers skidded out while speeding around curves. Others were sideswiped by trucks or flew beyond the end of the pavement where sections of road had been washed out. Passengers sitting behind the driver sometimes got their toes caught in the spokes of the rear wheel. When a nurse's aide came to get me to come see a new motorcycle injury case in the emergency room, our conversation might go something like this:

Dr. Phil McDaniel

Doctor: "What's the matter with the patient?"
Nurse's aide: "He was bitten by a Japanese dog."

"Be not unequally yoked."

This Bible verse (II Corinthians 6:14) gives advice about marriage. The metaphor is vivid for anyone who has observed a cart being pulled by two animals that are working at cross purposes. The team of bulls which pulled the mobile clinic's oxcart early in my time at the Kwai River Christian Hospital was literally unequally yoked. One bull was particularly aggressive. When pulling the oxcart, he would go faster or slower than the other bull. He also had a tendency to lean sideways into the yoke so as to push the other bull off the road. This caused some consternation on the part of the oxcart driver. Even when the bulls were not pulling an oxcart, they had a tendency to fight. They would butt heads until they became exhausted. Finally, one of the bulls would break away. These "bullfights" were rather entertaining for the schoolchildren and even for the hospital staff. However, they were not good for the bulls and with every fight, there was the danger of injury to the bulls or to the bystanders.

As these were fairly young bulls, the oxcart driver—who was also the hospital gardener—advised that we observe for a while and see if the bulls could sort out their differences. Unfortunately, the bulls continued to fight, and the oxcart driver reluctantly advised that the more aggressive of the two be castrated. A traditional veterinarian was called in to do a village style castration. With the help of the oxcart driver and a few others, the bull was hogtied very securely. The vet then used a hinged wooden instrument which, ironically, resembled an enormous nutcracker. He applied this across the bull's scrotum, above the testicles. He then used a large, blunt wooden chisel and a wooden mallet to hammer away at the tissue just above the "nutcracker". When the vet was satisfied that he had sufficiently contused the tissue supplying blood to the testicles, he removed his instrument and untied the bull. For five or ten minutes, the bull lay still. He must have been in some type of shock. When he finally struggled to stand up and walk, he staggered around more like a newborn calf than a full-grown bull. The castration had taken the aggression right out of him. Over time, he gained his strength back but, thankfully, not his aggressive attitude.

154

Adaptation and Perseverance

Burn creams

One day I was standing in the patient waiting area with one of the AFRIMS doctors when a burn victim was brought in. A white cream had already been applied to the burn areas. This very much resembled silver sulfadiazine, an antimicrobial cream used in burn units. We wondered if the patient had received some rather advanced first aid in his village. But no, it was just toothpaste!

Grandma spewing half-chewed rice

A treatment for burns that probably dates back to long before toothpaste, was grandma spewing half-chewed rice onto the burn. I don't know much more about this remedy beyond the fact that it was common. Did it matter whether the grandma was a maternal grandma or a paternal grandma? Did the grandma actually have to be the patient's grandma, or would just any old grandma do? If the patient's grandma was not handy could a parent or some other relative fill in?

Warm duck blood

Patients brought to the hospital with known or suspected ingestion of poison often had been treated in the village already with a local remedy to induce vomiting: warm duck blood. I've never imbibed it myself, but it's difficult to imagine that this wouldn't induce vomiting.

Slowly Come, Enormous, Famous, Fabulous, Snow White, Camera

What do the above have in common? They are the actual English names of local patients who received their medical care at the KRCH. "Slowly Come" was born after a prolonged labor. "Enormous" was presumably a large baby. The names "Famous", "Fabulous", and "Snow White" presumably reflect the hope the parents had that their offspring would be accomplished or beautiful. As for "Camera", I did ask once what the inspiration had been for giving that name. I was told that the name was chosen just because it had a melodious sound to it.

Long hours

My wife, Melba, wrote the following diary entry for May 23, 1980:

Dr. Phil McDaniel

Phil has just admitted his third case of cerebral malaria today. This patient, a young girl, was carried by stretcher from Songkalia (about 10 miles away) in the rain. It took the bearers most of the day to get here. Unfortunately, she arrived too late and died a few hours later, before the intravenous quinine had time to take effect.

For June 19, 1980 she wrote:

Phil went to the hospital to sleep and take call. Normally, one of the four nurses sleeps at the hospital, but this week one of the nurses is away on a [mobile] clinic trip, one is in Bangkok on business, and one is off sick with malaria. To relieve Jan Stretton, the fourth nurse [the only one left], Phil volunteered to take her place tonight. There were some pretty sick patients; consequently, he got very little sleep.

110 volts vs. 220 volts

"It ran great for a minute or so and then it quit!" Thus spoke a visiting medical student describing the behavior of a donated cast saw made for 110 volts when he plugged it into a 220 volt electrical outlet!

It quit because it had burned out. Standard electrical voltage in the United States is 110-120 volts. In much of the rest of the world, including Thailand, the standard voltage is 220-240 volts. This can cause a problem when someone unaware of the issue unwittingly plugs an item of equipment donated from the United States directly into a Thailand electrical outlet. We lost several items of equipment this way despite admonitions to staff and visitors to take care. We tried attaching large "110 volt only" labels near the end of the power cord. This worked most of the time, but it only took one person in a hurry to overlook the tag and burn out that item of equipment. A more effective

156

precaution was changing the plug on the end of the power cord to one that had a configuration of prongs that would only fit into a matching female plug on a 220-to-110 step-down transformer. With some items, we just soldered the power cord directly to the transformer so that wherever the equipment went the transformer was sure to go.

Dental forceps with slingshot rubber assist

I knew when I was getting ready to go out to Thailand as a missionary doctor in a remote post that it would probably be useful to know how to extract teeth. During my surgery preceptorship there was a dental surgeon who took me under his wing and taught me a bit about dental extractions on his patients who were under general anesthesia. He was not officially connected with the surgical group in which I was serving a preceptorship. However, he knew that I was planning to head out to a remote location as a missionary doctor and he went out of his way to help me prepare for that assignment. As I mentioned before, I also received some training and experience in the north of Thailand when I participated in a public health trip to a remote location called Baw Kaew. Hill tribe people came to get their vaccinations, family planning, and, in some cases, to have a tooth or two extracted. The Thai dentist on that trip encouraged me to pull some teeth under his supervision. This I did and the experience came in very handy later at the Kwai River Christian Hospital.

There is something especially miserable about a toothache and something especially rewarding about pulling out the offending tooth. As one stands there inspecting the extracted tooth, still in the grip of the forceps, patient and "dentist" can share a moment of satisfaction, knowing that at least THIS tooth will never cause pain again.

There was already a fairly good collection of dental instruments at the hospital when I began my time there. Armed with these and a pamphlet with clear drawings that described the technique of dental extraction under local anesthesia, I was able to pull many hundreds of hopelessly decayed teeth in my 23 years at the KRCH.

Most teeth could be removed without undue difficulty, but there was an occasional stubborn tooth, usually a molar, that did not want to budge. These required grasping the tooth firmly while patiently rocking it side to side tens of times to gradually loosen it up. I found that maintaining a firm grip on the tooth for a long time resulted in fatigue in my forearm muscles which were doing the gripping. This, in turn, could result in my getting impatient with the tooth and attempting the final extraction maneuver before the tooth was suitably loosened. The result was sometimes a broken root, and this could require additional work to remove. I thought how convenient power steering and power brakes are on a car and began looking for a way to create "power forceps". The nurses regularly used slingshot rubbers as tourniquets when drawing blood or starting I.V.'s. I tried winding one of these slingshot rubbers round and round the handles of the dental forceps during especially difficult extractions. This augmented the force of my grip on the tooth so that I could concentrate more on loosening the tooth and less on the grip itself.

I presented this technique in a serendipity session at a medical/dental conference for missionary doctors and dentists. The dentists at the conference did a skit about it on skit night. I came away with the feeling that in their opinion REAL dentists don't need slingshot rubbers!

Robberies

During the relocation period (about 1983–1986), there were a number of robberies in Sangkhlaburi District, including some armed robberies. Villagers being relocated had difficulty keeping their belongings safe while moving. The "new" hospital building in Huay Malai was only half finished when the hospital moved. The operating room and the delivery room were among the few rooms that could be locked. They had to be used as secure storage for medicines and equipment that had been trucked over from the old Lainam site. Meantime, operations and deliveries had to be done in a room nearby or in a wooden building behind the hospital.

On the compound of the Kwai River Christian Mission stood not only the hospital but also a school, a boardinghouse, teachers' houses, hospital staff houses, a generator shed, and various other support buildings. The frequent robberies in the area prompted the Kwai River Christian Mission Executive Committee to hire two watchmen. Every hour on the hour one watchman was to go ring the school bell. This was an old-fashioned clanging brass bell whose sound reached to every corner of the mission compound. The ringing of the bell demonstrated that at least one watchman was awake. He was then to walk around the compound shining a spotlight in various directions looking for robbers. After this inspection of the compound, he could return to his home base at the hospital. The other watchman was to stay put at the hospital to keep the nurses and nurse aides safe. When the nursing staff changed shifts in the middle of the night, one watchman would be available to escort them home. The ringing of the bell every hour on the hour followed by a brief walk around the compound created a fairly predictable pattern. Apparently, some local robbers worked out that if they waited for just a few minutes after the ringing of the bell, they could pretty safely burgle the school. They broke in undetected one night and took several items of office equipment. The Executive Committee of the Kwai River Christian Mission subsequently asked the watchmen to vary the time of their walk-around so that it was not so predictable. The hourly ringing of the school bell, however, continued every hour on the hour. This was annoying to some, reassuring to others. Either way, it had the dubious benefit of letting insomniacs know that they had endured yet another hour of sleeplessness.

Charcoal broiled laundry

For the first 30 years or so of the hospital's existence, all the hospital laundry was washed by hand. During the dry season, getting the laundry to dry was usually not too difficult. The linens could be hung on a line indoors or outdoors. If there was a large amount of laundry, some items could be spread out to dry on the top of the hedge near the laundry shed. In the rainy season, the rate at which laundry was washed often exceeded the rate at which it could be dried. This resulted in congestion in the laundry shed and shortages of some linens in the hospital. The laundry staff developed a low-tech way of hastening the drying of hospital linens. This involved lighting a small fire in a charcoal stove of the type used in village kitchens. This was placed under a huge inverted woven basket with the wet laundry spread over the top of it. Alternatively, the charcoal stove could be placed under an empty infant crib which had been modified to accommodate wet linens draped over slats that ran crosswise over the tops of the siderails. When surgical masks were dried using one of these methods, the next person to wear the mask could enjoy the aroma of charcoal, which persisted even after autoclaving.

Dr. Phil McDaniel

Bamboo in abundance

Bamboo is a mixed blessing and we had plenty of it. It is a nuisance to clear if one wants to plant a garden or build a building where there is already a stand of bamboo. It has a way of propagating through its root system. It has to be cut back from time to time so that it does not take over the surrounding area.

On the other hand, bamboo can be very useful. If, while making rounds, I determined that a patient in traction should have an additional cross piece on his traction apparatus, I could call in the gardener and show him what diameter and length of bamboo I needed. Before I was done with rounds, it would be ready. We used bamboo to make various struts and braces for orthopedic cases and skin transfer-flap cases. Bamboo could be fashioned into tongue blades and the stick part of cotton tipped applicators. A thin shaft of bamboo with a side branch could be used for an IV pole.

Bicycle-pump-powered nebulizer

Before we had regular daytime electric power, we were still able to create the air pressure required to make a nebulizer work. This was a boon to asthma patients because it meant that they could have a nebulizer treatment up and going within minutes. We were able to generate the air pressure required using a bicycle pump. This was a step up from the cheapest kind of bicycle pump. It could be used on bicycles or motorcycles. It had a little pressure cylinder attached which helped to even out the pressure between strokes. A nurse, a nurse aide, or a relative of the patient would be tasked with the pumping. Care had to be taken to pump fast enough to nebulize the medicine in the nebulizer but not so fast as to make the connections in the tubing blow apart.

"Gallons" for traction

Although Thailand is on the metric system (the only two countries in the world that are not are Myanmar and the USA!), there are still many carry-overs from the days of inches, pounds and gallons. In Thai, the term "gallon" refers not only to the liquid measure, 1 US gallon, it also refers to plastic containers that once held a gallon of something liquid. At the hospital we had many empty "gallons" because we bought many of our liquid medicines—for example, antacid and milk of magnesia—by the gallon. It turned out that "gallons" were a convenient way of obtaining just the right amount of traction for orthopedic cases. One "gallon" filled with water weighed approximately 8 pounds. If we needed less traction, we could pour some water out. If we needed more, we could add a second "gallon" filled with an appropriate amount of water. This was a convenient way of adjusting traction without resorting to expensive orthopedic weights.

Gigli saws (no, not "giggly")

In limb amputations, a wire saw is sometimes used. This has the advantage over a conventional handsaw in that one can cut and bevel the bone all in one pass. Beveling the end of the bone reduces the chance of a sharp bony protuberance at the end of the stump. This saw often goes by the name of its inventor, an Italian obstetrician, whose surname was Gigli (which sounds something like "jee gee"). A few of these saws came with some donated equipment. They worked well except for one thing: they tended to break before the bone was sawed through. Sometimes the backup saw also broke. I discovered that gardeners and arborists also use wire saws. The ones from the hardware store cut better and last longer than the ones from the surgical instrument store and are cheaper, too. We sterilized them along with the other equipment.

Library in the Operating Room

An atlas of anatomy as well as atlases of surgical technique in general surgery, orthopedic surgery, and ophthalmological surgery stood guard over the operating room from a shelf high on the wall. I could ask the circulating nurse to get one of these books down from the shelf and open it to the operation I was doing if I needed some guidance. Occasionally, I would get out one of those books before the operation began and open it up on a side table for reference. All this was done in plain sight of the patient, who was usually wide awake under some form of local or regional anesthesia. I don't think I ever heard a patient complain about the doctor looking things up. Perhaps they thought it was just as well that the doctor was doing things by the book.

Drifting Operating Room Light

When we moved the hospital from Lainam to Huay Malai, we took with us the operating room light. Because the ceiling in the Huay Malai hospital was built one meter higher than the ceiling in the original hospital, the carpenter installing the operating room light in the Huay Malai hospital had to build a box that extended down from the level of the ceiling one meter so that the base of the light assembly would be at its original height and the light itself would be within reach of the circulating nurse! The arm that held the operating room light to its base had various articulations so that it could be pushed and pulled and swiveled into a position where it illuminated the operative field. The carpenter who built the extension down from the ceiling was not our regular carpenter. He managed to get the base of the operating room light almost but not quite level. The light would occasionally drift during an operation. The circulating nurse would have to repeatedly pull the light back to the original position. Sometimes the drift was so persistent I would let the light drift to its own stopping place and then roll the operating table (with the patient still on it) under the light. My motto was, "If you can't put any light on the subject, put the subject under the light."

Passing out in the Operating Room

It can get hot in an operating room in the tropics. Start with a hot afternoon; add an operating gown plus cap and mask and latex gloves; then stand under a hot operating room light and you have a recipe for either the surgeon or the assistant passing out. When we first moved to the Huay Malai location there were no trees to provide shade on the operating room end of the hospital. One wall faced more-or-less south, getting sun most of the day. Nevertheless, I resisted the idea of installing air conditioning in the operating room because it seemed like an extravagance. Not only was there the expense of the air conditioning units themselves, but also the requirement to run a big generator to provide the power to run them. I thought we could all be good soldiers and press on through the heat without resorting to air conditioning. After all, we did have a fan in the OR. Then twice in the span of a few months, the nurse assisting me during an operation passed out. I decided then that we could justify air conditioning, though just for the operating room. At that time, I was still the only doctor at the hospital. One reason for the softening of my position on air conditioning was concern as to who would finish the operation if I should pass out.

Back-up to the back-up to the back-up

When I began my watch at the Kwai River Christian Hospital in 1979, our backup generator set was comprised of a single cylinder Yanmar diesel engine connected by belts to an alternator. This was rated at 5 kVA, which is rather meager for a hospital. This was a hand-cranked generator. I sometimes had to start it myself. This was especially so if the need for back-up power arose when the only other staff around were petite Thai nurses and nurse aides. The Australian missionary nurses—who were more robust than the Thai nursing staff —were usually able to start that old Yanmar generator. We used it for X-rays, operations, and backup power at night. When the Kwai River Christian Mission relocated to Huay Malai, we purchased a 15 kVA generator. I felt that this would surely provide adequate power to the mission compound for some time to come. This calculation was based on the assumption that residents on the compound would be using electricity only for electric lights. This turned out to be a foolish assumption (for which I take the blame). As soon as people obtained electric power in their homes, they started buying electric irons and electric rice cookers. Either one of these items uses many times the power of a 20 W fluorescent tube (the standard home light fixture in those days). Over the years we graduated from a 15 kVA generator set to a 40 kVA generator set and finally to a 125 kVA set. Each time we "graduated" to a more powerful generator, the previous one became the backup to the new one, albeit with some restrictions as to what could be run on the backup.

Even with all this redundancy, things could go wrong which would result in loss of electric power. This happened on one of my volunteer trips back to the Kwai River Christian Hospital in the early 2000's. I had just started an emergency appendectomy when the lights went out. For some reason, the automatic startup of the generator did not occur. I asked someone to find the maintenance man to start up the generator. I received word that he had gone into town on some errand or other, and it was not known when he would return. In the end, we used first a flashlight and then the watchman's spotlight (powered by a motorcycle battery). That got us through most of the operation. Just before we finished, the operating room light came on again: someone on the hospital staff had been able to contact the housefather at the student hostel, who knew how to start the generator.

"Toyatsun"

Around 1982 we had the opportunity to purchase a vehicle for the mobile clinic program. There was actually sufficient funding from the Baptist Union of Sweden to purchase a four-wheel-drive pick-up truck. I foolishly decided that a two-wheel-drive pick-up would be good enough, and the balance of the funds could be used for other expenses. My reasoning about the two-wheel drive was that in the dry season two-wheel-drive would work fine, but when the rains came, it didn't matter whether one had two-wheel-drive or four-wheel-drive, the vehicle wouldn't get through, and the mobile clinic would have to go by boat, oxcart, or on foot. There was some truth to this, but it did not take into consideration that there was a transition period going into the rainy season and a transition period coming out. During each of these transition periods there might be a few weeks when a four-wheel-drive pick-up could get to the villages and to Kanchanaburi, but a two-wheel-drive could not.

1984 is the year the Kwai River Christian Mission was moved from the original site in Lainam to the new site in Huay Malai. Ben Dickerson was in charge of relocation. He had a long history of driving Land Rovers and a Dodge Power Wagon. He was big on four-wheel-drive! He got word that in Kanchanaburi there was a mechanic who, for such-and-such a price and within such-and-such a period of time, could convert our two-wheel-drive Datsun to a four-wheel-drive vehicle by swapping out the Datsun undercarriage for a Toyota one. He gave the impression that this was fairly straightforward and that he had some experience doing it. Ben talked me into having this mechanic carry out this two-wheel-drive to four-wheel-drive transformation. There was delay after delay and problems with making things fit together. The project was over budget and behind schedule. Around this time, we learned that this was actually the first time that this particular mechanic had attempted this conversion. By then it was too late to abort. The end result was a vehicle of mediocre performance that we called the "Toyatsun."

Bugs on the sterile field

We had screened windows and screened doors around the operating room. This was to keep out bugs, but somehow, they still got in. This was especially true at night when bugs were attracted to the bright spot cast by the operating room light. Moths, gnats, and tiny winged creatures I do not even know the names of were attracted to the sterile field during nighttime procedures. If we were unlucky enough to be operating during a termite swarm, the flying ants (winged termites) could be very numerous and annoying. Whenever a housefly landed on the sterile field, we re-draped. If only moths, gnats, flying ants, and mosquitoes landed on the sterile field, we just shooed them away as best we could. It was not possible to re-drape for every bug. If we had tried to, we would have used up all our anesthesia time draping and re-draping.

Unforeseen benefits of donating blood

Melba entered the following news item for November 6, 1982:

> This afternoon the headmaster of our United Christian School, a 31-year-old Thai Christian, was married to Taow, a 19-year-old Thai village girl from Wangpato, one of the villages on the road south from Sangkhlaburi. At the wedding Kru (teacher) Weerasak, the groom, explained how he and Taow met. Several months ago, her father was admitted to the hospital, suffering from a ruptured appendix. He needed a blood transfusion and a message was sent to the school, asking if any of the teachers would be willing to donate blood. (The hospital has no blood bank, and sometimes the patient's friends and relatives are themselves unable to donate blood.) So, Kru Weerasak donated a unit of blood for the unknown

patient, and later decided to pay a visit to the man who had received his blood. While there, he met the patient's pretty daughter, Taow, and from then on was quite a frequent visitor at the hospital! Taow was not at that time a Christian— there are no Christians in her village—but she was apparently intrigued by what Kru Weerasak had to tell her about Christ. Her father was in the hospital for several weeks, and Taow sometimes attended the Wednesday evening Bible study class. Eventually, she made a commitment to Christ herself and was baptized.

Big fish in a small pond

Being the director and only doctor of the only hospital for miles around, I was "a big fish in a small pond". I was occasionally asked to give a speech or say a prayer at various functions or even to be a judge in a competition.

Once I was asked to be one of the judges in a choir competition. This was on the occasion of the annual meeting of the local association of churches. The choir of each church came dressed up in traditional Karen garb and sang the assigned song in front of an audience and a panel of judges. It was an honor to be asked to be one of the judges, but I protested that I was not qualified because I myself did not sing well and could not even read notes. I was assured that there was nothing to it. All I had to do was see how smartly the singers were dressed, how they filed in, how they filed out, the way they arranged themselves, their posture, and when they took their breaths. Yes, apparently good singers are not supposed to take a breath in the middle of a sentence or a phrase!

On another occasion, I was asked to be a judge in what could be called a "clothes washing contest". One of our senior nurses had taken some courses in human resources management and was in the process of screening several applicants for the position of assistant laundress. The nurse felt that the hiring should be done in an objective manner rather than based on the applicant's appearance or connections. To this end, the nurse arranged for the three applicants to wash some hospital linens by hand while a panel of judges looked on. I was asked to be one of the judges. I did not feel qualified to judge the technique of washing hospital linens, having no experience in this art myself. However, I was assured that no experience was required to judge. All one had to do was observe how much laundry detergent was used, how long and vigorously the contestant scrubbed the sample cloth and how much water they used to rinse. Unfortunately, I was not given clear guidelines as to how much laundry detergent was just right, how long of a scrub was enough to get the linens clean without spending an undue amount of time on the task, nor whether rinsing just once was better because it saved on water or whether rinsing twice was better because the linens ended up being less soapy! Despite the ambiguities, we judges made our selection. As far as I know, that lady is working in the laundry department to this day.

Every now and then, I was asked to give "the charge" at a wedding. The charge is not to be confused with the sermon that the pastor gives during the middle part of the ceremony. Rather, it is a short talk delivered by someone respected by the families of the bride and groom toward the end of the ceremony, admonishing the bride and groom to be supportive of one another through thick and thin, and that sort of thing. My Thai language skills are pretty good when it comes to talking about hearts and lungs and livers, but my vocabulary is meager when it comes to talking about love and marriage. Whenever I accepted one of these opportunities to "give the charge"—and it would have been rude to refuse one—I knew that I was accepting the risk of accidentally saying something comical or even risqué by mispronouncing a word or by unwittingly using a phrase that might have a double meaning!

"20 bed, 30 mat hospital"

"How big is your hospital?"

That's a question I got asked frequently.

Usually the answer to a question such as this is given in terms of beds.

For example, "50 beds". This would imply that the hospital could accommodate up to 50 inpatients at any given time.

KRCH was registered as a 10-bed hospital initially and later as a 20-bed hospital.

However, we did not turn away patients who needed treatment.

When we ran out of beds, we used mats. Many of the villagers were accustomed to sleeping on mats at home. So, it wasn't any particular bother for them to sleep on mats at the hospital.

At times we were a "20 bed, 30 mat hospital".

Curious remedy

I had gone for an outing with Olivia (head of the village health team) and some visitors from overseas. I cannot remember whether we had just visited a village church or if we had been sight-seeing.

In any case, Olivia suggested that we stop at the house of some friends to get out of the sun and have a little rest. As we chatted with the owners of the house the subject of natural medicines came up. They told us about one which from time-to-time oozed out of some rocks. They said it tasted vile but was reported to cure a number of ailments common in the area. They wanted to know whether I, as a doctor of modern medicine, thought the claims were plausible. Of course, I had no way to prove or disprove the efficacy of this "medicine", but they had gotten my curiosity up. I asked if I could see a sample. This they produced. It was a dark, almost opaque fluid. They once again reiterated how awful it tastes and, with barely suppressed laughter, invited me to try a little!

I thought to myself, "What harm can come from a little fluid that oozes out of a rock from time to time?" So, I tried a very small amount. It was more than enough to confirm that this was vile tasting stuff. I wondered if perhaps this was what crude oil tastes like, but having never tasted that, I could not say. I asked if it had a name. After a little discussion amongst themselves, they told me what it is called in one of the local dialects. I asked Olivia to translate to English. She said, "rock menstrual fluid!"

Memorable Patients

Uninformed consent for exploratory laparotomy?

In the days before CT scans and MRIs, it was not uncommon for a patient—even in North America or Western Europe—to have to undergo "exploratory laparotomy" for abdominal pain. The idea was that if the patient's abdominal pain could not be diagnosed after a thorough history and physical exam and after running tests on blood and urine and maybe taking some X-rays, the patient might have to be opened up and "explored". While this procedure may sound primitive, it does allow for direct visualization of the abdominal contents and the opportunity to feel the abdominal organs with a gloved hand. Now that's something that even an MRI doesn't let you do! Best of all, if the condition turns out to be a surgically treatable condition, the fix can usually be done right then and there. Exploratory laparotomies are occasionally done even today in hospitals with and without high tech imaging equipment.

A little old lady with abdominal pain of moderate severity was brought to the hospital by her son and daughter. After doing several basic tests, the diagnosis was still not clear, but a "surgical abdomen" was suspected. I explained to the son and daughter that I thought the patient had a condition that required surgery and that the only way to find out for sure which condition it was, would be to open up the abdomen and have a look and feel inside. They said to me, "It's up to you doctor. We put our trust in you."

I said, "Okay, I'll explain to the patient what we are about to do."

"Oh no, doctor! Don't tell HER! She might become frightened!"

Oddly enough, I do not recollect what transpired after that, but I'm pretty sure I did not operate without some form of consent from the patient!

A hunter too clever for his own good

The X-ray films I was looking at showed innumerable irregular metallic fragments throughout both thighs and both calves of the patient. He was a hunter. He had devised an instrument which, when

169

he blew on it, produced a sound similar to the squealing of a wild sow. His plan was to lure a wild boar close enough to shoot it. He had hidden behind a bush and blown on his instrument. He must have produced a fairly realistic sound because along came another hunter who shot into the bush. There were way too many metallic fragments to locate and remove. We took out the largest ones and the ones closest to the surface. The village headman was called in to arbitrate between the two hunters. He asked me how many metal fragments had been embedded in the patient. I told him there were too many to count. He insisted I come up with a number. I gave him a rough estimate, and I believe that he used that to estimate damages.

Cigar smoke as a diagnostic tool

A young lady came to us with an empyema (pus in the chest cavity) and a partially collapsed lung. I put in a chest tube and hooked it up to suction. We got out most of the pus, but the lung refused to re-inflate. This type of problem could be caused by a poor seal at the chest tube insertion site or sometimes due to a "peel" that had formed around the lung, preventing it from re-inflating. It could also be due to a bronco-pleural fistula: an opening between the bronchial tree and the surface of the lung, connecting the bronchial tree to the chest cavity and allowing the lung to collapse. These conditions are managed quite differently, and it is important to try to determine which one is the problem in a given case. It turns out that this lady smoked cigars, a very common habit for women in that rural setting. We had been discouraging this lady from smoking, but she had heeded our advice only intermittently. Compliance seemed to improve whenever she heard the doctor coming down the hall! One day I realized that we could use cigar smoke as a diagnostic tool. She was probably surprised when I asked her to take a long puff on her cigar and then hold her breath. I knew that if during this maneuver, cigar smoke appeared in the glass bottle that her chest tube emptied into, it would confirm that she had a bronchopleural fistula. The cigar smoke did appear in the collection bottle. She had a communication between her bronchial tree and the surface of the affected lung: a condition roughly analogous to a flat tire. The solution in her case was to increase the rate and strength of suction in order to outstrip the leak and coax the lung into re-expanding. Once the surface of the lung made contact with the inside surface of the chest wall, it began to adhere and after a week or so we were able to remove the chest tube.

On another occasion our receptionist told me that she had air coming out of her left ear. A quick ear exam revealed no obvious hole in the eardrum. I assured her that the "air coming out of her ear" was most likely just a sensation due to the accumulation of some fluid in the middle ear. She insisted that she really did have air coming out of her ear and that she could show me, too. She took a puff on a cigar while I looked down her ear canal with an otoscope. Sure enough! Here came a little puff of smoke, and closer exam revealed that there was indeed a small hole in her ear drum.

Buddhist monk motorized escort

A man in his 50s or 60s was brought to the hospital edematous, pale, and a little short of breath. He had end stage kidney failure and there was not much we could do for him. He was apparently a VIP at the big Mon temple in the town of Sangkhlaburi, about 10 miles from the KRCH in Huay Malai. I do not know if the patient had been a major financial contributor to the work of the temple or whether he had some other connection. He had a lay attendant and was occasionally visited by monks from his temple. I was told to take good care of him and not to worry about the expense. The patient's friends and relatives realized that the patient was in bad shape and might not make it, but they wanted us to do what we could and at least keep him comfortable. After a few days in the hospital he died. It was decided by the patient's friends and relatives that his body should be returned to his home temple where it could be accorded all the rituals due a man of his standing. They asked if the hospital truck could deliver the body. Our Toyota Hilux was probably in a little better shape than the average pick-up in that area. Moreover, drivers who used their pick-ups as taxis were reluctant to transport dead bodies for fear that their taxi would be viewed as a haunted vehicle thereafter. The friends of the deceased insisted on providing a Buddhist monk escort. This apparently was to honor the deceased and to make any houses we passed along the way safe from becoming haunted. I agreed to the escort, not knowing for sure what all was involved. The body was loaded into the back of the hospital pickup truck and off I went with Kyin Tun, one of the male nurse aids, in the passenger seat. I drove from the back of the hospital around the end of the hospital and was just passing the front of the hospital when Kyin Tun reminded me that we did not have our escort with us yet. I pulled over to the side of the road to allow the escorting saffron-colored pickup truck with a flashing orange light on top of the cab to get in front of us, and off we went as a two-truck convoy to the Mon Temple in Sangkhlaburi. It had been starting to get dark when we left the hospital and it was quite dark when we arrived at the temple. We drove around to the back of the temple and delivered the body to a cavernous hall held up by large concrete columns. There was no electricity that night. Kerosene lanterns and candles provided only feeble illumination. We left the truck lights on to supplement the light from the lamps and candles. Solemn figures moved around quietly, casting flickering shadows on the imposing cement columns. It could have been a scene from an Indiana Jones movie!

"Dry Baby" (from my mission newsletter dated December 1980)

"Please save it; I want to see it." Jun Tip was finally delivering her dead fetus. She had become pregnant 10 months ago but, unfortunately, the fetus had died at four months gestation. She was just now expelling it. "Don't throw it away; I want the father to see it."

"Sure, okay," I said, "No problem."

"Probably they want to bury the fetus or cremate it," I thought. "That's reasonable enough. She has carried it long enough that they probably feel a bit attached to it."

The fetus was dutifully washed and presented to the parents in a plastic bag.

I thought that was the last I would see of it. Not so. The next morning when I arrived at the hospital there was an air of excitement. Those "in the know" were excitedly telling those who didn't know. The couple, who I thought would be somewhat sad and disappointed, were actually proud and happy. They considered themselves lucky because they were now the parents of a "dry baby."

Dry babies are not buried or cremated but are allowed to dry out naturally and are "dressed" and "fed" and given presents. Dry babies are kept for years and are said to give guidance to the parents through dreams. Thus, a dry baby might indicate to its parents when to plant rice or where to build a new house. The babies are considered to be alive and to have feelings which can easily be hurt. Thus, it is important to give presents to the dry baby along with the other children, else the dry baby might become jealous.

Only small fetuses that have been in the womb a full nine months qualify as "dry babies". A miscarriage before term or even the birth of a term-sized dead fetus does not qualify.

The same day, another lady had delivered a healthy baby at the hospital. She was in the adjacent room. Of the two, certainly the mother of the dry baby appeared to be the happier.

[Editor's note: In medical terminology, the "dry baby" phenomenon is called "fetal mummification": shriveling of a fetus that has died in the uterus but not been expelled for months or sometimes even years. When the mummified fetus finally is expelled, it does not putrefy. This apparently is taken as "proof" in some cultures that the fetus is "alive," especially if the time of expulsion of the dead fetus occurs around the time of the "due date".]

Huge spleen

From my June 1986 newsletter:

> One Sunday evening in January [1986] a 17-year-old girl was brought in very short of breath, pale, and with abdominal pain. I had examined her several times before and knew she had a congenital blood disease called thalassemia major. Patients with this disease have markedly abnormal blood cells, which the spleen keeps filtering out and destroying. The patients are very anemic and require repeated blood transfusions. This girl's hemoglobin was down to about 40% of normal. That, in itself, is enough to make a patient short of breath, but further aggravating her problem was the fact that her spleen, now massive, was pressing up against her diaphragm.

> Her father said he wanted her to have surgery. He said he had been to several spirit doctors and diviners and they had all given the same verdict: the patient needed surgery at the hospital!

> In fact, splenectomy does often benefit patients with thalassemia major. It allows the abnormal cells to escape destruction a little longer. This way, they are allowed to carry the oxygen they <u>can</u> carry around to the body organs.

Her father had brought Nam Wan ("Syrup") to the hospital once or twice before, asking for surgery. I had declined to do it on the grounds that it would be a high-risk procedure and that the patient had been getting along reasonably well with an occasional transfusion.

Now, however, the situation was deteriorating. It had not been long since the previous transfusion and Nam Wan was already markedly anemic. She was also uncomfortable because of the sheer mass of her spleen and its pressure effects.

I noticed a peculiar thing as I examined this desperate young lady. She had little crosses for earrings. Now, it's not unusual for a young lady in the United States to wear earrings in the shape of crosses, but in this country that is 95% Buddhist and 4% Moslem, it is. I decided that this was not the time to ask her about her earrings, but I did make a mental note.

I decided to juice up Syrup with some blood over the next several days and then attempt a splenectomy. It was God's good timing that there was a volunteer work team from Australia here then. These good people were willing to give blood and we were able to get 6 units of blood from them for Nam Wan.

A few days before the surgery, I asked Nam Wan if she knew what the crosses she was wearing symbolized. We had a little chat about it, and she told me that she had been interested in the Christian God for some time. She said she had already decided that if she were cured, she would become a Christian. To this day, I don't know whether she was trying to make a bargain with God and the hospital staff or whether she was simply stating an intention.

In any case, I had to explain to her that the splenectomy would not cure the underlying disease, but would, if successful, make her feel more comfortable and allow her to go longer between transfusions.

Just before I made the incision, I explained to Nam Wan (who was under spinal anesthesia and still awake) that here in this hospital we pray for God's guidance before each operation. She seemed to like this idea. I prayed in Thai, and after each pause in which I asked the Lord for help, there came a soft grunt of affirmation from under the O.R. drapes.

The splenectomy was long and difficult and was accompanied by much prayer before during and after. The main spleen weighed 2.2 kg (4 pounds, 13 ounces). This is about 15 times the normal weight! There were also four tiny "accessor spleens" removed.

Nam Wan is doing well now. She has not required a single transfusion since surgery. She is still interested in the Gospel message. She asked for a hymnbook just the other day. She attends a Christian worship group in the town where she lives. Pray with us that she will continue to grow in faith and knowledge.

Adaptation and Perseverance

[Editor's note: I saw Nam Wan again in 2012. I was at the hospital on one of my volunteer trips and she came to say hello. She was at that time 26 years out from her splenectomy. She had only required a few transfusions in that 26 years. She looked a bit frail but was smiling and grateful.]

Warm blood on a cold night

I was awakened in the middle of the night to see a patient who had been brought to the hospital with heavy vaginal bleeding. She was weak and pale and barely conscious. She was having a miscarriage, but not all the tissue had been expelled and she had almost bled to death. She had a rapid, thready pulse. Blood pressure was unobtainable. She needed blood urgently. We had no blood bank, but I knew I had universal donor blood. I told the nurse to take a unit of blood from me. I had given blood to patients many times before, but this time was different. The patient was in such dire need of blood that there was some question whether there was even time to tap off a unit of my blood before the patient expired. To make matters worse, this was the cold season and the air was chilly. This made my veins clamp down and the blood flow slowly. I was in the exam room right next to the patient's and kept asking for updates on the patient's status. The reports were not good. The patient's level of consciousness was getting worse and death appeared to be imminent. The blood bag that my blood was running into was still only half full and the blood was coming very slowly. It seemed certain that the patient would die before the bag filled up! So, I ordered the nurse to take the half unit of blood that had been collected and to start running it into the patient. In my training I had been taught that any patient who needs a blood transfusion, needs at least two units. This lady could have used three or four! But here we were in the middle of the night, a hundred miles from the nearest blood bank with just half a unit. As the nurse hung the blood, I checked the patient again. She was unresponsive and her pupils were dilating. But as the blood ran in, she began to stir. Her pupils returned to normal and she showed signs of being aware of her surroundings. By now the watchman had fetched the lab tech on call and brought her back to the hospital. The nurses were looking for more donors. We cleaned out her uterus with a D&C and the bleeding stopped.

Dr. Phil McDaniel

Dangerous to operate; more dangerous not to

A twelve-year-old boy fell off the oxcart on which he was riding. One wheel of the oxcart ran over his head. He was brought into the hospital unconscious. External damage was surprisingly little: a contusion-abrasion on one side of his scalp. There was no obvious skull fracture on X-ray. Except for altered mental status he was neurologically intact. He reacted appropriately to painful stimulation. His pupils were equal and reactive to light. For a while he seemed to improve a little, but then he began to get worse again. His mental status deteriorated, and one pupil dilated and became unresponsive to light. The only relatives with him were his grandparents. I explained to them that their grandson was probably bleeding inside his head. He needed an emergency operation to open his skull and release the pressure. They asked if this would be a dangerous operation. I explained that yes, it would be dangerous to operate, but it would be even more dangerous— almost certainly fatal—not to operate. After some deliberation they decided that they did not want their grandson to undergo a dangerous operation; so, they refused permission for us to proceed.

Not long after we had finished making ward rounds and were getting ready to commence seeing outpatients, the hospital chaplain came to tell me that he had gone back to talk to the patient's grandparents after rounds and that they were now willing to give permission for the bur hole operation. I had mixed feelings about this news. I wasn't sure what assurances the chaplain had given the grandparents! Moreover, while I still believed that the patient urgently needed this operation, it was one I had never done before, nor had Dr. Jamie Rines, a visiting internal medicine doctor. The hospital did have a brace and bits for doing a bur hole operation, but we had no CT scanner or MRI to prove that the patient had a blood clot on the brain or to show its location. Thankfully, we had a two-volume book set called *Primary Surgery*. These were low-cost, soft cover books put out by Oxford Medical Publications for personnel working in the bush. The section on blood clots in the head gave a nice discussion on how to use various findings on physical exam to help localize the site of bleeding. The chapter ranked the findings in order of predictive weight for finding the site of the clot.

I went back to the ward to talk with the grandparents again. After explaining the crisis and the proposed intervention as fairly as I could, the grandparents reluctantly gave permission for us to operate, but then turned around and asked, "It won't be dangerous, will it?"

We prepared the patient and the operating room and began the procedure under local anesthesia. The patient was very cooperative because he was in a deep coma. With fear and trembling and much prayer I opened his scalp and made a bur hole using a special type of bit for opening craniums. We chose the region of his scalp with the contusion-abrasion as the most likely location of the clot. Thanks be to God; we found the clot right under the bur hole! Fortunately for us, it was an epidural—not a subdural—hematoma. While it was indeed causing pressure on the brain, it was not directly resting on the brain. A tough membrane called the dura was between the clot and the brain. This made evacuating the clot easy. As the operation progressed, the patient began to stir a little. He moaned and then he struggled. I had to have someone hold him down. While this movement made finishing the operation more difficult, it was an excellent indication that we had done the right thing. Over the next few weeks, the patient regained the ability to walk and talk.

Concluding Reflections

My time at the Kwai River Christian Hospital was not without its challenges. I worked long days and was often called down to the hospital at night. For my first 15 years or so, I was the only regular doctor at the hospital. It was wearing to be responsible 24/7 for patients who were seriously ill or injured.

"Ministering to the least" required keeping patient fees low enough so that villagers could afford care. But cheap fees meant meager receipts, which threatened to undermine keeping up with repairs and providing adequate staff salaries. Once there was a strike by most of the national staff over wages. Thankfully, it only lasted about 15 minutes. Even so, it was rather demoralizing.

Most of the time I was on good terms with everyone who worked in the hospital. The national staff, the missionary staff, and volunteers worked together well. They often worked overtime on emergency cases and not infrequently gave their own blood to help keep a patient alive.

Dr. Phil McDaniel

I count it a great privilege to have had the opportunity to work alongside all of these colleagues.

Next to helping very sick patients get better, the most gratifying experience at KRCH was working with medical students and residents from various parts of the world. In a typical year there would be a dozen or so of these students or residents. They were able to see and care for conditions that they would otherwise be unlikely to encounter in their home countries. At the same time, they sometimes introduced new ideas or methods to me.

In 2002 my family and I moved back to the USA in order to get help for our younger daughter, who is disabled both physically and mentally. She was at that time 14 years old and growing bigger and stronger and more difficult to manage. My wife, Melba, had worked with Melodie endless hours from the time she was less than a year old using various programs of intellectual and physical stimulation. However, Melba had reached the point that she did not feel able to give Melodie the help she needed.

We decided to settle in Oregon, which had good programs for disabled students. I did not have a job lined up yet. However, through a series of contacts that felt providential, I ended up working with a great group of family practice doctors at South Tabor Family Physicians in Portland. It was a big transition for me. At KRCH I had been called upon to treat malaria, leprosy, typhoid fever, do C-sections, amputations, appendectomies, extract teeth, and function as hospital director. At South Tabor Family Physicians, I was the most junior member of a family practice group.

Here in the US I had to study the fine points of managing chronic conditions such as hypertension, diabetes, dyslipidemia, obesity and heart failure. We did lots of annual physicals, school physicals, and camp physicals. Any major surgery was referred to a specialist. I spent as long documenting patient visits as I did in the actual care of the patients. This, because of the ever-looming threat of litigation.

My colleagues at South Tabor were very supportive. Several of them had done medical work overseas. I worked with them for almost 15 years, retiring at the end of 2017.

I made volunteer trips back to the Kwai River Christian Hospital every year or two while I was working at South Tabor Family Physicians and made two trips in the first year of my retirement. On return trips it was very gratifying to meet patients on whom I had done life-saving surgery or a C-section twenty or thirty years previously.

On one of my early return visits to Thailand, I was astounded to see a very tall cell phone tower on the other side of the road from the hospital. The sight was almost spooky. Gone were the days when we had no telephone connection at all and the mail was delivered once every week or two. Now people could use cell phones and internet.

One day I was evaluating an old man in the outpatient clinic. He was dressed in old faded clothes and was toting a hand-woven tribal shoulder bag. He looked as though the modern world had passed him by, and he didn't even care. As I was taking his history, I heard a little ring-a-ling-ling. I wondered whose phone was ringing. The old man didn't. He reached into his tribal shoulder bag and pulled out a cell phone, pushed the talk button and struck up a conversation as though he had done it a hundred times before—which he probably had.

Cell phones and internet access are just two examples of improvements in infrastructure. Roads have improved from rough jungle tracks to paved roads. Air-conditioned buses and vans now run where only Land Rovers and Jeeps could go before. Mail service is reliable and regular. The availability of medicines and medical equipment has vastly improved.

It has been fascinating to follow the changes of the last few decades and it will be interesting to see what happens in the next few.

Chapter 11

Non-Swimmer on a Sinking Ferry

Lea Lindero, RN

About the author of this chapter:

Lea Lindero, missionary nurse from the Philippines, served as a nurse and much more at the KRCH. She was a confidant of staff, a peacemaker, and a gracious host to hundreds of volunteers and medical students who rotated through the hospital over many years. At times she filled the role of head nurse. She was a blood donor in emergencies. She was a great organizer of celebrations, especially Christmas.

Span of service at KRCH: March 1984 to March 2015

I grew up in the Philippines in the Visayan region. I was one of 12 siblings. My father said there was no family planning then; so, they did "family planting". I grew up in a Christian family and I was baptized at the age of 16. I finished my general nursing degree at Saint Anthony School of Nursing and my Bachelor degree at Central Philippine University in Iloilo City. After I passed the board exam, I worked at Iloilo Mission Hospital as a Staff Nurse, then I was promoted to Head Nurse, Charge Nurse, and Supervisor.

I also worked at Kamput Refugee Camp in Thailand with Cambodian and Vietnamese refugees from 1981 to the end of 1982.

I went back to Iloilo Mission Hospital to work again after the camp was closed in early 1983. Then I decided to apply to go to the Middle East. I went to Manila to process my papers, but on the way back, the ferryboat sank. A fire started in the cargo area while we were still sleeping. When we awoke, half the ferry was on fire and the smoke was so thick that we could not see anything. We heard the captain of the ship ordering everyone to find a way down to the lifeboats. We finally found a rope and used it to jump into the lifeboat. I didn't have a life jacket and I didn't know how to swim. But thanks be to God, I was able to jump into the lifeboat. But my papers were all in my suitcase!

Someone threw the case in after me. The suitcase was wet and my diploma and other papers got wet, but at least I had them with me!

I had processed my papers in Manila, thinking of going to the Middle East, but it did not work out. Actually, my parents did not want me to go to the Middle East because it is not a Christian country. They asked me if I still wanted to seek for more money. At first, I had thought that by working in the Middle East I could earn more money to help my family, including my younger brothers and my one younger sister in their schooling.

After much prayer, I told my parents that I knew God had a plan and purpose for my life, and I said I will go where He wants me to go. A few months after that, I received a telegram from Bob Coats, Fellowship Secretary of the Thailand Baptist Missionary Fellowship, whom I had met while I was working in the refugee camp, asking me if I would be willing to help at the Kwai River Christian Hospital, with the Baptist Union of Sweden as my sponsor. Then I received a telegram again from Bob telling me to process my passport, and they would send me a letter of recommendation for the embassy and also a ticket.

So, I went back again to Manila. This time I took the plane because I was afraid to take the ferry again! It took a while to get all the papers ready. When my travel documents were finally in order, I resigned my post at Iloilo Mission Hospital where I had been working, and, in November 1983, I flew to Bangkok. I was met by Pat Coats at the Don Muang Airport. I stayed in Bangkok from November 1983 to the first week of March 1984. I was in Thai language school for those four months. At the end of that time, I traveled up to the original hospital location in old Sangkhlaburi with Dr. Phil McDaniel and his daughter Linette.

It was in 1983 that I accepted the challenge of being a missionary nurse in Sangkhlaburi. At first, I was hesitant since the language barrier and cultural differences would be a great hindrance to fulfill my mission in the field.

I had doubts and fears during my first year in the ministry. There were times I felt pressured to meet the expectations of the people around which led me to question my capability. Truly God is omnipotent. He's been there for me to give a guiding light and courage to serve Him faithfully. He blessed me with true friends and family at KRCH. Although we've been through floods and natural calamities, still my faith serves as my strong foundation to rise up again, go on and show everyone that God is stronger than any storms.

In 1986 my mission as a missionary nurse continued as God gave me an opportunity to go to Sweden for six weeks. I visited churches for deputation, telling about the work and vision of KRCH. I felt overwhelmed by the positive feedback of the people from different churches about KRCH. It was a great honor to be appointed not only to represent KRCH but as God's servant to spread His goodness. The Baptist Union of Sweden helped with the Under-Fives Program, the School Health Program and a charity fund for those patients who could not afford to pay their bills.

In 1989 I went to the States to visit my friends for a month in Seattle and in Vancouver, Canada. I did not see it as an opportunity for relaxation and pleasure but a great avenue to have a clearer view of God's purpose in my life. I met new friends who share the same faith as me and was moved by their stories of events that had touched their lives in mysterious ways.

After missionary nurse Jan Yawan and husband Jit Yawan had left to go back to Australia for a seminary course in 1994, I was assigned as head nurse of KRCH and continued in that role up to 2008. I helped to run the hospital by scheduling all the workers. I also helped with some administrative work. Although working in this role was sometimes tiresome, I took it as a challenge: not as a step closer to the fulfillment of my dreams, but as a promotion of my faith in God.

I couldn't possibly tell how many sacrifices we nurses have had to endure. But at the end of the day, when I know that somehow, I contributed to piecing together the life of our patients, being a nurse is the best feeling in the world.

In those days the equipment at the Kwai River Christian Hospital was mostly quite low tech. I still remember using a gadget that resembled a hand-held bicycle pump to develop the suction for the vacuum extractor used to assist mothers having difficult deliveries. If a patient with asthma needed a nebulizer treatment, the pressurized air needed to make the nebulizer work was apt to be generated by a hand-operated motorcycle pump. But the lack of equipment did not hinder me and other hospital staff in rendering service to the people. We tried our hardest to make people feel better about their situation. Because there was no blood bank, when a patient needed blood, we sometimes had to donate our own blood before we could proceed with an operation. Surgical cases from land mine explosions were common. Malaria, TB, parasitism, and malnutrition were the most common diseases.

In 2001 when Keith Tennis invited me to go to the States, I never hesitated to accept it. On that trip I was commissioned at Green Lake, Wisconsin as an International Ministries associate missionary. It was a nice feeling to be called for the glory of God to serve, to care, and to love. I was in the States for 7 weeks to visit churches in order to do deputation and then came back to Sangkhla.

In 2005 Dr. Anchalee, our Thai lady doctor, and I went to Kerala, India for 7 weeks for palliative care training. We were assigned dying cancer and HIV patients.

In 2009 I was given an opportunity by my 3 boards (Baptist Union of Sweden, International Ministries of American Baptist Churches, and the Australian Baptist Missionary Society) to have a yearlong break, so I went home to be with my family, especially my mom, who was in her 90's.

Unfortunately, I got sick and underwent an operation. Sickness took my strength from me and the means of serving Him, but it didn't jeopardize my relationship and trust in Him.

While I was home in the Philippines, I was still watching the progress of KRCH with interest. I was certain that they would all go on to achieve far better things than I did. If my legacy to them was time spent building the hospital up, their legacy to me was companionship, faith in teamwork, and an abiding passion to serve the Lord.

I came back to KRCH towards the end of 2009 to manage the TB program for 3 years. During this time, we accomplished our mission to provide compassionate support and quality service to patients with TB, HIV/AIDS and their families. I also gave a helping hand whenever needed to support the public health program. Besides an HIV/AIDS clinic and a TB clinic, there was an Under-Fives clinic (giving immunizations), prenatal care, and post-natal checkups. I delivered babies and helped examine OPD patients if the doctor was not around. Along with the KRCH staff, we also followed up our TB/HIV patients at the town of Three Pagodas with a mobile clinic.

I was humbled by the dedication of our volunteers. It is a privilege and honor to work with such a conscientious group of caring people.

For many years I was responsible for hosting volunteers and [other] guests of KRCH from different countries. I always tried my best to provide for the needs of the volunteers out of appreciation for their humble service to the hospital. [Editor's note: Lea's hospitality became legendary among volunteers to KRCH!]

Throughout my entire journey, I have been aware that my desire to become a missionary nurse was truly a blessing, and my rewards are many, often being the kind that await in the afterlife. I may not have been given the opportunity to preach to bring in crowds to the faith, but I hope my kindness and compassion will bless those who see in my actions a true glimpse of who Jesus is as I reach out to them in practical ways.

Becoming a missionary is a great way to serve the Lord. However, following God's call requires not only a passion for service, but also a pure heart and strong commitment to serve and honor Him despite all the negativities and difficulties along the way.

My 31 years at the Kwai River Christian Hospital and my 3 years at the Christian Center for the Development of People with Disabilities (CDPD) in Maesariang in the north of Thailand rendering joyous service as a missionary nurse have been a great journey full of fantastic adventures.

Chapter 12

From Nanny to Registered Nurse

By Eiam Eiamchan, RN

About the author of this chapter:

Eiam Eiamchan, RN served at the Kwai River Christian Hospital 1986-1990. Here she recounts her remarkable journey from poor village girl to RN at the Kwai River Christian Hospital.

Span of service at KRCH: 1986–1990

I was born on February 2, 1956 in Minburi District of Bangkok, Thailand. I was born into a poor family.

Minburi was a rural area of Bangkok, so I received only a fourth-grade education. My parents were farmers. When I was 14 years of age, my older sister, who worked with a missionary family, arranged for me to come and work for Dr. John and Mrs. Nancy Freeman. They were new missionaries in Thailand in 1970. At that time, they had two boys (4 years old and 3 years old). After I had worked with the Freemans for one year in Bangkok, they moved to Bangkhla, Chachoengsao Province because Dr. John had started working at Bangkhla Hospital. I followed them to take care of their children. They had a baby girl born in Bangkok before they moved to Bangkhla. They had a second girl born at Bangkhla two years later, for a total of four kids. The Freemans had a big family at that time.

In 1974, Dr. John and his family decided to move to the jungles of Sangkhlaburi, Kanchanaburi to work at the Kwai River Christian Hospital (KRCH). I followed them because I loved them and the kids.

In 1976 I became ill. I had developed painful blisters in my mouth. Dr. John tried to treat me with medicines, but I did not respond. They took me to Bangkok to a dermatologist for treatment and I went home during treatment. My diagnosis was pemphigus. A few months later I developed blisters in my mouth again. My parents' money was gone. It had been used up on my treatment. I could not eat. I was very thin and waited for the end of life. One day Dr. John and his wife came to

187

Bangkok and tried to find the way to my house. They met my mom and came to see me inside the house.

They took me to the Institute of Dermatology in Bangkok to see a young Thai doctor who had just completed his dermatology residency in America. He explained the tests and treatment to Dr. John and admitted me to the hospital. I was in the hospital one month.

After about one month, I was normal but continued my medications. I returned to Sangkhlaburi and stayed with Dr. John's family and worked again. I cooked and took care of the children.

When I was a little girl, the government regulation was that all children 8 years old and up had to attend school at least through the 4th grade. Families in rural areas often did not want their children to go to school. They needed them to help in the fields. I studied grades 1–4 at a rural school about 2 km from my home. I walked through farm country to get to school and back in the dry season. In the rainy season, I went by wooden canoe along the canal. I was the only person in my village who continued school beyond 4th grade. Dr. Freeman's family in Sangkhlaburi encouraged me to continue my studies. I was able to skip 5th grade and begin in 6th at the United Cristian School in Sangkhlaburi, on the same compound as the Kwai River Christian Hospital. (My grades had been good in 4th grade and by now I was older and bigger than the girls in 5th grade at the United Christian School. So, they let me start in 6th.) Mrs. Nancy Freeman helped me learn English at her house.

Two years later I moved to Sammuk Christian Academy (SCA) at Bangsean, Chonburi Province. I lived in a dormitory at school. Dr. John and his family left Sangkhlaburi for America about that same time. I thought that Sammuk Christian Academy (SCA) had a lot of Jesus' love because the teachers were friendly with all students. They taught Bible study every morning before going to the classrooms. At last I became a Christian and was baptized by Rev. Dick Worley in the sea at Bang Sean beach.

In June 1980 I graduated from 10th grade at Sammuk Christian Academy (SCA). I then went back to Bangkok to complete the last two years of high school before attending university. I applied to Wattana Wittaya Academy (WWA) [Thailand's first boarding school for girls, established in 1878 by the American Presbyterian Mission—Editor]. I passed the entrance exam and enrolled.

From Nanny to Registered Nurse

In 1982 I completed my studies at Wattana Academy. I was already 27 years old—too old to enroll in a government university, where only applicants 18–25 years of age were being accepted. I wrote a letter to Payap University, a private institution, asking if I would still be eligible to apply at age 27. I said that even if I could not attend Payap University, I would not feel sad that I was unable to continue my studies, because I believed that God would open some way to me. One week later, I received a letter with an application form from Payap University as well as information on the date and time of the entrance exam. The university informed me that it accepts students up to 30 years of age.

Thank you, Lord! I was so happy. He had answered my prayers! So, I filled in the application form and sent it back to Payap. Soon after I graduated from Wattana, I bought a train ticket to Chiang Mai [where Payap University is located]. The train left Bangkok for Chiang Mai at night and arrived in the morning. When I got off the train, I was met by Dr. Edwin McDaniel and his wife, Kathryn. They had come to pick me up! Kathryn smiled at me and introduced herself. They took me to their house and encouraged me to pass the exam.

They knew me because Mrs. Nancy Freeman and Mrs. Pat and Rev. Bob Coats arranged for me to continue my study at McCormick Faculty of Nursing at Payap University. Dr. Edwin and Mrs. Kathryn McDaniel took good care of me while I stayed in their house. They took me to Payap University for the entrance exam and interview by a nurse teacher. I was very, very lucky because the nurse teacher who interviewed me was a graduate of Wattana Academy in Bangkok, the school from which I had graduated! She recognized my Wattana Academy uniform which I had decided to wear to the interview. She laughed and talked about Wattana events and did not ask me any questions. I felt sure that I had passed the interview!

One week later, Dr. Ed and his wife took me to Payap University to look at the results of the entrance test on a bulletin board at the university. We looked for my name. When I saw it, we were so glad! I had passed the entrance test and the interview! Dr. Ed told me about a Scholarship to McCormick School of Nursing from the Kwai River Christian Hospital (KRCH).

Eiam Eiamchan

In 1982 I enrolled in McCormick School of Nursing of Payap University. Dr. Ed said that I had received a scholarship to McCormick Nursing School for 4 years. When I finished, I would have to go and work one year for each year that I had received scholarship funds. I agreed to this as it was already my intention to become a nurse and work at the Kwai River Christian Hospital. It is the reason that Mrs. Nancy and Dr. John Freeman arranged for me to continue my studies because I wanted to be a nurse to take good care of sick and poor people like everyone I saw at KRCH while Dr. Freeman was working there [1974-1977].

Dr. Ed and Mrs. Kathryn McDaniel were my guardians while I studied at nursing school. I lived in the nurses' dormitory across the street from McCormick Hospital.

In 1986 I completed my training in nursing and midwifery, earning a Bachelor of Science Degree in Nursing and Midwifery from Payap University. I came down from Chiang Mai [to Bangkok] and went up to KRCH and started working immediately with Dr. Phil McDaniel, who was the director of KRCH. He was the only doctor in the hospital and worked hard day and night.

On March 30, 1987, I went up to Chiang Mai again for the formal graduation ceremony of my class and to receive my diploma.

The University allowed only the students, teachers, and VIP's into the auditorium. Most friends and relatives had to sit or stand outside. I told the Director of Nursing that Dr. Ed McDaniel and his wife would like to come to see me graduate because they were my guardians. She agreed and gave me a VIP card to show to a teacher at the front door to go inside. Rev. Bob and Pat Coats, Dr. Frank Curry and his wife, Beryl, (who both were volunteering at KRCH), came up to Chiang Mai to surprise me. They would like to see me also! I told the teacher at the front door that "Maw Mac" [as Dr. Ed McDaniel was known in Chiang Mai] had many guests and, "Could you allow them all to go inside together?" He said, "Yes, they can go without a VIP card."

Following the graduation ceremony, Dr. Ed McDaniel and his wife, Kathryn, Dr. Frank Curry and his wife, Beryl, plus Rev. Bob Coats and his wife, Pat, and I all went to a restaurant in Chiang Mai to celebrate. Pat said to me, "Eiam, you are like a daughter to us. We are so glad that we were able to attend your graduation ceremony. When our children in America received their degrees, we were unable to attend because we were in Thailand."

I was so proud and happy because I was finally a professional nurse able to help sick people. I had long wanted to be a nurse or a doctor. Thank you, Lord! He made my life successful. He gave me brainpower, knowledge, and skill. He also gave me opportunities which came by way of Dr. John Freeman's family. The KRCH staff worked hard and the doctor was on call 24 hours per day when I was there. I was happy and had a good relationship with the rest of the staff. Dr. Phil McDaniel was very expert for everything and was a teacher for the staff nurses, medical students, and visiting doctors. He showed kindness to everyone, particularly patients, and served Christ always, like his father, Dr. Edwin McDaniel. I had a very good experience working at KRCH.

In 1990 I resigned from the Kwai River Christian Hospital and began working at Bangkok Nursing Home Hospital (BNH) where I had many friends from McCormick School of Nursing. (BNH Hospital is a general hospital, not an old people's home as the term "nursing home" would mean in the USA. It is an international hospital. Patients come from many countries to use its services.)

In 2017 I retired but still work part time.

Eiam Eiamchan, RN
July, 2019

Chapter 13

From Orphan Boy to Hospital Director

By Dr. Sakda Netek

About the author of this chapter:

This is the story of an orphan boy who became the first Thai doctor (and later, the director) at the Kwai River Christian Hospital. He attended the United Christian School on the Kwai River Christian Mission compound while living in the Christian boarding house on the same compound. After completing grade 6 he transferred to Sammuk Christian Academy in Chonburi for grades 7-12 (matayom 1-6). From there he went on to medical school and then a year of internship in a government hospital before returning to serve at the Kwai River Christian Hospital in 1996. He took extra training in surgery at Ramathibhodi Hospital in Bangkok from May 2000 to April 2003 and then returned to KRCH. He served as director of KRCH from 2004 to 2010.

Span of service at KRCH: 1996–2010

In 1978, 6 years after my father had passed away, my mother got sick and then also left me forever. I was 8 years old then. My grandparents were now burdened with three orphan boys: my two brothers and myself. They considered the importance of our education and also the difficulty of raising three of us. In the end, they kept my youngest brother with them, but handed over my older brother, Satja (nicknamed "Kung"), and myself to a lady evangelist, Kru Sai Kham, who visited our village. Then in late April of that year, the district of Sangkhlaburi came into my consciousness.

Travelling from my village of Suanpheung in Ratchaburi Province to the town of Sangkhlaburi at that time took 2 days. We stayed overnight in the city of Kanchanaburi. Then early the next morning we headed to the small town of Sangkhlaburi. We took a Land Rover from Kanchanaburi over a long and bumpy road for hours and hours. Thick, powdery red dust stained our hair and faces. We passed small rivers and climbed many hills. Bamboo rose high on either side of the road most of the way.

We arrived in Sangkhlaburi in the evening with Kru [Teacher] Boonchom accompanying us. We stayed in his house for a couple of days, then moved to the mission hostel when school opened.

I attended the United Christian School beginning at grade 2. I enjoyed the classes very much, but the English lessons were difficult for me. In 1978, most of the government schools did not start teaching English at grade one. I had finished grade one in the government school in Suanpheung. Therefore, I had no background in English at all. It was terribly stressful.

Malaria was very common in Sangkhlaburi. In November 1979, I got sick for the first time with Pf (Plasmodium falciparum) malaria. Later I got both Pf and Pv (Plasmodim vivax) malaria for 3 consecutive months: on December 12, 1980, again on January19, 1981 and yet again on February 28, 1981. I got treatment from the Kwai River Christian Hospital. It was Dr. Philip McDaniel who gave me the medicine. Quinine was the only effective drug at that time. It tasted horrible. It was more bitter than anything I could imagine. About a quarter of an hour after taking a dose, my mouth and saliva became bitter. The quinine also made my ears ring as though I had a cricket sitting beside my head and making annoying sounds nonstop for an hour. During high fevers, my body temperature was very hot, but I felt very cold deep into my bones. My whole body started shaking uncontrollably. My teeth chattered. Ten layers of blankets covering me were not enough to make me feel warmer. But after 15–20 minutes, I began sweating all over and finally my temperature dropped back to normal. The next day this sequence of fever, shaking chills, and sweats repeated itself and kept repeating itself day after day. That was quite terrible, and I was surprised that I didn't die.

I studied in this school [United Cristian School at the Kwai River Christian Mission] for 5 years. The first 2 years, I couldn't go back home for summer vacation as no one came to get me. Although I didn't have my father and mother waiting for me at my village, I still missed my home very much. The fathers and mothers of other students came to get their children, and most of my friends went back home. Fortunately, Olivia [who headed up the village health program at the

Kwai River Christian Hospital] took an interest in me. She had nephews, "Singto" and "Suriya", who lived nearby the school. I was able to play with them during summer vacations. There were some books at the hostel and in the school library that made me happy with reading and also alleviated my homesickness.

Sangkhlaburi is a very beautiful and quiet place. This was especially so before the Khao Laem hydroelectric dam was constructed. The rain forest was green almost all year round. Only for a few weeks in the hottest part of the dry season did the forest become dry and brown. The rainy season is longer in Sangkhlaburi than in many other parts of Thailand. It starts about the middle of May each year and ends by the last week of September. Some years in July or August, rain will keep falling without stop for more than 2 weeks. When this happens, the sky is obscured by clouds or fog the whole time. There may be no sunshine at all for some weeks. The humidity can become oppressive.

The nearby Ranti River was a favorite place for the boarding house kids and the local village kids to have fun. The water was very clear and clean. The river was our swimming pool. We could play the whole day in the river.

After completing grade 6 in Sangkhlaburi, I left for a new school in Chonburi: a small Christian School named Sammuk Christian Academy. Someone had told me that Dr. Philip funded me to attend this school and expected me to study medicine in the future. It seemed like I had set up my goal to study medicine from that point on. I studied 6 years at Sammuk Christian Academy before commencing medical school in Hadyai, Songkhla Province. During my six years of studying medicine, I was always thinking about coming back to work at KRCH.

I came back, starting work at KRCH in 1996. Many of the patients were villagers living nearby, but many of them also came from Myanmar. They were poor and lacked health insurance. Some were refugees, having escaped from war in Burma. I was so proud to be serving at KRCH.

"Thank you" to Dr. Douglas Corpron. He is the pioneer in medical service in this area. He ran the hospital from the beginning from nothing to a building that showed the love of God whom he served. Dr. Corpron had a few cows [that he raised for beef].

When Dr. Roy and Dr. Gill Myers came, they added more services at this hospital. Dr. Roy was also interested in farming. He supported villagers to raise pigs.

Later, Dr. John Freeman, besides his medical service, loved gardening. He grew a lot of trees and vegetables. Dr. John also initiated a public health program and mobile clinic. These greatly benefitted the villagers in Sangkhlaburi District.

Dr. Philip McDaniel replaced Dr. Freeman a few years later. Dr. Phil worked with the KRCH longer than any other doctor. He made significant additions to hospital services. He was also involved in the relocation of the hospital to the current place in Huay Malai. Dr. Philip does not have an agricultural bent, but besides his medical work, he facilitated water projects for the 5 villages around the hospital. His work had a great impact for community health. Water projects provide clean water that can prevent most of the village from diseases like diarrhea and cholera. Dr. Philip McDaniel has electrician skills; therefore, whenever the hospital had electric problems, he fixed them himself. Many students received scholarships funded or facilitated by doctor Phil to study nursing and medicine, including myself.

Dr. Anchalee was the first Thai doctor to be director of KRCH. She helped the TB treatment program run more effectively. I followed her as the next hospital director. It was my privilege to work at this hospital and to follow in the footsteps of the doctors before me who served God with all of their hearts.

Part 2

Expat Family Life at the

Kwai River Christian Mission

Chapter 14

Memories of a Missionary in Thailand

By Helen Corpron

About the author of this chapter:

Helen was born in the USA and obtained a BS degree in home economics. She was the mother of 7, including one set of twins. Helen worked alongside her husband, Dr. Doug Corpron, to establish the Kwai River Christian Hospital.

Mrs. Corpron served at the dispensary and, later, the Kwai River Christian Hospital in various capacities, including nutritionist and bookkeeper. She also kept busy homeschooling her children.

Period of service at KRCH: March 1961 through June 1967. She died in Yakima, WA in January 2009.

Editor's note: Doug Corpron thinks Helen wrote this memoir in about 1985. She intended it for her children, but her writing captures so beautifully what the earliest days were like, that Doug thought it would be a nice addition to this collection of letters and memoirs.

Introduction

For many years my daughters have asked me to write about what it was like to be a missionary with my husband in Thailand. Much is written about the men's work, but little of the women's work.

When I married Doug, I knew I would be spending time in a foreign country. Where, we were not sure. I knew it was his dream to return to China where his parents had served for 25 years as missionaries.

Preparation

After his internship, Doug decided that a year in a surgical residency at the V.A. Hospital would be very helpful no matter where we went.

During that year, we were called by our mission board and offered a post in Thailand to begin a hospital in the remote hills among a group of people known as the Karen (pronounced ka-REN). The communists had taken over China so we could no longer go there. They had also suggested that we could go to the Belgian Congo, but that was not something we wanted to do. Nor did we want to go to India. After some deliberation, we agreed to go to Thailand. At least it was an Asian country and had so many medical needs we felt that we would be happiest there.

One of the reasons we were interested in working with the Karens is that they had an interesting folktale about the white man coming to save them. It went like this: Yahway, the Karen god, was about to go on a long journey, but before he went, he called his sons to him and gave each of them a book of life. To the eldest son [the ancestor of the Karens] he gave the Golden Book of Life. To the rest, he gave other Books of Life. The younger white brother took his book and went away to the west and was not seen again. The Karen brother took his book, and as long as he read and followed it, his life was happy and his soul was at peace. One day he left it on a stump in a field he was clearing. When he burned off the field, the book was nearly destroyed. The pigs and chickens ate the charred remains. After this, his quality of life grew worse and worse until all he knew was hardship, persecution, and suffering, even as the Karen people now endure. The Karen people believed a prophecy that the white brother would return and share his Book of Life. The prophetic words are as follows:

Book of Silver, Book of Gold

Book that Pah K'sa Yahway told;

Lost, it will again appear

When a white man brings it near.

Traveling to Thailand

We left the United States in July 1958 and traveled through Europe for a month with three young children (Bill 6, Ken 4, and Cathy 2). Along the way, Doug attended meetings of the United Christian Missionary Society in Stratford-on-Avon, England, while the children and I visited parts of London, mostly the parks and our hotel.

First Year in Bangkok

In August 1958, we flew into Bangkok for the first time. As we stepped off the airplane, we were greeted by a hot blast of air like nothing we had ever known. We were glad to be met by a friendly group of fellow missionaries, including the McAnallens, Sams, Carlsons, and two Chinese doctors, Dr. Chen and Dr. Chek-ling. We had no knowledge of the language and couldn't even ask for a drink of water. They took us to a house on 199 Hicks Lane that was to become our home for the next two years while we were learning to speak Thai and learning about the culture of our new home.

Our home was sparsely furnished until our own goods arrived from the States. We had carefully packed all our belongings including beds for all of us, a refrigerator, dishes, pots and pans, some clothes we thought would be suitable for Thailand's climate and anything else we thought we could use for the next four years. We planned on buying dressers and other furniture that we might need. We found that our new home had three upstairs bedrooms, a bathroom, and a sitting porch. Downstairs we had a living room and a dining room. Our kitchen was in a separate little house with cupboards, a charcoal stove, a sink with running water, and a table for workspace. There were also several rooms for servants' use.

Next, we had to find household help while we were in language school. This was something I definitely was not used to doing. Again, our friends, the McAnallens, came to our rescue. They came with two girls and a man and told us that these people had previously worked with foreigners. The man was to become our gardener; one girl, Somjit, was to cook; and the other, Mena, did laundry. Together they would help out with our children. They turned out to be good help.

Helen Corpron

In addition to having servants, there were many other things to get used to in Bangkok. A canal, or klong, filled with foul-smelling water was right across the street. The city was filled with new sounds: the three-wheeled pedicabs, or samlo, were everywhere ringing their little bells; taxis honked all day and night; people sold their wares on the streets and shouted to passersby; even the colorful lizards, called tokgays, called out in the evenings. Thailand was so much warmer and more humid than we were used to. We slept under fans and had them going much of the day, too.

One of my first tasks was to learn what I needed to do to prepare and shop for food. When we visited the local open-air market, we saw many different fruits and vegetables. We also saw all the flies swarming about the market and on raw meat hanging on hooks waiting to be sold without any refrigeration. We decided it would be best to let our young cook shop early every morning for fresh foods. A nearby Chinese-owned grocery store had lots of American-style cereals and canned goods—if we didn't mind paying their high prices! I had to learn to cook on the charcoal stove, so I was glad that the only meal I had to cook during the week was breakfast!

Once we began language school, I was not prepared to learn all the tonal variations of the Thai language. Each sound had many meanings, depending on the tone one used. After about 6 months of language study I found out that I had been hanging "tigers" in the closet instead of "shirts". We studied language with our Thai teachers for four hours every day, five days a week. It was intense and intimidating, but we finally learned enough to get around.

While we were in language school, Bill went to the International School for English-speaking children; Ken went to a private kindergarten; and Cathy stayed at home with our helpers. As the year went by, I also began teaching English as a second language at a Chinese boys school. I also went to a girls reformatory to teach them some food preparation, how to set a table properly, some easy crafts, and some English. Most of these girls had not actually committed crimes themselves but were at the scene of a crime. If the person who actually committed the crime (such as her father, brother, etc.) was arrested, they were too. It was hoped that some of these skills would help them find work when they were released.

I also found myself in charge of the Sunday school program at the International Church here in Bangkok for kindergarten-aged children, including Ken. In spite of all these activities, my first responsibility was always to my family and to caring for my children. We always wanted to put them to bed ourselves, to read their bedtime stories, and hear their prayers.

We were so glad when all our things did arrive from the States. It was good to get out our own beds and other furnishings such as towels, sheets, books, and games and toys. Do you remember what it was like to find some of our home canned Yakima fruit in the barrels? Ken, you almost cried when you dropped a quart jar of Bing cherries and they splattered all over the cement driveway. We were just getting used to all the tropical fruits, so it was a treat to have some of the familiar tastes of peaches and pears once in a while.

At this time Bangkok was showing signs of growing. Pedicabs were banned, so our cheapest and most dangerous mode of transportation disappeared. We decided we needed some form of transportation of our own. We bought a Vespa scooter with a sidecar. We could get our whole family on it if Bill stood in front of Doug and the other two sat in the sidecar with me. We scooted all over Bangkok in it. New buildings were going up everywhere we looked. New streets were being made and old ones paved. Beautiful old trees were being torn out so that streets could be widened. Canals were being filled in for the same reason.

While living in Bangkok, we joined the Bangkok Royal Sports Club. This meant we could go swimming any afternoon that we were free from other responsibilities. This was a place the kids really learned to love. They all became good swimmers, and Doug played tennis with some male missionaries early on Saturday mornings while it was still cool. Some days we would go there as soon as we were all home from school and spend the rest of the afternoon there. It was one place we knew we could cool off when the temperature was over ninety and the humidity about the same.

Shopping in Bangkok was an adventure, and I did love to shop! Hundreds of little shops lined the narrow streets. One shop sold baskets of all sizes and shapes for any use you could think of; the next shop was lined with bolts of fabric; another had nothing but sewing notions such as buttons, lace, and zippers. The second story of the shop usually was the proprietor's home. Open air food markets had fresh fruit and vegetables in great abundance and variety. There were all kinds of bananas, oranges, mangoes, guavas, pineapples, custard apples and even imported Washington apples! Some markets also sold an abundance of fish, poultry, beef and pork. The main food for Thailand was the same as for other Asian countries: rice. Another place that was fun to shop was called the Thieves Market, because stolen items were bought by the merchants and then sold to anyone who would buy them. What a store of treasures that was! You never paid the first price given to you by any merchant or peddler; they would start high and you would start low and if you still thought it was too high you would pretend to walk away and usually they would come after you and offer a good price and you came to an agreement on the object you wanted. I still treasure some of the bronze trays that we have in the family.

We wanted all of you to remember and celebrate the American holidays. When you went off to school on Halloween, you all dressed up in costumes. The first year Ken won first place because he was most symbolic of Halloween with a witch costume and green face. After Ken looked in the mirror, we could hardly convince him to go to school looking that way.

Thanksgivings were celebrated with our fellow missionaries complete with turkey and all the trimmings, including pumpkin pie. While the missionaries met to discuss mission business and have fellowship, all the missionary kids had fun playing games together.

Our first Christmas in Thailand was different in many ways. We didn't have the same kind of tree as in past years, but one made from big branches of a type of saltwater cedar which we tied together. After decorating it with Christmas tree lights, ornaments and tinsel we had brought with us, we had a very pretty tree. You children were just as excited as in past years. According to a song Bill learned to sing, Santa came by boat on a klong in Thailand. In December of that first year I discovered that I was pregnant with Pam. For the most part, this was a good time for me. The most difficult time of the day was when I had to go out to our kitchen to fix breakfast. Our Thai neighbor would be in her kitchen, which was back-to-back with our kitchen, fixing their breakfast. The smell of garlic cooking would almost make me sick to my stomach. I'm sure you girls would understand that.

Memories of a Missionary in Thailand

Pamela Marie Corpron was born on July 18, 1959. She weighed 6 lbs. 7 oz. She had very light hair and blue eyes. We were not expecting our new baby to arrive until August 13th, but she couldn't wait. Cathy couldn't understand why Pam wanted to sleep all the time, because she wanted to play with her. She asked me one morning if Pam had a tricycle. When I told her she didn't, she said, "That's okay, she can share mine. We can take turns." By that time, Cathy was attending a nursery school and had learned more about sharing.

In October 1959, I was appointed to help audit our mission's books. I spent a month going over them many times, trying hard to figure out someone else's bookkeeping methods. I was very glad to turn them over to the CCT when I was finished!! I also helped Doug make tapes to go with the pictures he took of our work and of fellow missionaries. These were sent to many churches that helped to support the work we were doing. Doug was able to do other things too. He was able to do some medical work and took his Thai Medical Examination and earned his lifetime license to practice medicine in Thailand.

Preparing for the Mission at Sangkhlaburi

Throughout our first year of language studies, the Church of Christ in Thailand continued to search for a site for our missionary work. After many trips, your dad and the mission board selected a village at the headwaters of the River Kwai, an area that was inhabited by many ethnic groups, including Pwo Karen, Sgaw Karen, Mon, Burmese, Chinese, and a few Thai (mostly government border patrol). At that time, you had to travel one day (ninety miles) by train and one to two days by boat or Land Rover (ninety miles) depending on the season. The exact site was selected because it was an old graveyard, and the local people would not build near there.

While arrangements were made for legal possession of the land by the CCT, shipments of materials were shipped up for the original mission buildings of the Kwai River Christian Hospital. Two residences, a generator shed, and a work shed were built. Getting two different families and two different missions to agree on plans for all this was somewhat difficult and took a lot of time. We had to decide how many bedrooms and how many bathrooms, whether we would have showers or tubs, the floor plans, etc. We decided all those between our two families and then the plans had to be submitted to two different mission boards. We held our breath on this and were pleasantly surprised when they both agreed on them as submitted. Later we could make minor changes on our own.

In April 1960, Doug went up to Prae (about 500 miles north of Bangkok in central Thailand) to make use of his new Thai medical license while I stayed in Bangkok. In May, I learned that my mother had passed away. This was a hard time for me because I could not go home to be with my family. I packed up the children and their schoolbooks, and we joined Doug for the rest of the time he was up there. We stayed with the Roadarmels, who had been good neighbors on Hicks Lane while finishing their language studies. This was the first time I had to teach any of you. We got along very well, and we were very happy to be together as a family again.

After we returned to Bangkok, I was becoming so busy with my many tasks that we decided that we had to simplify meal preparation. We created a kitchen inside the main house with somewhat modern cooking facilities. We talked our landlady into putting in an indoor sink, and we bought a kerosene cook stove with three burners and an oven. This worked out well and I was able to teach the cooks to use it with some degree of efficiency.

We [missionaries] all looked after one another and each other's children. When one missionary family entrusted their children to another missionary family, they usually sent some of their help over to ease the workload. That way everyone was happy; including our help. I was studying language fifteen hours a week and teaching at the Chinese boys school four hours a week, so I was very busy.

In August 1960, Doug and I had a nice trip to Singapore so that he could study tendon transplants in leprosy patients. We were able to place Bill and Ken with one set of friends and the girls with a couple that helped at a Thai student center. It was fun for us to travel without worrying about any of our children. We stayed in a fairly nice hotel, ate American food, and spoke English wherever we went. We would take drives into the country sight-seeing, stop whenever we wanted and visit markets and buy fruit or whatever. During that stay, Cathy went to a festival with a cartoonist that drew a picture of her titled, "Little Orphan Cathy." For years she was convinced that she had been adopted.

As soon as we returned to Bangkok, we began packing to move up to Sangkhlaburi. Then Doug came down with dengue fever and was in bed for five days. I packed most of seven barrels and several wood crates by myself. When he was able to be up again, we started on the furniture, crating all the beds, four dressers full of linens and all the clothing except for the bare minimum we needed for travel. We crated the stove, refrigerator, lamps and anything else we wouldn't need until we arrived in Sangkhla. We were able to borrow enough furniture to get along until we left. In all, 75 tons of things went up the river to Sangkhla. This included a lot of building materials needed to finish our house. During this time the children had returned to their respective schools.

When we returned from Singapore, I found that I was once again pregnant. This turned out to be Danny. This was not a very good time to be pregnant as it was so hot, and my big tummy made it hard to lean over to fill barrels. There were so many decisions to make, and Doug wasn't always there. It all had to be done in a short length of time as we were soon to leave for Sangkhla. I can remember Doug and John Sams shoving me out of the door to go get on the train even though there were a few more things to pack into the last box.

During these final months, I had to fire our cook, Somjit, because she became very hard to get along with and would not follow orders regarding Pam's care. This left us without a cook at a very difficult time, and it was hard to hire a cook for just two or three months. We asked Mena, our laundry helper, if she would like to become our cook for that period of time. She surprised us by saying she wouldn't mind it at all for that length of time. Her one condition was that she could not handle or cook pork as she was Muslim. Mena was not a cook by training, so I had to spend time teaching her how to cook our American food. She was a great Thai cook, so we enjoyed Thai meals at lunch and our familiar foods for dinner. She was also helpful in finding us a new laundress, her younger sister Pian. In all it worked out very well, and we were all happier.

I knew when we got to Sangkhla I would have to start all over again in hiring and training help. We understood that there were a lot of Chinese in the area, so I hoped we would be able to find a good

Chinese cook! We decided that we would hire an additional helper to look after the younger children.

Bangkok had a very nice zoo and it was always fun to take you children there. We would spend a lot of time just walking around enjoying all the animals. I wonder if Cathy remembers the time when a giraffe stuck its head over the fence and smiled into her face? She was very startled but didn't move. It was as if the giraffe had to have a closer look at her. Before we went to the zoo that day, we had all had our cholera shots. This was kind of a reward because all of you were so good about it. We took a picnic lunch and had a long day of it. Even Pam, who was less than two, enjoyed it.

At that time, Pam was a little dickens, and we had to watch her constantly. She would get away from all of us sometimes. She would escape through the gate, and we would find her across the street sitting on the bridge over the klong happily eating fruit and rice with a group of old men. They knew where she belonged, but they were too fascinated with her fair skin, blonde hair and blue eyes to make her return home. Another time she disappeared down the lane to see some spirited and high-strung racehorses. I was scared to death, but she stood very still just watching them.

We were walking down our lane one day when she decided to dash across it to see something on the other side, and I had to grab her arm to keep her from getting hit by a car. I pulled so hard that I dislocated her elbow and she was in a lot of pain. As usual, Doug was out of town. Fortunately, another missionary doctor lived on the next street, and he was able to put it back in place. She would never stay in one place for very long and needed constant watching! At Christmas time that year, we waited until the last minute to put up the tree because we knew she would have it all torn apart.

One of my jobs while we were still in Bangkok was to keep track of all our food purchases so that I could estimate what to order for the next year's food supply in Sangkhla. Of course, after we had been in Sangkhla for a while I found we needed to adjust these amounts. We found that some things didn't keep well for long periods of time, particularly flour, which attracted weevils. We learned to purchase flour and similar items more often to be shipped up in smaller loads. Because there were no markets in Sangkhla, we resorted to eating some canned vegetables part of the time. We had a large storeroom off of the kitchen. Here we kept our food supplies. To keep the insects down, we stored items such as powdered milk, sugar and flour in big fifty-five-gallon drums.

Holidays in Hua Hin

Some of our happiest times were our annual two-week vacations with other missionaries in the Gulf of Siam at Hua Hin. Our love affair with that place began the very first year we were in Thailand when our missionary group held a retreat there. We were able to stay in the beach home of a Chinese doctor who worked in Nakon Pathom. It was close to where another mission group had their vacation site. As a result, we spent a lot of time in fellowship with them. The first year we celebrated Cathy's third birthday with the help of all the missionary children and homemade ice cream and cake.

We spent hours combing the beach for all kinds of seashells. In those days there were shells everywhere. We also spent time reading and just resting. In the evening we would build bonfires down on the beach, and everyone from the different mission groups went down to the beach to sing and enjoy popcorn and cold pop. Another favorite activity was to chase and capture the little sand crabs, which were tasty when you fried them in oil. April was also mango season and not a day went by when we didn't have mango and sticky rice.

Eventually, the CCT and the Baptist mission developed cottages right on the beach in Cha Am. It was a very restful and beautiful place and the cottages were usually full. Ken loved to find one special shell that we called the "rainbow mussel," because it came in all the colors of the rainbow. He spent many hours combing the beach for them, and we still have that collection to this day. At the end of every vacation, we all spent hours deciding which shells we had to take home with us.

On to Sangkhlaburi At Last!

On March 4, 1961 we were finally ready to leave for our new home in Sangkhlaburi, though much later than our original plans. We packed up our remaining belongings and prepared to leave Bangkok. The first day we traveled by train to the end of the line at the village of Wangpo. We spent the night in a little hotel. There was a restaurant downstairs and sleeping rooms above. It was the only hotel there at the time, but I cannot remember its name. It was probably the Wangpo Hotel. Some of you may remember it because we stayed there many times over the years coming and going between Bangkok and Sangkhla.

After breakfast the next morning, we all headed down to the river where our hang yaw ("long tail") boat for the next leg of the trip was docked by a bamboo raft. It was a long day's journey to Takanun, and we arrived at supper time. As we went along the river there were several small villages with raft houses tied up along the way. You could almost always find a coffee shop of sorts that also made glasses of chocolate Ovaltine for you kids.

After settling into the little river bamboo guesthouse at Takanun, we went and found some dinner. Afterwards, we were resting and Pam, as usual, was running about when she tripped and fell with her face against the hot Coleman lantern, receiving some pretty bad burns over her sweet little face. It is hard to say who cried longer, Pam or her mother. Doug found some antibiotic ointment in the village and applied it to the burns, and over time the burns healed without leaving any scars.

The third morning we started out early in our mission Land Rover for the last leg of our trip. We had to ford several rivers and, in the afternoon, we were hit by a torrential downpour. We had to use the winch on the front of the Land Rover to pull ourselves out of the many gullies. It was dark by the time we arrived in Sangkhla. The Dodges, our coworkers, had arrived several months earlier [the Dodges had arrived just the previous month, February 1961] They fixed us a nice supper. We were all very ready to settle into our empty house for the night. We were sleeping in sleeping bags on the bare floor, but we were so tired that it didn't matter. We were in our new home!

The next few days were spent in unpacking some of the things that had already been sent up and kept in storage awaiting our arrival. All you children were as happy as we were to be sleeping in our own beds. The next day, quite a few local people came to us looking for work. We finally settled on three girls for our household help. Tiw would clean house and look after the children, mainly Pam; Sa Mon would be the wash girl and had to wash our clothes down at the river until we had running water up at the house. Wan would be our cook. I had fun teaching her to make American food, such as salad, roasted meats, and baked bread. We decided that we would still have Thai food at noon, American food in the evening, and I still fixed breakfast. Our cook would look around the village to see what kinds of vegetables she could find for us as there was no regular market.

We were somewhat limited in the variety of things that were available, but we did very well and had plenty of food. Our vegetables were mainly cabbage and long green beans. We also had fish, poultry, pork, some duck, and deer. Fresh fruits were available here, and at this time of year there were bananas, papaya, and jackfruit. We had brought some pomelo (a large citrus fruit like grapefruit) with us on our trip. Rice was our main staple, but we were able to find a few potatoes.

We could not get over the nice cool weather. It would be quite warm in the daytime but would cool off nicely at night. We were sleeping under blankets for the first time since coming to Thailand. All of you children were getting used to your new surroundings. You went swimming in the river every day, as much as you wanted. The water was clear and safe since there were no villages upstream. The boys tried their hand at fishing. You all had fun exploring in the jungle surrounding us. We let you play all day until the rest of our things came, and I had your books for school.

Our first night we had a bit of excitement when the village headman came to tell us that a fire was burning over the hill in back of our house. Doug and Paul Dodge had to hurry out and start a backfire before the other fire got too close to our houses. There is nothing like the sound of bamboo burning; it explodes like a hundred 4th of Julys all rolled into one. We could hear it all night long, but at least we knew our homes and other buildings were safe. We had electricity because we used a generator each evening from about 6:30 PM to about 10 PM. The plumbing was not finished so our gardener had to haul water up to the house from the river for cooking and washing dishes. We couldn't use our nice bathroom upstairs in our house yet, but we did have a Thai style toilet we could use downstairs because it took less water.

We bathed in the river so our need for water in the house would be less. Eventually, we had a well and could pump water from the well to the two big tanks behind our house on the hillside. There gravity took over and brought water into our homes. Before we could use the water for drinking or cooking, however, it had to be boiled. It was nice to be able to take showers once again and to be able to use our flush toilets.

Our homes were two stories high with a lot of open space beneath plus a Thai style toilet room, a servant's room and two storerooms for supplies. Upstairs we had a kitchen, dining area, living room, schoolroom area, three bedrooms, a study, and a bathroom. The house was open and airy with lots of windows which had louvered glass that could be open most of the time but closed when it rained. We also had a large porch area next to the kitchen where we had our charcoal cook stove.

After about two weeks we discovered that our cook's husband had active leprosy, and we couldn't take the chance that she wasn't a carrier of the germ. We were sorry to let her go because she was a good cook and really clean about her work. We hired a new cook, La Miat, and I began teaching her to cook American food for our evening meals. She could also read and write Thai, and we made a cookbook in a notebook that she could follow. She also taught me to cook a lot of Thai dishes. She became a very good cook and stayed with us until we left Thailand in 1967. La Miat did not like to walk home by the cemetery after dark because she feared the evil spirits waiting there. She sometimes rushed us through dinner almost taking our plates while we were still eating.

The Dodges

As you all know, Paul and Winnie Dodge were our coworkers in Sangkhla. Paul was an evangelist and planned that part of the program. He would preach in Thai and Olive Pa would translate it into Karen. As a nurse, Winnie assisted Doug with patient care and surgery and was also responsible for the training of the nurse aides. When she wasn't there, I stepped in to do a lot of those things. I also helped in sorting the many medicines for the pharmacy and sometimes in dispensing them to the patients. Both Winnie and I taught school for our own children, which took a lot of time and planning. Bill was a third grader; Ken was in second grade; Cathy was kindergarten aged. In all, they had four children: Sherwood, Glen, Forrest, and Brooks. These boys were your constant companions. Most of the time you got along very well, but like most cousins or siblings, you would need to be separated when you weren't getting along with one another.

Dan's Birth in Sangkhla

At 6:40 A.M. on May 1, 1961, Daniel Raymond made his entrance into the world. He was delivered by his dad and assisted by our co-worker Winnie Dodge. He was the first white baby ever born in this area. It was interesting to watch the local women's reaction to the fact that I was up and about so soon after delivery. They believed that a woman had to stay by a hot fire for the first ten days and to eat only rice and salt. It was a miracle that they could still nurse their babies successfully.

Dan and I spent a lot of time in our funny bamboo rocking chair. For nearly 18 months, he was a very colicky baby and holding him seemed to be the only way to make him comfortable. Every recording we made to send to the States had Danny crying in the background.

Doug became very busy within the first month of being there. He soon had over a hundred patients. He had several serious surgeries, and several patients who did not survive because they came in too late for help. He lost one young fisherman who blew off both forearms and blinded himself in both eyes after failing to throw a homemade stick of dynamite into the river fast enough. [This method of fishing brought up many fish at one time.] We thought patients would slow down after that, but they continued asking for medical help.

At first Doug was seeing patients under our house. Soon we realized that having crowds of sick people under the house wouldn't work very well, so we turned one of our storage sheds into the clinic and built a little Thai-style lean-to for the waiting room. Doug hired two workers: Sudah, a young woman he trained to help in the office and dispense drugs and Surin, who we trained to do lab work and do anesthesia. Surin later became our X-ray technician, too. Dad's first major surgery was on a 21-year-old young man, Jute, with an obstruction at the end of his stomach that was slowly starving him to death. With the Dodges and I assisting him, Doug performed the surgery. A month later Jute was up and about and able to eat solid food for the first time in three and a half years, and he had put on fifteen pounds.

I was quite often called upon to help at the clinic where we were seeing patients with malaria, tuberculosis, malnutrition, anemia, and skin diseases, including leprosy. We were finding that one of our biggest jobs would be public health education, and we needed a well-baby clinic to serve a great many people in the area. The local mothers did not realize that for a few baht (one baht was five cents then) a month their baby could have soap to prevent scabies, vitamins to resolve avitaminosis-related problems, and an antimalarial medication. For a few more baht a month, they themselves need never have malaria again. To them our simple operation in the jungle was "modern medicine". We could only think how wonderful it would be when the hospital was built, and we could provide even more medical care for these people.

We found that the village police officials were appropriating aid from UNICEF and selling the products to people. On our next trip to Bangkok, we talked to the UNICEF people, and they assigned us to oversee their program in Sangkhla. Guess who got that job? The mothers and children came once a month to a temporary clinic under the house where we would weigh and measure the babies and young children. I talked to them about the children's diet and the need to keep them clean. Then I would dispense cod liver oil (from Australia), soap (from England) and whole milk powder (from America) all free from UNICEF. It was fun to see how much better they became over time.

Keeping House in Sangkhla

Because our house was directly in front of the footbridge that crossed to the main Thai and Chinese village, I was always on the lookout for someone that would sell us any food they were carrying. One time it was two baskets of ducks, and we could use any eggs they might produce and later eat them. They were so beautiful, I always hated to kill one. Another time it would be baskets of vegetables or eggs or chickens. We learned how to raise our own chickens for their meat and eggs. After we discovered how hard it was to raise our own beef and pork, we made other arrangements for that. The villagers did that for us. We had what we called the pork queue. People would sign on to raise pigs or cows. Whenever we needed meat, we would call upon the person at the top of the list to kill their animal and bring to us any portion we thought we could use, whether it was all or part of an animal. We paid about twenty dollars for a whole animal. For this we could get four hams or roasts, two slabs of bacon, two dozen pork chops, and spareribs. The rest of the meat, fat, and entrails we sold back to the villagers that wanted such things, making our cost for meat even less.

The process of cutting and curing our meat was my job. The freezer in our kerosene-run refrigerator held a week to ten days' worth of meat. I made hams, bacon and sausage. Sometimes Doug would go over to the Mon village to make house calls. They usually paid him for his services with eggs, fish or various kinds of fruit. Occasionally someone would bring us a large lizard whose meat tasted a lot like chicken. A couple of times Doug was paid with a big basket of frogs, and I had to pith and cut off their legs which were fried like chicken and very good to eat. One time we were without any kind of eggs for over three months because a chicken cholera killed all the chickens in the area. I really had to think hard about what kind of American desserts I could make that didn't call for eggs; chocolate pudding was our standard substitute.

We were able to plant our own garden and eventually had a lot of things to eat from that. We had radishes, corn, peas, green beans, tomatoes, onions, cucumbers, and pak bung (a native spinach) among other things.

Our cook also taught us about a number of edible plants that grew in the jungle. Did you know that the flower of the banana tree is good to eat? One ground flower, dok din, looked like a small orchid and was edible too.

Eventually we built two more buildings, including a home for the Burmese Karen couple (evangelists Olive Pa and Olive Mo) and their family who came to work at the mission station. The other was a student hostel for boarding students, particularly during the rainy season when the rivers were too big to cross. The hostel also served as the first classrooms for our Christian school. I became the math teacher for the early grades. That was fun to watch their faces light up when they learned a few easy ways of doing math that was not in their sing song way of memorizing facts. Pam became a student at the Thai school in the afternoon and soon came home sing-songing what she had learned. She learned a lot about the Thai language and tried to teach Dan what she knew.

Helen Corpron

Furlough in 1962

In June 1962, we began packing and getting ready for our return to the States for a year's furlough. After visiting family and friends in California, we decided that it would be best to settle in Yakima for the rest of our furlough. While in Yakima, we needed to speak in a lot of churches and at other organizations about our work to help raise money for that work. Doug did more of the long-distance speaking while I did a lot of speaking closer to home. We were fortunate to have Grandma and Grandpa Corpron living close by to help with all of you children when we were away. We lived in a house on Chestnut and 40th Avenue about a block away from them. We were able to furnish our home with beds, dressers and linens from the White Swan Christian Mission Boarding school. Friends and family provided whatever else we needed.

Bill, Ken, and Cathy went to Whitney Elementary School that year; Pam and Dan stayed at home with each other for company. Dan was my little shadow and followed me everywhere I went. Sometimes I would change my mind about where I was going, turn around, and knock him down when I turned around. The house we were in had an attic that was just big enough for you three older children. That was your room in the winter months, but it became so hot in the summer that we made a room for you in the basement where it was nice and cool.

A friend from church, Dick Vandiver, loaned us a car for the year. In all, people were very generous and we got along quite well. I enjoyed doing my own cooking and laundry once again and babysitters were in abundance when we needed them. While we were home, we collected whatever medical supplies we could to take back with us, including sample medicines from doctors' offices. We packed these in quart jars, which I would later reclaim for canning fruits and vegetables when we were back in Thailand again. One morning I had a phone call asking if I thought Doug could use a hundred pounds of rubber gloves. Without thinking I said yes. When they arrived, I was surprised at how many rubber gloves were in a pound, but we packed them all up and distributed them all over Thailand. The year went by in a hurry and we were eager to get back to Thailand. Once again, we were busy packing boxes, barrels, and suitcases for the return trip.

Return to Thailand, 1963

In July 1963 we left the USA. We had a brief rest stop of ten days in Hawaii. Our friend and minister of the Christian church there, Rev. Jacobs, had arranged for us to have a little cottage, right on Waikiki Beach at none other than the Royal Hawaiian Hotel. We had two bedrooms and a porch where the boys slept. There was also a kitchen and dining room. Dan fell and injured his arm and had to spend two days in a sling. It was completely well by the time we left on Sunday evening. What fun that was and how very much we needed that rest after all the scurrying around that we had been doing! Traveling with five children was challenging, but you were all very good travelers. The older children helped with the younger ones and kept them entertained. We left Hawaii at 6:00 P.M. and you children slept most of the way. We flew to Japan by way of Wake because there was a strong head wind and we had to refuel. This took an extra five hours and we arrived at the hotel in Tokyo about 11:30 P.M. Since the kids had had a fair amount of sleep already, they only slept about 4 hours and they were ready to go again. They were all hungry, so we finally had to go out to an all-night hamburger stand called "The Hamburger Inn" at 5:30 A.M. where we got them all fed. It was a real chore to keep them all quiet until breakfast time at the hotel.

Back to Bangkok

We were concerned about bringing all our purchases into Bangkok, but we didn't have any problems and didn't have to pay any duty. Once back in Thailand, we wrote the hotel in Tokyo and they sent the case of Barbie dolls which had been left behind. Were you ever excited about that!

When we were in Bangkok, we purchased our necessary food supplies for the coming year. We also bought a little three-burner gas stove with an oven to use for cooking in Sangkhla. This meant that we also had to figure how many butane gas cylinders we would need for the coming year. I was excited about this, for it meant that it would be so much easier to cook and bake our bread and cookies. Another useful purchase was a treadle sewing machine as I always needed to make or mend clothes. Since we did not have electricity most of the time, a treadle machine meant I could sew whenever I wanted. We also intended to make all the original hospital bed sheets, sterile cloths for surgery, and other such items. Again, guess who was going to have to do all the sewing? We bought many bolts of white sheeting material.

The boat with our personal goods from the United States did not arrive on schedule, so we decided to go on without them. We were also trying to get Pam and Dan through immigration. The Thai government only admitted a certain quota of American citizens who were allowed to get permanent visas each year. Since they were both born in Thailand, this created a bureaucratic problem that took two weeks to solve. We decided to leave Bangkok and go as far as Nakon Pathom to stay with the McAnallens for a while. Doug arranged for a boat to take all our supplies on up to Sangkhla. We had a nice two-week rest and caught up with our missionary friends in the area, including the Estoyes (who also worked in Nakon Pathom) and the Eubanks (who were working in Sam Yak). Those visits were few and far between, and we liked to get a feel for each other's work.

Upriver to Sangkhlaburi

The big Chinese junk finally arrived and after loading all our goods onto it, the seven Corprons also loaded onto the same boat. We then began the slow trip up the River Kwai, which was quite swollen with the heavy monsoon rains. The trip took six days and I must admit that I would never choose to travel this way again. We were all enclosed in one small boat, sleeping on top of our supplies, and trying to keep the kids from falling overboard or getting in the way of the boatmen. Our hang yao boats could have made the trip in three days, so we lived and we learned!

We were very happy when we reached Sangkhla on August 13th and we were able to stretch out on our own familiar beds to sleep again. The next month found us in the process of going through all our stored things, as well as sorting and putting away all our new supplies.

Doug found himself busy immediately with patients who were very happy to see him back. They had been without any medical facilities for almost two months as the Dodges had already left for their furlough to the United States. It was obvious from all we saw and heard that they had put in a very busy year in our absence. We missed them in so many ways.

Our personal goods from the United States finally arrived in Bangkok at the end of August. This meant that Doug would have to make a trip back down to Bangkok to get them through customs. This could be, and usually was, a very trying experience, but our things went through with very little effort on our part and only cost about one hundred baht (approximately US$5 at that time). We were short-docked only one piece and that was the motor for our speed boat, which was probably stolen. This was reordered and arrived a few months later. We felt very fortunate when all of our things finally arrived in Sangkhla in mid-September along with Doug.

As soon as I could locate the kid's schoolbooks, we began lessons for Ken and Cathy. Bill had gone down with Doug in August and entered a missionary boarding school in Chiang Mai, the Chiang Mai Children's Center in Northern Thailand. They had an excellent boarding home with kind American house parents to oversee the children. We felt that it was very important for all of you children to have a good education and to have the opportunity to socialize with children of your same age and background. Bill would be home again in December for Christmas.

We had pretty well decided that Ken would be joining Bill in Chiang Mai after the first of the year, as his educational needs were not being entirely met in Sangkhla. I was finding that my services were needed more and more at the hospital because of Winnie's absence. I was not able to devote as much time as needed to teach two children and keep up with all my other responsibilities. I was also the bookkeeper for the mission books, which took quite a bit of time. The boys would return for two months of vacation in the middle of March, during the hot season, and then return to their school in the middle of August.

Whoever wrote the book *What to Do Until the Doctor Arrives* certainly did not have my situation in mind. Some of the suggestions might have been fine for an hour or two, but Doug had to make frequent trips to Bangkok for weeks at a time. I found that I had to do a little research in his absence to learn enough to manage the hospital while he was gone. By law, I was limited from doing a lot of things, and there were plenty of things I would not even try to do. But I could diagnose some diseases common to our area, like malaria, and take care of some stomach aches, headaches, and some forms of diarrhea. Much of this became routine treatment and by following the little book Doug had prepared, I could be of some service at the hospital. The people knew that I was neither a doctor nor a nurse, but they still came hoping for help. Some would stay until he [Doug] came back from his trip.

Our hospital unit was still not finished when we returned from furlough. Much remained to be done before it could officially be called a hospital. In the meantime, we ran a clinic while the final installation of electricity, screening, plumbing, and painting were being finished. We were able to use the building and it was so much more adequate than the old storage building converted into a clinic. We could take care of "inpatients" when absolutely necessary. Doug could perform necessary surgeries in the present facilities, even though they were not ideal. Even without all the modern facilities found in a hospital in the States, much could be done. We never felt like we needed to apologize for what we were unable to provide. We had an adequate laboratory, drug department, surgical unit, and X-ray unit with people to run each adequately for our needs.

We had brought back a lot of vegetable seeds and it was our desire to share them with the people, so that it might lead to improving their diets for the whole area. This was made possible because of a generous gift of seeds from Harold Adams, a friend in Yakima. We were planting our own garden as the rainy season had passed. We had people coming daily to ask for seeds in order to plant gardens to provide food for their families. We made a kind of demonstration garden planting lots of corn, beans, beets, carrots, potatoes, cantaloupe, and watermelons. We had pretty good results, though a lot of the melons and cantaloupes disappeared during the night. In my kitchen garden closer to the house, I had asparagus, several kinds of lettuce, tomatoes and spinach.

Later in this year, we found that there had been several people traveling with us on the supply boat who had active tuberculosis. Bill, Cathy, and I were found to have converted from negative to positive skin tests for tuberculosis, and we all had to go on drug therapy. Cathy developed a synovitis of the hip joint which caused a lot of pain for her.

One of our projects every year at Christmas time was to hold a big celebration. As a part of that we showed films on a big screen that we had made of unbleached muslin stretched between bamboo poles.

When the films were shown on this screen, they could be viewed from either side. The films came from different sources in Bangkok, including topics such as healthcare, the Christian faith, and entertainment. People would come from as far away as three hundred miles and every year the crowd grew larger. In the early years, the children put on a play about Christ's birth. In later years the village children and some adults formed a large group singing songs in native dialects that were well received.

It's Twins

In February 1965, I was once again pregnant and after several months we discovered I was going to have twins! I remember well the day Doug was examining me and said, "Oh, oh!" Alarmed, I asked him what he meant, and he told me he had heard two heart beats. I refused to believe him until I used the stethoscope and heard it myself. Because twins are often born early, Doug decided it would be best if I went down to Bangkok at least six weeks before my due date. I sat in the Bangkok Christian Guest House with Pam and Dan until two days before they [the twins] were due. Karl Gordon was born at 3:05 A.M. [on September 23, 1965] weighing 5 pounds and measuring 19 ½ inches long. Karen Grace was born at 3:22 A.M. weighing 5 pounds 10 ounces and measuring 18 ½ inches long. Both had light hair and blue eyes. What a relief to have these two finally delivered! They were born in the Bangkok Seventh Day Adventist Sanitarium and Hospital. When Bill came to visit me in the hospital, he could hold both twins at the same time with his big teenage hands (one in each hand, that is).

Bill, Ken, and Cathy were enrolled in the International School for English speaking children in Bangkok for this year. This was a large school with eighteen hundred students in the student body. It was for grades one through twelve. You all found that the standards were a lot higher and the homework was harder, but you did very well. This was a very modern school and their graduates did very well in colleges around the world. You all lived in a new boarding facility that the missions provided. The house parents were a Burmese couple whose names were Nu Nu and Spencer Zan.

When it became time to return to Sangkhla, Pam, Dan, and Doug went up the river by our speed boat and Helen and Karl and Karen went home in the Border Patrol helicopter.

Helen Corpron

Progress at the Kwai River Christian Mission

By this time, we began the building of the new Christian School in Sangkhla. While it was being built there were work crews to be overseen and a program to develop. The Dodges had returned from their furlough and a lot of this became Paul's responsibility.

There were Christian teachers to be found and interviewed who would be willing to come to this remote part of Thailand. The hospital buildings had to be completed, and the school building was started. By December of 1966 the school had classes expanded from one to five grades. A new seven classroom school building was underway. The cement slab floor was poured and the soil-cement block walls and concrete posts were being erected. The soil-cement block units were made on site with a mixture of one-part cement and nineteen parts laterite. (This was a clay-like soil, red in color, with a good sprinkling of gravel in it.) It was the same kind of building block that had been used to build the hospital walls.

Elephants were hauling twenty logs to the site where they would be sawed into timber for the roof supports and other needs. We often had elephants working on various projects. The Mahouts very often let the kids have rides on the elephants when they weren't working. They all really loved that. The current classrooms were bursting at the seams. We had four fine Thai Christian teachers on the staff.

The medical work was expanding every month. We were seeing more people from the Burma side as well as the Thai side from down river. As things were deteriorating in Burma and medications became unavailable, people were looking elsewhere for care. We had a Karen man who came by wagon from deep in Burma who had an old gunshot wound. He became a paraplegic from bruising that didn't sever the spinal cord. With physiotherapy he would be able to walk again. It was the end of the rainy season and most of our patients were coming upriver by boat, some on foot, and often by elephant. We felt that as time went on, we were being increasingly depended on by the people of our valley. They were finding that half of their babies did not just "naturally die" as fate's method of family planning. Women didn't have to lie by a fire for three weeks eating only rice and salt after childbirth and were coming to doubt many of their old superstitions.

Memories of a Missionary in Thailand

The church program was growing, though slowly. We had a number of new members join the church. Many interested people were inquiring into our faith. The children were coming in large numbers for the Sunday School program. Mary Thadin, one of the Christian evangelists, had a children's choir and they had memorized over sixty songs in seven languages. My, how those children loved to sing! We had a Karen Christian evangelist, Na Htoo She, in one of the outlying villages for the first time. We had land and the capital for a Christian Witness Center across the river in the main part of the village. We hoped to see that program get underway in the next year with a young Thai man who was a graduate of the School of Theology to head it up.

Bill, you were fourteen that year. You were as tall as I was and weighed about as much as I did. You were in the ninth grade. You were playing baseball, the guitar, and clarinet. In December you were singing as Amahl in the Bangkok Music Group's production of *Amahl and the Night Visitors*. We were hoping that your boy's soprano voice would not change before the program.

At this time, I was having more health problems with a lot of pain in my right side. After many medical consultations it was decided that they would do exploratory surgery to see just what was going on with me. When they finished the surgery, all they could determine was what it was not—not what was causing my problems. After that, everything seemed to get better. We spent that Christmas in Bangkok without Karl and Karen, who would remain in Sangkhla with the Dodges. I was given permission to sneak out of the guesthouse just long enough to attend Amahl for the night you were singing that part. It was very good and I've never forgotten that story.

One of our projects when we returned to Sangkhla in 1963 was to bring with us the plans and equipment for a walk-in freezer unit. Doug saw to the building of the unit which consisted of two small rooms. One was a cooling room and the other actually was a large freezing room. Our hope was to be able to keep larger quantities of meat for all on the mission station. We had to have large tanks of Freon for the freezing part of the unit. One evening while I was getting you children ready for bed, Cathy and Pam turned up missing. We searched all over the mission from the hospital to our house and down to the river where you children often played, without finding you. I even sent Bill and Ken over to the immediate closest part of the village, but no one had seen

223

you there. I was beginning to panic when Doug recalled being called to the hospital on an emergency and remembered that you two girls had been playing in the freezer. (This was before we had had a chance to install a two-way door opener.) We rushed down there to find both of you shivering in the freezer section. Fortunately, we were just turning it on to see if it was ready to run full time and it was not cold enough to really hurt you. That two-way door opener was installed immediately after that. Doug felt so bad about what had happened.

Our days were filled with many things to do and we felt fulfilled in many ways. New doctors had been found who were to take our place and we felt that we had done what we had promised our mission board that we would complete. It was time to move on in our life. Once again, our days were filled with the packing up of any of our things that we needed to take with us. We sold most of our furniture to the Myers, our replacements. We needed to return to the United States to prepare the way for all of you to complete your high school years and for us to put aside some funds for your college educations.

There was a wonderful celebration, and we were presented with a beautiful Tiger Skin. Beautiful dances were performed by the Thai teachers from the school and some of the children (including you, Pam). There were speeches from the village headman, and other officials and that was followed by a wonderful banquet. We said our goodbyes to all our faithful workers not knowing if we would ever see any of them again. The final scene that nearly blew our minds was all of the displaced Karen soldiers standing on an island as we passed by saluting us! Our boat made its way down the river and each of us had feelings of our own about the place we had called home for so many years. I knew in my heart that we had really made a difference in a lot of people's lives and that we had started something very worthwhile and meaningful that would be there for many years to come—and that has been proven to be true. I was looking forward to being reunited with our families in the States but was sad to be leaving so much of myself behind.

This, my children, was what our life in Thailand all those years was all about.

Chapter 15

Tested

By Melba McDaniel

About the author of this chapter

Melba McDaniel, wife of Dr. Phil McDaniel, grew up in Ashland, Kentucky. She held a master's degree in microbiology and worked at the University of Illinois Hospital bacteriology lab during the early years of their marriage while Phil was finishing medical school at the University of Illinois. On the mission field at various times she served as hospital bookkeeper, payroll officer, mission accountant, fill-in pharmacist, tabulator of statistics, English teacher, and homeschool teacher.

Span of service at KRCH/KRCM: April 1979 to June 2002

I was almost 29 when, in the summer of 1978, I moved to Thailand with my husband and two-year-old daughter, Linette. Phil and I had been married almost 6 years at the time and he had finally finished all his medical training. Now at last he was ready to fulfill his dream of returning to Thailand as a missionary doctor. Phil had made it very clear to me before he asked me to marry him that Thailand was his eventual goal. I had never felt any particular "call" to be a missionary myself, had never traveled out of the United States, and had no particular ambition to travel the world, but I was willing to go where God directed, and so said "yes." When Phil and I first visited Thailand in 1973 after we were married, I experienced a fair amount of culture shock, but after seeing the poverty and need of the hill-tribe peoples, I also began to look forward to living there. However, I never did really consider myself a missionary. I was a missionary wife and mother who made it possible for Phil to work at a remote hospital. I was happy to help out in various ways, but I never felt completely at home there and would not have been heart-broken if we had had to leave. (In our early years there were rumors of Communist take-overs and also rumors that the government intended to expel all missionaries.)

One reason I never felt at home was the language difficulty. Because Phil could already speak some Thai when we began language study, he was able to skip over the first three months of the curriculum. The usual curriculum was nine months, and when he finished his study [after six months], we left immediately for the Kwai River Christian Hospital, which had been without a regular doctor for many months. Thus, my language study was incomplete, and although I tried to study some on my own, my reticence in speaking and the fact that my work didn't require my speaking Thai, meant that my language never progressed beyond "survival level." I was comfortable traveling alone but could not have anything other than a very superficial conversation with native Thai speakers. Thai is a tonal language with five different tones, and I never did master the differences between them, nor could I tell when I was or was not pronouncing them correctly. People were always gracious to me when I tried to speak. "You speak Thai very well" they would say, when I knew I was butchering the language. I once tried to preach in Thai at church. My Thai was not only translated into another local language, Karen, but was also translated into Thai. I never again tried to give a talk in Thai!

The Kwai River Christian Hospital is located in a very rural part of Thailand. In the early years, getting there could be quite an ordeal. There was no paved road all the way, and in the rainy season much of the trip had to be on the river in a long-tail boat. In our first newsletter, Phil wrote about our very first trip to visit the location:

The Land Rover, crowded with eleven passengers and numerous boxes, gave a sudden lurch and nearly tipped over. The driver managed, without too much difficulty, to get it straightened up but soon thereafter ran into another problem: the car became stuck in the mud, and all his best efforts only succeeded in making the right rear wheel sink deeper and deeper. The passengers climbed out, into drizzling rain and picked their way gingerly through the thick, gooey mud. For nearly an hour the passengers stood around in the mud and rain or helped try to push the car out of the mud.

Keeping a two-year-old occupied and reasonably clean outside in the rain for an hour was not fun.

[Phil continued] After an hour, word came that the car was ready to start—heading back in the same direction it had come! In the midst of valiant efforts to push the car out of the mud hole, it was discovered that the back wheels were not responding. With only front-wheel drive it would be impossible to make it up the hill. They were a twenty-minute drive away from the boat landing to which they had been heading. Now they would have to travel two hours back to the nearest big town. On the way back, the car became stuck again: what had been passable in four-wheel drive became impassable in front-wheel drive alone. Again, everyone hopped out and waited around in the mud while the car was freed.

We climbed back into the car dirty, hot, and disheveled. We spent our second night in the relatively primitive hotel in Kanchanaburi. (We had traveled there by bus from Bangkok the day before.)

[Continuing] The following day by 11:00 am …[we] were sitting on a boat traveling up the river. Our wooden seats were only four inches from the floor and uncomfortable … [We] wore lifebelts in case by chance the boat should tip over and spill us out into the swollen, muddy river. We traveled through forested hills and caught glimpses of elephants and kingfishers along the riverbank. Six hours and two rest stops later our boat driver suddenly pulled over to a sandbar along the side of the river for an unscheduled stop. The rudder needed replacing! We all got out of the boat, thankful for a chance to stretch. After only about thirty minutes we were ready to travel on. Darkness found us still on the river, an hour away from our destination. We plowed on, once nearly running into an unlit raft, and another time nearly running into some branches sticking up from the water. Eventually, the boat driver turned on a light and passed it up to one of the passengers in front. It cast an eerie glow on the river ahead as he shined it alternately from shore to shore. It helped some, but the boat driver still had to rely heavily on his familiarity with the river.

When we finally reached the boat landing below what would be our house, we climbed up the steps from the river and then up a small hill and up more steps into the house. The electricity was very dim, and entering the large house with wooden floors and walls reminded me of entering a cave. I assume we took showers or perhaps dipper baths (if the water wasn't running) after the trip, in cold water. I don't remember where Linette slept; there was no reason the house would have had a crib.

What Phil didn't mention about the boat ride in the letter quoted above was that although there was an awning over the top, the sides were open, and the rain came in on us. All our luggage was wrapped in plastic to keep it dry, and we had on rain ponchos. The only bathroom stop I remember was at a small restaurant built over the water, with the toilet opening up directly into the river. The beautiful scenery, though, almost made up for the discomfort.

Tested

Not long into our second term, the road from Kanchanaburi to Sangkhlaburi became passable by jeep, and the river rides were soon a thing of the past. There were advantages and disadvantages to traveling by jeep. The trip was quite a bit shorter by jeep, but there was no air conditioning, of course, and no seatbelts or assigned seating. As many people as possible crammed into the Jeep and once settled down, it became difficult to move for the rest of the trip. The forest scenery we traveled through was always brown and dusty along the roads, and we would arrive at our destination covered in dust.

By the time we left Thailand in 2002, there was a good paved road all the way to the hospital, and we could take the hospital truck and drive directly from our house to the Bangkok Christian Guest House in about six hours. If we wanted to go by public transportation, we could take an air-conditioned bus from Sangkhlaburi (the district capital) south to Kanchanaburi, and then an air-conditioned "tour bus" (which served free bottled water or soda pop and sometimes showed movies) from Kanchanaburi to Bangkok.

Rainy season began soon after we first moved up to the hospital after language study. In a newsletter, written about a month after our arrival at the hospital, I wrote:

I never tire of looking out our front windows onto the dirt road that runs past the house, with the river beyond, and then hills and mountains on the other side. With the frequent rain, the tops of the mountains are often shrouded in mist, causing them to look slightly different from day to day. Just across the road is a poinsettia tree bearing masses of pink blossoms and adding a bright splash of color to the predominant greens, blues, and browns. The Lord knew of my great love for hills and mountains and graciously allowed us to begin our mission work in such a spot of beauty.

Linette [almost 3 years old] … has really been enjoying the sights and sounds of the country. She runs to the window whenever she hears the bells of an oxcart going by, and once she saw an elephant walk down the road with a man, woman, and little boy on its back. ... We raise our own chickens here, and she was thrilled to see two little brand-new baby chicks that were hatched last Sunday. Already Linette has learned to recognize and imitate the sounds of various animals and birds she hears: the chickens that wake her up in the morning; the gecko, a large house lizard with a distinctive call; a gibbon that one of the school teachers has for a pet; and a common local bird known as the coo-caw. She has watched entranced as "hundreds and thousands and millions and billions and trillions" of ants quickly collect whenever any food has dropped ...

We have, of course, had various minor problems to contend with since our arrival here. Our tap water is pumped directly from the river and after periods of heavy rain it often comes from the tap quite muddy and sandy. The electricity, which we only have in the evenings, is supposed to be 220 volts current. In fact, it has varied between about 70 and 200, never quite getting up to the prescribed 220. Our house, though quite well-built, does have numerous small cracks in it which allow various insects to enter at night and buzz around the lights. Usually this is only a very minor irritation, but on days when the flying termites swarm, the insect population inside the house increases considerably. That is nothing, however, compared to the problems caused by the winged termites inside the hospital operating room. The circulating nurse is obliged to spend most of her time trying to keep the termites away from the sterile operating field…

One fun thing about having a house with "holes" in the floor is that a tree grew up through a hole in our bedroom. I always enjoyed sharing our bedroom with a tree!

Usually the termites would swarm only one or two nights a year at the end of the hot season after the first big wind and rainstorm. After briefly flying around and mating, they would drop their wings, and the next morning the whole house would be covered with termite wings which had to be swept up. One year, instead of termites, we had "glue bugs" come. These bugs would fall to the ground and die, excrete some sort of sticky substance that would dry like concrete and have to be scraped away. Fortunately, these bugs were bigger than the termites and only a few got inside the house.

Besides the flying termites, we had to contend with ants and cockroaches inside the house. The ant problem could be solved by having the legs of our tables and food storage cabinets set in "ant cups"—containers filled with water except for a dry area in the middle where the table leg would go. To deter cockroaches, I would make what we called "cockroach balls," a concoction of flour, sugar, boric acid, and milk molded into balls that I would put in the cupboards. More troubling were the scorpions that one would occasionally find in the house. Their sting was very painful. Fortunately, we only once had a centipede in the house. I went into the bathroom one time and there in the sink was a centipede, that had evidently crawled up through the drainpipe. Centipedes in Thailand can be 6 to 8 inches long, and their bite is so painful it is said that "you cry for three days." Once there was a snake in the house, which our gardener killed, and once our cat brought us a "present" which she fortunately left on the porch outside the door: a newborn poisonous snake still wrapped in its amniotic sac. Rodents were a constant problem, but by keeping a cat we could keep the rodent population under control. We had small, harmless house lizards that liked to gather around the window screens (it was always fun to watch them catch the flying termites). Sometimes a much bigger house lizard called a "tookay" would take up residence.

The temperature in the rainy season was always about the same, day and night, and was, in my mind at least, the most comfortable season, temperature-wise. In the early part of the season, it would rain intermittently every day, but by the middle of the season it wasn't unusual to have several days or a week of constant rain day and night. The muddy walks and the need to constantly carry an umbrella were a nuisance. The clothes (which were dried on a line) sometimes took several days to dry, and mold grew everywhere: on books, leather shoes, audiovisual equipment, and clothing. We had to keep the camera and any videos in air-tight plastic containers with silica gel at the bottom. When the silica gel was new, it was bright blue. After becoming saturated with moisture, it would turn pink and have to be recharged: by baking it in the oven a short time, it would regain its blue color. Floods were also a frequent problem toward the end of the rainy season. Our houses were built up high and therefore flood-proof, but a few times the flood waters came almost all the way to the concrete slab the house was built on.

Neither the hospital nor the church was built on stilts, and occasionally they flooded. That didn't stop us from having worship services. Linette wrote about one such church flood in a letter in 1996:

Since the floor of the church is concrete and the benches are wood, the water couldn't do much damage, so we were able to enjoy the novelty of wading to church through knee-deep water and cooling our feet and ankles during the service. The normal sounds of the Sunday service were punctuated by the children splashing their feet and, for me, by Melodie [age 8 at the time] whispering urgently into my ear, "I wanna swim!"… The stray sandals floating between the pews were a nice change from the dogs that usually wander into church!

Nobody seemed upset about the water—the choirs sang and the ushers took up the offering standing in water.

Tested

The cold season succeeded the rainy season, starting in about October and lasting until about mid-February. In this season, there was almost never any rain, but everything was still lush and green, and the skies were often a bright blue. The mornings and evenings were cool and usually required us to wear sweaters or light jackets. Locals would huddle around small fires they built outside their houses. The afternoon temperatures often got up into the eighties. Churches sent us sweaters and jackets to pass out to the local people who needed them, and all the hospital patients were supplied with a blanket for use while they were in the hospital. Since our house was open to the air at the top (with wire screen) the temperature inside the house was as cold as outside, and we slept under several blankets.

The hot season followed the cold season and lasted from about mid-February to mid-June. This was my least favorite season, especially during April, the hottest month. By the time the hot season came around it hadn't rained significantly in several months. The vegetation was brown and the drought-deciduous trees had shed their leaves. Although the early morning and evening temperatures were tolerable, as soon as the sun rose, the temperature began to rise, often reaching over 100 degrees by afternoon. We had ceiling fans which helped a lot to keep us cool, but once the temperature in the house reached 100 degrees, the fans no longer seemed able to mitigate the heat.

During our first term, we had no fans in the house because we did not have electricity in the daytime. I would cool off in the afternoon by filling the bathtub with water and lying down in it with a book. This seemed to amuse the locals. Linette and her friends spent much of the afternoons at the local river. Many of the fruits of Thailand are seasonal, and Phil said that the only good thing about the hot season was that was when mangoes got ripe. Whenever possible, we would take our annual vacation in April, staying in cabins on Khun Tan mountain where the temperature was usually pleasant. Occasionally on Khun Tan, there would come a cold rain and hail and we would light a fire in the fireplace.

When we first went to Thailand, I didn't have a good idea as to what my particular work would be. It seemed logical that I might somehow use my bacteriology training in the hospital, but the lack of daytime electricity made it impossible for the hospital to run an incubator, and the lack of an incubator meant I couldn't culture out any bacteria.

My first job was recording the hospital statistics—daily, monthly, and yearly: numbers of outpatients, inpatients, deliveries, surgeries, and cases of malaria (the latter statistic required by the government). This didn't require a lot of time and I soon volunteered to fill another need—supervising and correcting the work of the local hospital bookkeeper. She was a diligent worker but not very skilled at correcting mistakes when the books didn't balance.

I had no training in bookkeeping but was good in math and the basics were easy enough to learn from a book; so, for the first two terms this was my primary job. Eventually, the local bookkeeper moved on to other things, and I did all the bookkeeping myself by hand (no computers at that point), not only for the hospital but also for the mission work in general. Sometimes I was asked to audit the school or boarding house accounts as well, and I helped prepare periodic financial reports.

Because of the accounting work, I was the person in charge of the hospital safe where all the money was kept. There was initially no local bank, so we missionaries would have to transport money up from Bangkok any time we traveled there. It was always a little disconcerting to be carrying around the equivalent of thousands of dollars in Thai baht on public transport, but fortunately, no one was ever robbed bringing cash up from Bangkok. When hospital pay-day came each month, the hospital manager would bring me a list of how much cash each employee should receive—broken down by 500, 100, 20 and 10 baht notes and 5- and 1-baht coins as well as the smaller 50 and 25 satang coins. (The smallest coin, 25 satangs, was worth about a penny.) Sometimes it was challenging to have enough small bills and coins in hand to pay everyone the exact amount they were owed.

People would come to me at all times of the day or evening to get reimbursed for legitimate expenses. Our house doors were always open when we were home, and it was the custom for people to just walk in without knocking and come and stand quietly behind me or call my name softly. This was a courtesy so that I wouldn't have to get up and go to the door and let them in, but it was sometimes a bit disconcerting to look up from my work and find someone (occasionally even a stranger) standing behind me in the house. I was also responsible for paying the salaries and subtracting the fees (retirement account, water and electricity fees) for the various mission workers. I still occasionally have nightmares about forgetting to pay people their salaries at the end of the month.

Besides homeschooling our children and doing the financial work, I also sometimes taught English—both to hospital and school staff who wanted to learn or improve their English, and, for a short time, at the local high school, about a mile's walk away from where we lived. I enjoyed the teaching but it didn't last long due to pregnancy-related nausea I was having at that time. After the villages relocated, the high school was in a different village from the hospital; so, I did no more teaching there. For a few years I worked with the "Candlelight Program" for children with disabilities, and tried to teach the Thai alphabet, among other things.

Our first term was challenging for me. Phil worked long hours at the hospital and didn't always make it home in time to eat lunch or dinner with Linette and me. We frequently had medical students or resident doctors living with us, and at times they tended to monopolize our mealtime conversations.

Phil and I were the only married missionaries at Sangkhla (there were several single women nurses and an evangelistic worker) and I didn't have anyone to talk to about my child-rearing questions. ("Does your four-year-old act like this?") Mail service was erratic, and it would sometimes take six weeks to receive the answer to a question I had asked. We seldom traveled anywhere because the journey to Bangkok was so exhausting, especially with a little one along. Not infrequently, there was no electricity even in the evenings because the city generator was broken. When there was electricity, it was often very dim. I remember once seeing a brighter than usual light in another room, and when I went to see what it was, I discovered it was a candle. There was running water in the house, but no hot water (until Phil installed a water heater in the bathroom, an early priority for him). Sometimes debris would clog the pipes leading from the river pump, and we would be without water and have to use the large storage jars in the bathroom and kitchen that were always kept full of water. But the inconveniences soon became part of normal life, and I was usually content.

One of the events I remember most vividly from our first term was a murder that happened in a house next to the hospital. A well-educated Karen refugee from Burma, named Kya Doe, had lived there with his Karen wife, her children from a previous relationship, and their joint baby. Kya Doe had graduated from Sandhurst in England and served in the British army as a Brigadier General during World War II. After the war, he returned to Burma, married, and started a family. For some reason (I'm not sure I ever knew the exact details) he became implicated in the Karen independence movement in Burma, and was suddenly exiled from the country and forced to leave his wife and family behind. He escaped across the border and settled down near the hospital. Because he was an illegal immigrant, he was not allowed to travel freely in Thailand. After some years it appeared there was no chance he would ever be allowed back into Burma, so he married a local Karen woman.

When I knew him, he was elderly, spoke excellent but very formal English, and was receiving a pension from the British government for his war service. Unexpectedly, the Burmese government suddenly issued an amnesty to some of those who had been exiled, and he decided to return to Burma and his first wife. He made provisions for the support of his Thailand family by leaving two gold bars behind for his wife: gold bars which were stored in the safe in our bedroom. The story I heard later was that the wife had been bragging about having the gold bars, and some people broke into her house to steal them and also murdered her and her sons. Kya Doe's son, who was two, was left unharmed (and later went to live with Kya Doe in Burma). Phil was called to the house to officially pronounce the deaths and take pictures for the police. (The murderers were never caught.) Before long, a rumor went around that the murderers, now knowing that the gold was in the doctor's house, were going to hit that house next.

A June 1982 newsletter reports what happened next: "In less than a week we learned of two more murder incidents, both within ten miles of our house. These events set everyone's nerves on edge. For a while the local army branch patrolled the area, but when there were no more murders for a while this patrolling was discontinued." A man followed me home one night after my teaching at the hospital. I didn't recognize the man and was a bit apprehensive when I noticed he was carrying a gun. I realized it was probably just one of the watchmen but all the way home, kept imagining what I would do when I got home if he wanted to follow me into the house. Fortunately, just as I turned onto the path leading to our house, he called out some friendly greeting in Thai and continued on down the road.

Linette was nearly three when we finished language school and moved to Sangkhla. We began hoping for another child, but month after month went by, and I was never pregnant. Linette was over five when I finally became pregnant again. My pregnancy this time was much harder on me than my first one. I usually felt OK when I awoke each morning, but as the day went on, I would become more and more nauseated and would have to retire to bed after only a few bites of supper. I was being seen monthly by a midwife at the hospital maternity clinic, and as far as she (not always the same midwife) could tell was progressing normally. The hospital had no Doppler ultrasound at the time, and although the baby's heartbeat could not be detected with a stethoscope, that could have been just due to its position in the womb. Nobody but me seemed worried, but I couldn't shake the strong premonition that something was wrong. About half-way through the fifth month, I woke up one morning and realized that I was bleeding slightly. The doctor (Phil) prescribed complete bed rest. It was the middle of the hot season and our bedroom faced west and was the hottest room in the house. As I lay in bed hour after hour, I kept a basin of cool water next to the bed with a washcloth to periodically wipe off my sweaty face and neck. Sometimes the bleeding would stop for a few hours, but it always returned, and after a week—and a negative pregnancy test—Phil decided to do a pelvic exam to see if I was having an inevitable abortion (miscarriage). It appeared that I was, and he proceeded immediately to a D&C. I had not been given any anesthesia [Editor's note: I think she had a paracervical block], but only some Demerol to act as an analgesic. As the D&C proceeded, Phil began removing partially decomposed fetal body parts and it became evident that the fetus had been dead for several weeks. The procedure was painful, but not excruciatingly so, and I remember praying over and over, "Please, God, don't let him perforate my uterus" (always a danger during a D&C). Suddenly I felt intense waves of joy and peace washing over me, and I knew God was there in the operating room with me. I only half heard Phil counting out the various body parts as he removed them: "arm, leg, torso, leg, arm, leg —wait a minute, that was 3 legs," and it was only then we realized I had been pregnant with twins. I never looked at—or had any desire to look at—what was being removed from my uterus, but my biggest regret (other than their death) was that we could not tell the sex of either baby, because of the decomposition.

After it was over, two medical students who were staying with us at the time wheeled me home from the hospital in a wheelchair. There was a Thai church official from Bangkok arriving that day who was scheduled to stay at our house. I begged Phil to have someone else house him (it would have been hard enough to entertain a stranger speaking English, but I didn't feel like straining to understand Thai), but there really wasn't anywhere else he could go. Phil did agree to leave the guest alone at the house later in the evening so he and I could go for a walk and privately grieve.

Before this, whenever I thought about miscarriages, I assumed the grief would be minor compared to losing a child at or shortly after birth. Perhaps it is, but it was much more devastating to me than I had expected, and lasted for months. It didn't help when a few months later another missionary gave birth to two healthy twin boys. I never blamed God or myself because I knew I had done everything I could to have a healthy baby. One thing this experience taught me was that whatever happened to me, God would be there, and there was no reason for me to fear.

Not long after this incident, our first four years were up, and we returned to the United States for furlough. I remember my mother being a bit shocked at our appearance, saying we all three looked like we were suffering from anorexia. But we soon fattened up. We spent our furlough year in New Orleans, with Phil studying tropical medicine at Tulane University. Linette began first grade. Our October 1982 newsletter opened like this:

"Mommy, when black children talk to each other they speak in English!" Linette said to me one day in a surprised but delighted tone of voice shortly after we moved to New Orleans. Her experience in Thailand had been that people of a different color spoke a different language—at least when they talked to each other. … There were many things about her own country that were new to [Linette]. One of the things she had had no experience with in Thailand was television, and because of her previous lack of exposure to commercials, she believed without question every word the advertisers spoke.

She would argue with us in the grocery store when we weren't buying the "correct" product. She had never heard of "Pac Man" before and I had to laugh when she brought home an arithmetic paper saying that the greater than (>) and less than (<) signs were Pac Man's mouth, always pointing to the largest number. When her class played musical chairs one day, Linette was the only one who didn't know what to do when the music stopped.

About six months into our furlough I became pregnant again and began seeing a local obstetrician.

Because twin pregnancies have a higher percentage of problems, I asked for an ultrasound before we went back to Thailand to make sure I wasn't pregnant with twins again. I wasn't, but the doctor still told me that if I went back to Thailand, "I would be playing dice with my baby's life." Phil's father, also, thought it might be best if we remained in the US until after the baby was born. After a lot of prayer, however, we both felt peace about returning to Thailand, but decided I would take the precaution of staying in Bangkok until after the baby was born. The birth was still almost four months away, so Phil went alone to the hospital to work and Linette and I remained behind at the Bangkok Christian Guest House, where I began homeschooling her in second grade. The plan was that Phil would return in August for two months to take some advanced Thai studies and thus would be with us when the baby was born. The baby's due date was Sept 25, but my bag of waters broke on the 9th and I walked the two blocks or so to the Bangkok Nursing Home Hospital to give birth.

Nathan was born at about noon on September 7, 1983, and seemed to be perfectly healthy, except that Phil noticed he was breathing a bit faster than normal. He was taken to the nursery, I went to sleep, and

Phil went back to the Guest House. When I woke up, I called down to the nursery to have them bring the baby to me, but they said he first had to be checked out by a pediatrician. After waiting about an hour, I got up and walked down to the nursery to see him. There were two babies in the nursery and two mothers looking in the window at them. There was another baby out in the hall surrounded by white-coated medical personnel. "Is that your baby?" one of the women asked, and I realized it must be. I started to walk closer to see what was wrong but was shooed away, and someone said they would be with me soon. When she (or he—I don't remember) finally came over, I asked what was wrong, but instead of answering, I was asked where my husband was. She said she would explain to both of us together when he arrived. I frantically called the Guest House, only to be told that Phil wasn't there, but was at a restaurant with some guests who had just arrived. I think someone went to find him, for he arrived at the hospital not long afterwards. We were told that Nathan had hyaline membrane disease and a pneumomediastinum (air in the middle of the chest from a small hole in the lung or bronchus) and was having difficulty breathing.

Eventually, Nathan's pediatrician, after consulting with one of her former pediatrics instructors, decided to send him by ambulance to the nearby Chulalongkorn Hospital, a university hospital, where he was admitted to the Neonatal Intensive Care unit. It was about midnight, and Phil went with the ambulance through the flooded streets of Bangkok while I stayed at the nursing home. We learned afterwards that Nathan was essentially "smuggled in" as the NICU was supposed to only be for babies born at that hospital. He was hooked up to a CPAP machine, and Phil was told that the next three days would be critical. I have a hazy memory of someone estimating his chances were about 50-50. Nathan was assigned his own special duty nurse to watch over him. Phil gave me [at the Bangkok Nursing Home Hospital] a report on what was happening and then went back to the Guest House to try to sleep. The next day Nathan seemed about the same—certainly no worse—and we were beginning to feel optimistic he would survive. On the morning of September 9, our wedding anniversary, we were told the pneumomediastinum had spontaneously closed.

That afternoon Phil got a call from another nearby hospital, the Bangkok Christian Hospital, and was told that Dr. Lois Visscher from the Kwai River Christian Hospital had just been brought in via border police helicopter and had been rushed right away to surgery. The previous evening some men had broken into her house and stabbed her multiple times. Then they fled without taking anything from the house. The abdominal puncture had penetrated her liver and perforated her stomach and diaphragm. She had emergency exploratory surgery to repair the wounds. She was then admitted to the intensive care unit and put on a respirator.

A few hours later we got word that Nathan had developed bilateral hemopneumothorax. The slight positive air pressure had blown holes in his lungs and they were leaking blood and air. Our November 1983 newsletter reported:

> At the time we learned of this new complication, the Bangkok missionaries were having their every-other-week fellowship meeting. Phil called and told them the news and was assured of their prayers. Later we learned that those present agreed to participate in a continuous 24-hour prayer vigil for Nathan and Dr. Lois, each person signing up for one hour of the twenty-four. Others—in America, Australia, and northern Thailand— were also praying.

By the next morning, I checked myself out of the hospital and went to view him through the NICU window. With the CPAP machine, a needle in his scalp dispensing antibiotics, two chest tubes and a catheter, I thought he looked terrible, but Phil said he was looking a lot better than he had earlier. They were soon able to remove the CPAP machine, and Nathan was released to the Bangkok Nursing Home on the 14th, and then discharged from the hospital to the Guest House on the 21st. Phil went back to the Kwai River Christian Hospital to take over Dr. Lois's work, and Nathan, Linette, and I stayed at the Guest House and took Nathan to weekly doctor check-ups. By early November, Nathan was considered stable enough to move to Sangkhla, and Phil returned to pick us up. Dr. Lois's recovery was more complicated and involved a medical evacuation to the United States, but she, too, eventually recovered completely and even returned to

Thailand to work as a volunteer in one of the refugee camps a year or two later.

Not long after we moved back to Sangkhla for our second term, the active phase of relocation began.

For years we had been hearing about the proposed dam that was to be built across the Kwai River south of us that would flood the whole upper River Kwai Valley. Our August 1980 newsletter showed some of the uncertainty everyone felt:

This will affect all departments of the mission here: the school, hostel, hospital, and evangelistic work. Will we disband or relocate? And if we relocate, where will it be? … We are to some extent going to be dependent on the Thai government in terms of amount of compensation received for the property and relocation sites available.

Three and a half years later, the title of our April 1984 newsletter was "It's Actually Happening." The newsletter continued:

Three weeks ago, we moved out of our old house so it could be dismantled. … The six missionaries still at the old site [including our family of 4] have all moved together into the last intact missionary residence, a duplex originally designed for 2 single nurses.

After talking about how the stress of relocation was affecting the local villagers by causing an increase in suicide and violence, the letter continues:

Our family is facing our second relocation-related move in 3 ½ months (and 5th total move in 13 months) next week to our newly-rebuilt house at one of the relocation sites. Even then, we will not be able to become fully unpacked and settled for another 4 to 6 months, as we share our home with two missionary nurses and a pharmacist until their home can be torn down and rebuilt.

Our relocation site was not as scenic as the old site on the river, and we missed our fruit trees. At first, there were feelings of disorientation and uncertainty among both the local villagers and hospital personnel. For example, in a 1985 newsletter, Phil writes:

The cornerstone of our public health program has been the mobile clinic. But who wants to go out into the jungle with a mobile clinic when there are robbers all over the place! No sooner had I gotten home after that night-time drive through the mud [described earlier in the letter], when I was told about the recent attempted armed robbery of the little store just across the road from the mission compound. Only a few nights earlier, five or six men armed with a carbine and some shotguns came to the shop in the dead of night and demanded that the two fellows inside (who slept in the shop to guard it) open up. When they didn't, the bandits began shooting through the doors of the shop! Luckily, they didn't hit either of the men inside, both of whom are good friends of ours. [They had climbed up into the rafters to what was a safer spot.]

Later I heard about robberies along the road in broad daylight: a lady's gold earrings and another lady's cash, just received from the sale of fresh pork. These two episodes were told to me by the manager of our public health team. She said she didn't want to go out on any mobile clinic trips as long as there is this kind of trouble going around. I really can't blame her. Twice in the last week a wounded bandit has been brought to the hospital... The first one had been shot in the right groin by a policeman as he was reportedly lunging at the policeman's head with a knife. The second man had been shot in the face while eating his supper. This was apparently an act of revenge or "justice" on the part of the assailant. ... Somebody came by at midnight the next night and, reaching through one of the temporary windows of the hospital, shot the already wounded man while he was sleeping in his bed. Miraculously, the patient survived this second gunshot wound with only minimal damage to right shoulder and chest wall. I told the man as I did his dressing today, "You have now been shot twice without dying. Perhaps God has a special plan for your life!"

Eventually, the new site became familiar and we were able to appreciate the advantages. Travel was easier and instead of owning an oxcart for travel, the hospital now had a truck. Instead of walking several miles to the main village area to buy fresh produce, we could now take advantage of a food truck that stopped at the hospital almost daily. The water system was improved and there was no more muddy water in the pipes during the rainy season. The government-supplied electricity was much improved and when it wasn't working, the new mission generator could be started up. So, we now had 24-hour electricity and could use fans during the daytime: a real improvement! We were able to replace our former kerosene refrigerator with an electric one and were able to buy a VHS tape player to show videos. (We were not able to get any TV channels.) It didn't take long for the new place to feel like home, and that is where we lived for the remainder of our time in Thailand. It is the only home that either of our two younger children are able to remember. Our new house was the same size and shape as the old one except that we now had a second bathroom and a somewhat larger porch. The main beams had been numbered one-by-one as the house was dismantled and most were able to be used in the same positions as before. After the overgrowth of bamboo had been bulldozed away, new trees had been planted around the mission area which had first been rather barren. We missed the river but did have a small creek that ran just back of our house.

Although there were some advantages our children missed by not living in the United States, one of the good aspects of their growing up in rural Thailand was that they had more freedom to roam around and explore their surroundings than they would have had in a city. As a preschooler, Linette especially enjoyed wandering around the village, visiting people she knew. When she was very young, she would often escape from the house before breakfast and go next door to play with our cook's children. She was even the one who suggested the English name they gave their first daughter. (Some of the local Karen people had three names: one English, one Thai, and one Karen.) She also liked to visit the pastor's house where she would beg for sugar cubes! She wandered down to the hospital often to talk with her friends, the nurses, or to visit the little store next to the hospital. One time she asked our cook for money to go to the store, and he handed her the package insert from a box of medicine and told her it was "Karen money." She was surprised and disappointed to learn that the "Karen money" was not accepted at the store. I also can remember her going around selling snails to the other missionaries, saying they would be good for their gardens. One day Linette came home with a gibbon from the porch of one of the schoolteacher's houses, which we promptly returned, but we kept the kitten she brought home another time, the runt of a litter. (Because of rats, we always kept one or more cats at home. They were inside-outside cats and ate table scraps. It was always fun to play with a new batch of kittens.)

Nathan was even more adventurous than Linette. He would sometimes wake up in the middle of the night, unlock our house door, and wander around outside for a while, before returning, relocking the door and going to bed. We were unaware of these nocturnal adventures until the night he escaped earlier than usual, and either Phil or I noticed the door was not locked and locked it. He had to knock on the door to get back into the house, and that ended his nighttime excursions. (It was really rather dangerous for him to be wandering around, because there were watchmen with a rifle guarding the property at the time, and he might have been mistaken for an intruder and shot.) One day Nathan brought a little goat into the house that he had seen grazing outside somewhere. He told me about it, but I thought he said "little girl" instead of "little goat."

"That's nice," I said, glad he had a playmate.

But then he added, "I put it under the table."

"Wait a minute," I said. "What did you say you brought home?"

As they got older, Linette and Nathan became comfortable exploring the area beyond our village. One time, Linette, age about 13, was walking on a circle walk, part of which was out in the country where there were no houses. The village headman told Phil it was not safe for Linette to be wandering alone in such an area. So, after that she always stayed closer to home. When Nathan learned to ride his bicycle, he often took a road outside the village that led to another village called Yakadee. He also would ride over to where the Australian volunteers and villagers were putting in a gravity-fed water system and watch them work.

Of the three children, Melodie probably spent the most time with the villagers. She would be accompanied by her babysitter. Because she could speak their Karen language well, she was always popular and not infrequently when I was out walking with her, someone I didn't know would call out her name and say something to her in Karen which I didn't understand, but she did. She and Nathan would occasionally stay overnight at the home of A'Nong, their babysitter, and Melodie was also not infrequently invited to stay overnight at the home of one of the Candlelight School teachers. Nathan was so comfortable at A'Nong's house as a preschooler that he would immediately greet guests and offer them her supply of betel nut, which almost all local adults, especially the older ones, chewed. This gesture was a bit like offering tea or coffee to a guest in some other cultures. Nathan and Melodie enjoyed the fried insects that their babysitter shared with them.

Partly to keep Linette home more, I began teaching kindergarten to her when she was only four.

Home-schooling was uncommon at the time, and the only curriculum available was from the Calvert School. I used their regular kindergarten program, only slightly simplified, and by the next year had to make up my own lessons, since I didn't want to start her in first grade early. She already knew the alphabet and sounds, so I made up reading lessons for her. I would make worksheets with a true-false simple sentence ("Yes or no: A fish can swim. The sun is hot. A man has 4 legs.") or draw pictures and have her match the words to the pictures. Each day I would write a new story on the whiteboard about "The Adventures of Linette" for her to read. Nathan wasn't quite as interested in schoolwork as Linette had been, so he didn't begin kindergarten until he was almost six. Unlike Linette, who never did learn much Thai or other local language (partly because the children she played with spoke several different languages), Nathan as a preschooler spoke the Karen language of his babysitter more fluently than English. At least, I was told he spoke it fluently. When he didn't know I was watching he would sometimes talk to himself in Karen when playing with his toys, but any time he saw me he would immediately stop. As Linette and Nathan grew older, there were more school curricula from which to choose, and my lessons were often eclectic, using materials from several different curricula. I think I actually enjoyed preparing the lessons more than teaching them, since the kids weren't always as enthusiastic over their lessons as I was. But in general, they were cooperative and we had fun together. When they went away to school when they were older, we had already established such a good relationship through daily schoolwork that I didn't feel overly deprived of their presence.

Once they were school age, neither Linette nor Nathan played much with the local children, who were all in school during the day. In order to provide more socialization for the kids (since there were no missionary children living in Sangkhla), Phil's father and stepmother, who lived in Chiang Mai, in northern Thailand, invited them to stay with them and attend the Chiang Mai International School. Linette was there for the last half of fourth and the first half of fifth grade, and Nathan spent the last half of seventh and all of eighth grade at the school. In a letter to Phil's sister Carol written when Linette was 9 and had been in Chiang Mai a month or two, I wrote:

Linette seems to be really enjoying school in Chiang Mai. ... I

talked with Linette's teacher ... and she said Linette had done fine academically from the start … and was making progress socially but still had a bit of a problem. At first, she tended to play only with the younger children (kindergarten and first grade) at recess but now she was beginning to associate more with the kids in her class. … She was unfamiliar with the games they played in PE and would usually be chosen last of the six girls in 4th-6th grade. … The teacher said at first, she had trouble adjusting to other kids in the classroom. For example, if someone didn't give the right answer to a question, Linette would say something like, "No, that's not right. I read that it was such and so," not meaning at all to be arrogant but coming across that way. So, the teacher had a little talk with her once and told her in a sort of joking way that she had the tact of a steamroller…" Incidentally, Linette had a similar problem when she started high school. She did a lot of reading, and at first would use "big words" in her conversations that the other kids didn't understand and thought she was showing off. She had to learn to keep her "big words" for writing and not for conversation. Both Linette and Nathan eventually made good friends their own age in Chiang Mai, and both had birthday parties there with their friends, a new experience for them. Nathan participated in soccer for a time while he was at school. He was often assigned to the position of goalie and then got blamed when the other team scored!

Linette went to public school in the 6th grade while we were in Ashland, Kentucky on furlough, and went to boarding school for grades

9–12 at Stony Brook School in Stony Brook, New York. Those years she did not come home for Christmas, but did come home most years for summer vacation. On furloughs, Nathan went to public school in the States for a few months of first grade and for all of fourth grade. He went to Christ Church Episcopal School in Greenville, South Carolina for ninth grade.

Instead of going to Stony Brook for high school as Linette had, Nathan chose to go to Woodstock School in India. He found India to be very different from Thailand and quite a culture shock. But he was able to be home each year not only for summer break but also for a long Christmas/winter break. I went with him to school when he enrolled and was there for his graduation, but Phil was unable to go either time. He had fully intended to attend Nathan's graduation but came down with pyelonephritis and was too ill to travel. Nathan graduated at the height of a Pakistan-India conflict, when US nationals and other westerners were encouraged to leave India. I was one of only three white people on the plane going over, and the planes returning were booked solid for several days. When we left Woodstock School we were in a taxi where the driver spoke no English. The original driver had stopped along the way and we were handed over to another driver. He took a different way to the airport than I was familiar with and as the time got closer and closer to departure time and it didn't look to me like we were anywhere near the airport, I began to get worried that we wouldn't arrive in time to catch our plane, and then what would we do? But we arrived in plenty of time.

The first time we had gone to India, I had foolishly taken an unregistered taxi at the airport (something we routinely did in Thailand because it was cheaper). The driver said the way to our hotel was blocked, and he took us on a rambling journey through Delhi, eventually dropping us off at a small restaurant. The restaurant owner kindly drove us to our hotel (without experiencing any roadblocks) and warned us in the future to only take registered taxis. I don't to this day know if the taxi driver had originally planned to harm us or not, but I thank God for keeping us safe!

When they began college, neither Linette nor Nathan had any trouble adjusting academically. Both were more sophisticated in their understanding of world events than their peers, but somewhat behind socially. However, they did well and eventually made good friends and did not experience much of the turmoil missionary kids sometimes feel when starting college in their "home" country.

When we went to Thailand, we knew Phil would be the only doctor at the hospital, but the mission board assured us they were looking for a second doctor to help out. Unfortunately, that second doctor never materialized (until about twelve years later). A newsletter written in 1985 stated:

> In the last several years we had known of three doctors who had
>
> applied or inquired about coming to work, but for various reasons
>
> none of the doctors had been appointed to help out.

Rightly or wrongly, I felt somewhat betrayed by the mission board. My resentment increased when the mission board, without asking us, paid for two medical students to come over for six weeks or so. Medical students were sometimes as much a hindrance as a help, since there was only a limited amount they could do on their own and required a lot of time from the doctor to help them find things they could do. These two were especially troublesome to me. They complained about their food and lodging, monopolized Phil at mealtimes, and I felt took advantage of the local villagers by stopping by to visit them, often at mealtimes when they would be fed. One evening when they were supposed to show up at our house for supper, they didn't come. They had borrowed motorcycles from someone and were out riding around. We waited a bit and then ate without them. Sometime after the table was cleared and I was at work at my desk, I heard them coming into the house. I was so annoyed at them I felt like telling them to warm up their own food (on the stove, as we didn't have a microwave until later), but God told me clearly to get up and serve them. As I did, my resentment disappeared. It turned out that after they left the hospital, they persuaded a resident doctor they knew to come work there for a stint, which he did. He was very helpful and recruited some others to come serve after him.

The 1985 newsletter continued:

Tested

Sometime early in 1984, Loes de Vos, one of the Australian missionaries here, had been sharing with us (at our weekly Sunday evening gathering) how overwork and pressure were causing her to become tense, easily upset, depressed, and joyless. She said she felt God had been telling her that this was not the way He wanted her to live and that such overwork, even for a seemingly good cause, was nothing more nor less than sin—specifically the sin of pride, of feeling oneself to be indispensable. All of us at the meeting identified with the pressures of overwork and a discussion followed on the solution to the problem… A volunteer who was present at the time suggested that we just pray to God to send more people to help in the medical work. I must confess to having felt just a bit cynical at this point. It seemed as though we had prayed and prayed during our first term here that God would send a second doctor to help us. Although we did get a doctor in time to allow us to go on furlough, and she had agreed to stay on an extra year after our return, a brutal attempt on her life forced her to discontinue her work here as of September 1983. [This was the same doctor who was rushed to hospital in Bangkok around the time that Nathan was born, described by Melba earlier. For more detail, see the account by Jan Vertigan/Yawan of the attack on Dr. Lois Visscher in chapter 8.] … We didn't know of any more prospects in the near future. I was very discouraged at the thought of another term with no (or only very sporadic) help for Phil. Maybe the others prayed in faith that night, but I confess my own faith was weak. Nevertheless, our prayers were answered. True, we are … no

251

nearer to having a second missionary doctor to help us here, but a continuous stream of medical help has been provided from that time on, with the exception of the rainy season last summer when weather conditions (essentially impassable roads) prevented large numbers of patients from appearing daily at the hospital anyway.

The rest of the newsletter details 7 volunteer doctors or medical students who appeared one after the other more or less out of the blue.

The newsletter also reported on several volunteer nurses who came as well as a short-term volunteer bookkeeper:

We hadn't known any of these people might be coming at the time we prayed. Their help has been of tremendous benefit to our family. In addition to a lighter workload, we've been able to arrange vacations last year and this for the time we wanted [the hot season so we could take advantage of some cabins in the mountains where it was cooler]... and Phil has had time to help supervise the relocation of the hospital at the new site. And later this month, he will for the first time be able to attend a medical conference to acquire the continuing medical education credits that he needs to keep his US medical license current. Truly our God is able to do exceedingly abundantly above all that we ask or think (Ephesians 3:20).

Although that newsletter ended on a triumphant note, I still had not completely learned my lesson about God's ability to provide for us. More and more patients began coming to the hospital as the years went by and I feared the constant work pressure would be bad for Phil's health. My heart became bitter towards God and the mission board for not doing more to help us, and I resolved to keep a daily record of exactly how many hours Phil spent daily on medical work at the hospital so I could document that he was overworked. I diligently kept track of when he left in the morning, when he came home for lunch, when he went back, and when he was done for the day. I also tried to record the amount of time he spent there on evenings, nights, and on Sundays. This required Phil's cooperation since I was often asleep when he was called out. I became an added stress to Phil by bugging him about how many hours he had been gone each time. I don't remember how long I kept the record, but I do remember the weekly totals were often near or over eighty hours a week. I think the longest time was 83 hours. Eventually I was able to repent of my bitterness and quit my obsessive record-keeping.

At first, when we had volunteer medical people, they lived with us and shared in all our meals. Later, they were given a place of their own to stay, and only ate breakfast and the evening meal with us. They then became a real source of pleasure to me, not only for the help they provided but also for the opportunity to learn about their backgrounds. One had worked on a nuclear submarine before enrolling in medical school. One had been a competitive figure skater in Japan and shared the practice rink with the Japanese Olympic champion. One had donated her bone marrow to her brother who had leukemia. One, son of missionary parents, had lived hidden in the jungles in Burma for years after the missionaries were told to leave the country. Others had been in the Peace Corps. A medical student from northern England wrote in advance of coming, asking what kind of English the hospital people spoke: was it American English or British English? She had a strong northern English accent, but did not appear to have any trouble understanding our "American English." Phil, however, sometimes had trouble understanding her accent.

A Japanese eye doctor came to the hospital to teach Phil some eye surgery. He could remember as a boy during World War II watching Allied bombers drop incendiary bombs on his homeland. Partway through his volunteer stint at the KRCH, a group of Dutch former prisoners of war stopped by at the hospital for an unannounced visit. They were old men by this time. They had worked on the Siam Burma

Railway ("Death Railway") during World War II as forced laborers under their Japanese taskmasters. The ex-POWs' interest in the Kwai River Christian Hospital probably lay in the fact that the hospital had originally been built at a site not far from the bed of the old Death Railway and bore the name of the river along which the Death Railway had been built. All sides were gracious and forgiving at this potentially awkward encounter.

Since several of the missionaries were from Australia, we became quite conversant with the "Aussie" way of saying things. When Nathan was in first grade in the United States, he spoke in what his teacher called a British accent.

I loved to listen to the two women who visited from Northern Ireland speaking in their delightful Irish lilt. There was a Jewish woman who fixed special Sabbath bread for us each Friday evening, and medical students who taught us some Scottish dances. Several volunteers brought musical instruments with them. There were volunteer doctors, medical students, and nurses from Canada, England, Ireland, Scotland, Australia, New Zealand, Singapore, Sweden and India, and from all parts of the US. Our children also enjoyed the chance of getting to interact with people from many different backgrounds. The volunteers often participated with us and the other missionaries in periodic movie nights or game nights. Several volunteers came more than once, and it was always fun to see them again.

Christmas time in Thailand was an interesting experience. December 25 is not a national holiday, so schools and businesses are open that day. In our early years, there weren't many Christmas decorations up at the stores in Bangkok. Earlier in December, in honor of the King's birthday, buildings all over the city displayed colored lights, many more so than for Christmas.

By the end of our time in Thailand, stores had large Christmas displays and played Christmas carols over the loudspeaker systems. We heard more Christmas songs with a gospel message in stores in Buddhist Thailand than we do now in "Christian" America. December was a busy month in Sangkhla. On the last night of November, there would be an evening church service that lasted until midnight to celebrate the start of "Sweet December." Various groups would go caroling around the mission and in the villages around Christmas time. Phil was never particularly happy to be awakened from sleep by the carolers, but the village people seemed to appreciate it. Each department of the mission would have its own Christmas celebration on a different day, so we often went to several celebrations. On the evening before the mission-wide celebration, someone would slaughter a pig and volunteers would stay up all night cooking rice and packaging it up in banana-leaf bundles, and roasting pork, and making preparations for the curries to be served. It was interesting to see them using a boat oar to stir the food in huge woks over a fire. Nathan and Melodie really enjoyed watching the pig-slaughtering. The whole village would be invited the next day and everyone would be fed lunch. Sports and games would follow. Christmas was always celebrated together as a community, rather than family by family. Sometimes it was hard to find time to get together as a family and open our gifts from each other. In 1994, Phil wrote to Linette, away at school, about the hospital Christmas celebration that year:

Christmas at the KRCH was a marathon of a celebration as usual. We picked the 20th of December as a suitable day to celebrate Christmas: suitable mainly because it was a day that no other department was planning to celebrate Christmas, nor was it a prenatal clinic day or an under-fives clinic day. The day began with a 6:30 AM sunrise service on mats in the front yard of the hospital. This was followed immediately by a hurried breakfast of coffee, tea, and … fried kanoms [sweets]. Scarcely had we downed our fill of these when Lea [head nurse] summoned us with her bullhorn to assemble for the parade. The drummers began thumping away on their drums as the red team fell in on one side and the green team on the other. [The hospital workers were divided into two teams to compete in games later in the day.] The procession began at the front of the hospital and…ended at the back entrance of the hospital. … Christmas at the hospital continued with presents for the patients [practical gifts such as soap or toothpaste, handed out by one of the hospital workers or a visiting medical student while the rest of the staff sang Christmas carols with gusto to the patients in each ward], then games for the patients, a gift exchange for the staff, followed by a dinner for the staff, and finally the evening program, which started about 7:45 pm and continued until sometime after midnight. I only stayed until about 11:30 pm! In fact, a good part of "Christmas Day" I was busy in the hospital taking care of patients.

The evening program was a "talent show" with participants from the hospital and village communities. Some of the entries were really good, some were terrible, and many were funny. I always looked forward each year to the "talent show."

Some of my fondest memories are about Christmas. There was the time when Linette, as a 2-year-old, saw a manger display in a hotel in Bangkok and spontaneously picked up the baby Jesus and kissed him. There was the time I was not feeling well and was alone in the house while Phil and Linette were at some sort of Christmas celebration, and I heard the carolers stop underneath the house and sing several songs. There was the time two of the neighbor kids happened to see the lights on our Christmas tree and gazed at them in wonder, even trying to blow out the lights like candles. There was the time we hadn't received any mail for about six weeks until the postman happened to bring all the accumulated mail on Christmas Day. My best present that day was opening all the many letters we had been sent. And there was the year Nathan carefully recorded all the different caroling groups and made cassette tapes of the songs for all of us to remember.

Tested

In a 1986 newsletter I wrote about a young baby our family took turns taking care of. "Jenny" was born in the hospital weighing a pound and a half, and her mother decided she wouldn't be able to care for her. Until she was about 14 weeks old (and had attained a weight of over 4 pounds) she stayed at the hospital in an incubator, was given an enriched oxygen atmosphere to breathe and was fed by feeding tube. At that age she was strong enough that it was no longer necessary or desirable to keep her in the hospital, and various members of the hospital staff, including our family, took turns keeping her in our homes for a night at a time. Linette loved having a young baby at home (Nathan not so much) and begged to adopt her. According to Thai law, however, that would not be possible, since families with two or more children were ineligible to adopt. We had hoped a local family could be found to care for her, but no one chose to accept that responsibility. She was eventually processed through the Holt Foundation and adopted by a Lutheran minister and his wife from the United States. Her family kept in periodic touch with us, and after her high school graduation she and her adoptive mother returned to her birthplace to meet her mother and grandmother and siblings. She has by now graduated from college with a degree in graphic arts.

The Kwai River Christian Hospital was located in western Thailand, not far from the Thai-Burma (Myanmar) border. During our early days there, several of the ethnic groups in Burma were fighting against the Burmese government. The two main groups that lived in the Burmese territory bordering our area of Thailand were the Mon and the Karen. After some years, both the Mon and the Karen armies signed a truce with the Burmese government and the fighting lessened. No longer were land-mine injuries coming to the hospital every month. However, in about 1988, when our children were about 12 years old, 5 years old, and 7 months old, the Mon and Karen soldiers began fighting each other. ... One of our prayer requests in our September 1988 newsletter was about this situation:

As in so many other parts of the world, there is political unrest in this otherwise peaceful "jungle" area. ... Until recently, the fighting was confined to Burma and affected us only in that the hospital was often called on to treat "war injuries" involving Karen and Mon soldiers as well as civilians unlucky enough to step on a land mine left in their fields by one or another of the warring armies. Recently, however, the fighting has taken a more ominous turn. Some of the Karen and Mon soldiers have begun fighting each other over control of Three Pagodas Pass, the town about twenty miles from here that is situated right on the Thai-Burma border on the trade route between the two countries. Some of this fighting has taken place on the Thai side of the border, and the Thai police have now blockaded the road south from the area, not allowing anyone to enter or leave. A patient who with difficulty managed to make his way through the blockade to the hospital said there is a lot of suffering among the villagers of the area. Many have left their homes and are living as best they can in the fields— and this, in the middle of the rainy season. Many are sick with malaria or other diseases and are unable to leave to receive medical care…

The guns [artillery] from the fighting could be heard from our house, and the mission organization discussed contingency evacuation plans for the missionaries in our area should the fighting escalate. We were told to always have a suitcase packed and ready to grab with essential papers and other things we would need in it. If we did have to evacuate, the hope was we could follow the road south into the provincial capital, but there was some talk that we might have to escape (illegally) through Burma and so we were advised to have several hundred dollars in American money with us, which might be more useful in emergencies than Thai money. Fortunately, the fighting died down after a few weeks and we never had to put the plans into action.

Sometime during our second term, I believe—I don't remember the exact date—I faced a mental health crisis. For several years I had occasionally experienced short-lived bouts of depression that seemed to come out of the blue. I learned how to manage the depression so that it didn't significantly affect my life. But one time I developed a much worse major depression that I could do little to control. Although nothing was particularly bothering me at the time, one morning when I woke up, I couldn't seem to get out of bed. When I would finally get up and try to interact with people, the smallest irritation, which normally wouldn't bother me, would set me off and I would break down in tears or express myself in anger. I knew I was acting irrationally but couldn't seem to stop. I felt like I was a failure as a missionary, wife, and mother, and no amount of reassurance or encouragement from anyone helped me feel better. I spent most of my day in bed dozing or reading a very light romance novel or murder mystery—that was the only kind of reading material I could at all concentrate on. I was able to do my bookkeeping work for up to 30 minutes at a time, but no more, and then, only if nobody talked to me. I didn't feel particularly sad, but just had no pleasure in doing anything or imagining doing anything. I couldn't seem to read the Bible or pray. God seemed very distant, but I couldn't think of any particular sin I needed to repent of. This went on day after day with no lightening of my mood. Our household help were able to look after the children, as I had no patience with them at all. I didn't want anyone to talk to me; I just wanted to be left alone. There was some thought that we might have to leave Thailand, but I didn't want to do that because it would just make my sense of failure worse. I felt as though Phil and the children would be better off if I were dead, but I was too lethargic to seriously consider suicide. Phil was not at that time very well-versed in psychiatry and didn't know what was wrong with me. I remember telling him one day I wanted him to devote thirty minutes a day thinking about my problem. He could pray or read his medical books or whatever he thought might help, as long as he did something to help me because I was desperate.

He ended up studying his psychiatry books and came to the conclusion that I had clinical depression. That didn't seem right to me, because I didn't feel sad, but I agreed to try taking an antidepressant and after a few weeks began to feel better. Because this episode was not my first history of depression (although all the others had been minor), it was decided that I needed to continue the medication for life. It has now been over thirty years since that time and I have been essentially stable ever since except for a few minor flare-ups from time to time.

By 1987 we had a daughter and a son and considered our family complete. We were scheduled for a furlough in 1987 and Phil planned to get a vasectomy then. As we were preparing to leave, we gave away all our baby supplies. Another missionary was then pregnant with her first child, and happy to take what we no longer needed. After my menstrual period was more than a week late, I turned in a urine specimen to the hospital but was somewhat relieved to find the pregnancy test was negative.

However, my period didn't start and a week or so later I submitted another specimen. This one was positive. The next morning, I woke up feeling sick. I thought it was psychological morning sickness now that I knew I was pregnant, but as the day went on and I developed a fever and headache, I realized I was ill. We were supposed to leave Thailand for furlough in a few days and had hotels booked in Italy, England, and Scotland on the way back to the US. We couldn't postpone the trip because our visas were due to run out the day after we left. A lab tech from the hospital came to the house to take a blood sample to test for malaria. It was negative, but I took a dose of quinine just in case. The next day I started spotting. I went to the hospital to have a pelvic exam to see if it looked like I was having a miscarriage. If so, I wanted to have a D&C before we left, so I wouldn't have to worry about aborting on the airplane or in a foreign country. One of the doctors taking over for Phil during his furlough did the pelvic exam and decided that the pregnancy might still be viable so he didn't do the D&C. I breathed a sigh of relief when we left Italy for England, knowing that now if I miscarried, at least I wouldn't have to deal with a foreign language! The spotting continued for about a week and then stopped. When we got back to the US, I had an ultrasound done and everything looked normal. I began to get excited about having a new child.

Tested

This was not the first time we had traveled from Thailand while one or more of us were feeling ill. I remember one time when Phil was just starting to get over some kind of sickness and I had just become sick when we had to leave. Riding in an airplane on a long trip and going through customs, etc. is no fun when you are feeling ill! On the way to Europe, Linette also became ill on the airplane, but she recovered much more quickly than Phil or I did. We had been scheduled to spend a few days in Italy, but neither of us really felt like much sight-seeing. Nonetheless, either Phil or I would take Linette with us for a few hours each day to see some important site, and the other one would stay home in bed and look after Nathan.

Fortunately, we escaped many of the endemic diseases of Thailand. Phil and I did both get malaria (once each) but neither we nor the children got dengue fever or other tropical illnesses.

Melodie was born in 1988, in Ashland, Kentucky, where we were living on furlough. She ended up being an unusual brow presentation and labor was slightly prolonged. Because she had swallowed some meconium, she went to the neonatal intensive care unit as a precaution but was brought back to me the next day. When the pediatrician had examined her, he told me her head circumference was at the fifth percentile. I thought he said fiftieth percentile and wasn't concerned. When subsequent measurements were done, it became obvious that her head was indeed small, but at first it seemed to be growing at a normal rate, so we didn't hesitate to return to Thailand when she was three months old. At first, she seemed to be meeting all the usual baby milestones, and was even earlier than Linette and Nathan in such things as turning over and looking toward a voice. But by 6 months her growth and development had slowed. She seemed to have a cold frequently, and I hoped that her delayed development was just because of that. But we took her to Bangkok at about seven months to be examined. The doctor did various tests to rule out known causes of microcephaly (small head), but was unable to say what had caused the problem or what the prognosis would be. Melodie was referred to an early intervention program at one of the Bangkok hospitals and we took her down there every few months to get re-evaluated and get guidance on how to stimulate her development.

Melba McDaniel

When Melodie was 10 months old, my father in Kentucky had a stroke and died about a week later. Because of problems with communication, I didn't even learn about the stroke until some days later when Phil brought word back from Bangkok. The next morning, we drove to the nearest city where there was a telephone, and I called and learned he had died shortly before. There was no way I could return to the US for his funeral, but we agreed I would bring Melodie with me for a visit with my mother as soon as I could get a ticket. Having a new granddaughter to play with helped lessen my mother's grief some, and I was able to help her with some of her post-funeral responsibilities. Since I planned to be in Kentucky for a month, we arranged to have Melodie seen by the early intervention team there. We had noticed that although none of her limbs was paralyzed, she seldom used the left side of her body. For example, when picking up a block she would always use her right hand even if her left hand was closer to the block. And when she took a bath, she would kick only with her right foot. The team tested Melodie in four areas: gross motor, fine motor, speech, and social development and she was behind in all areas, but not by more than a month or two. At that time (when Melodie was about 11 months old) she could neither stand nor crawl. She could scoot forward, pulling herself forward with just her arms but not using her legs at all. The interventionist suggested certain things I could do to help stimulate her, and we returned to Thailand and tried to put into practice the suggestions from both the Bangkok and Kentucky teams.

Around this time, a volunteer from Australia came to supervise the installation of a village water system that was being funded by the Baptist Union of Sweden. He had a daughter with Down Syndrome, who was at that time in a regular high school class and doing satisfactorily. As a baby, she had been extremely behind in her development. The family spent some time in the United States at the Institutes for the Achievement of Human Potential in Philadelphia, Pennsylvania. The staff there taught her parents an intensive and time-consuming program of neuro-developmental stimulation to do with her daily, which her parents (with the help of volunteers) followed for months and months back home in Australia. She made tremendous strides on the program. I had earlier heard about the Institutes in some

262

library books I had read before we went to Thailand and thought their program would perhaps help Melodie.

I made an appointment at the Institutes to take a one-week course there designed to teach parents how to evaluate and design a program to work with children with neurological disorders. We couldn't do the program they recommended twelve hours a day, but we probably managed to get roughly half of each day's work done. One key part of the program, which the Australian volunteer had already taught us about, was called "patterning." With the child in a prone position, her head and limbs would be moved rhythmically in a simulated crawling pattern. It took three people to "pattern" Melodie: one to move her head, one to move her right side, and one to move her left side. As we patterned her, we sang Sunday school songs and nursery rhymes. Phil and I utilized medical volunteers and Linette (then thirteen years old) as the third person. Patterning had to be done 4 to 6 times a day. Right away we noticed improvement in Melodie's ability to crawl, although she never did learn to do it perfectly.

The most time-consuming part of the program was having her practice crawling on her tummy (and later, crawling on hands and knees, walking, and running). I would start her in the back bedroom and have her crawl (on a wooden floor) all the way across the house diagonally into the kitchen and then turn around and crawl back. Naturally, she often resisted the crawling, and so we constantly had to invent new ways to motivate her and to crawl along with her giving her constant encouragement along the way. For a long time, one of her favorite motivators was eating a raisin at the end of each crawl. As she got older, Phil would sometimes ride his bike down the dirt roads and have her run after him.

Another part of the program that required a lot of time-consuming preparation was "picture cards."

We would buy pre-cut pieces of poster board about twelve inches square and then glue a single large picture on the front of each card. The pictures were often cut from magazines or calendars in such a way that all the background detail was omitted and just the object itself was glued to the card. These picture cards were organized into groups (breeds of dogs, flags of countries, presidents of the United States, paintings by Renoir, etc.), and she would be shown ten pictures at a rate of about one picture per second while I named the object or person in the picture. When the first set was finished, another set would be shown, until 5 or 10 sets were shown at one sitting. After each showing, the picture sets would be shuffled so that the next time she saw them, the pictures would be in a different order, and after she had seen one picture several times a day for a week, it would be removed and replaced by a different picture in the same group.

After a couple of months, the original pictures would be shown again, this time adding one fact for each picture, and later two facts, etc. Collecting the pictures and cutting and pasting them took hours of my time (and the time of many volunteers). Eventually, I ended up with over a thousand picture cards. The picture cards were especially valuable to Melodie in helping her learn to speak. Most of her early words were names of the picture cards. One of the cards was a picture of Georges Clemenceau, the French leader during World War 1. For some reason she especially liked this card (people were usually her favorite objects to look at) and she is probably the only toddler in the world with "Clemenceau" as one of her first hundred spoken words! Speech—which in early evaluations had been one of her weakest areas—became one of her greatest strengths. She had both a good vocabulary and good enunciation and could form sentences appropriately, although we realized later, she didn't always understand what she was saying. She was very good at parroting other people, and in addition to English, could speak Thai properly, Karen properly, and Thai with a Karen accent, depending on who she was speaking to. Of all our children, she was the most gifted at speaking the local languages.

Two areas where she did not improve much were in fine motor skills, especially with her left hand, and in reading. Despite hours of effort, she continued to have left-sided weakness and did not learn to read or write.

A 1993 newsletter explained how I was able to spend so much time with Melodie:

Nathan was ready for kindergarten, and Linette was in the seventh grade. With teaching them and doing the hospital bookkeeping, I didn't see how I was going to be able to work with Melodie, too. I envisioned perhaps having a volunteer come out to help with

Melodie, but when I walked into the mission office [one day] ...
the mission secretary asked me first thing if the hospital would
have any need for a volunteer who knew bookkeeping and office
procedure! A woman from Australia with those qualifications had
applied for refugee work, and since there was no need in that area,
he wondered if he might offer the Kwai River Christian Hospital
as an alternative. We and she were happy to accept the offer, and
in the summer of 1989, Maureen Feaviour came to Thailand as a
volunteer. She soon succeeded me as hospital bookkeeper, and I
was free to devote more time to Melodie's needs. Maureen's
original commitment was for one year, but at the end of that time
she agreed to extend for another two years in order to set up the
bookkeeping work on computer and to train a national to take over
the bookkeeping on her departure.

As Melodie became school aged, I began trying to homeschool her.
I felt quite competent in homeschooling my older children, but I had no
experience at all in working with a child with special needs. I was able
to use a regular curriculum for some things, and obtained workbooks
for skills in which she was subpar but had to heavily modify other
lessons. Sometimes I would get discouraged and run out of ideas on
what to do for her, but it seemed that whenever that happened, before
long the Holy Spirit would inspire me with new ideas to try. She
seemed to mostly understand the concepts of history and science that I
taught her orally (at least in the primary grades), but reading was
always a struggle. She could recognize many words by sight and
seemed to be just on the verge of reading and then lose interest. I would
wait for a time and then try a new approach, but nothing worked. Also,
it seemed as though her abilities to do things would come and go. Some
days she could do something fairly easily, and other days she seemed
not to understand at all how to do the exact same task. In retrospect, I

wish I had pushed less hard on trying to teach her to read, and concentrated more on things in which she was more interested.

Melodie and I were fortunate enough to have volunteers work with us from time to time. Several times doctors who came to help out at the hospital would bring their wives with them, and the wives graciously agreed to help out several hours a week with Melodie. Also, in the summers, Linette was a huge help. As Linette wrote in a 1996 newsletter:

Since I have been spending four or five hours a day teaching my sister, Melodie, and my brother, Nathan, on my summer breaks since I was 15, I have sometimes thought that I really do have a summer job; I just don't get paid for it! But few summer jobs could give me the same kind of reward that I get from being an instrument in my siblings' development, particularly Melodie's. Since Nathan has recently started Chiang Mai International School in the north of Thailand, and Melodie is attending a local special education school half-time, they both needed less home-school attention this summer term than previously. So, when I was offered the chance to teach English to a group of local high school students four times a week, I was pleased to be helpful outside of my immediate family.

Melodie was able to profit from the local program for special needs children for several years. She was taught in Thai and wore a typical Thai school uniform with her name (in Thai) embroidered on the front of her blouse. But as she got older, the school was not able to be very helpful for her, and she was back with me teaching her full-time again. The following is from our April 1999 newsletter:

Tested

Phil, Melba, Nathan and Melodie plan to return to Thailand for four more years on or about June 10. We hope that Linette, who is now working on her master's degree in linguistics at the University of Oregon, will be able to join us in early July and stay for the remainder of the summer. We would appreciate your remembering in prayer: Melodie, that she may learn to enjoy her academic exercises and her developmental therapy; Nathan, as he goes off to Woodstock (boarding school) in India toward the end of July to begin tenth grade; Linette, as she tries to decide on a research topic for her master's thesis; Melba, as she perseveres with Melodie's schooling and developmental stimulation program. This requires almost superhuman patience even when the weather is fine. On hot, muggy days, the challenge can be ferocious; Phil, as he resumes patient care and administrative responsibilities at the Kwai River Christian Hospital. The known challenges are great; the unknown, likely greater still.

As you can see from the above quote, we fully intended to spend another four-year term in Thailand. But circumstances made that undesirable. As Melodie grew older, and especially as she approached puberty her "meltdowns" (behavior she exhibited when she was frustrated) grew both more frequent and more violent. She could go almost instantly from a calm demeanor to an explosion of fury, usually over things that seemed trivial to me. For example, one time while we were at a conference and were carrying our dinner plates to the tables to find a place to sit down, she decided she wanted to sit in one particular location where the table was already full, and began screaming and hitting me because I wouldn't let her sit at the table. In her meltdowns, she would hit, kick, pinch, bite, pull hair, throw things and/or tear things up. Trying to reason with her did not help at all, nor did rewards for good behavior or penalties for bad behavior make any discernible difference in her propensity for meltdowns. Eventually, she would calm down and often apologize, but I don't think she actually could remember much of what she had done. When asking her why she was saying she was sorry, she could give only vague responses. As she became physically stronger, it was harder for me to subdue her and I would often go around with bruises. I was afraid if we didn't do something soon, she would be impossible to control as she got older and would get in trouble with the law for assault. Reluctantly, we began to think about leaving Thailand and trying to find some special education programs she could attend in the United States.

When we first went to Thailand, our intention was to stay there until we retired, but now it didn't look like that would be possible. Everyone I talked to about Melodie's situation, including a psychiatrist we met at a medical conference, recommended that we return with her to the United States. And so, in 2002, shortly after Nathan graduated from high school, we left Thailand on an early furlough, not planning to return. It was especially hard on Phil to leave the country he so loved and to envision the very different ways of practicing medicine in the US, but he was willing to make the sacrifice for the well-being of his family. When we left Thailand, we had no home in the US and no immediate prospect of a job for Phil, but we trusted God to provide and he has done so abundantly.

Part 3

Hospital History in Photos

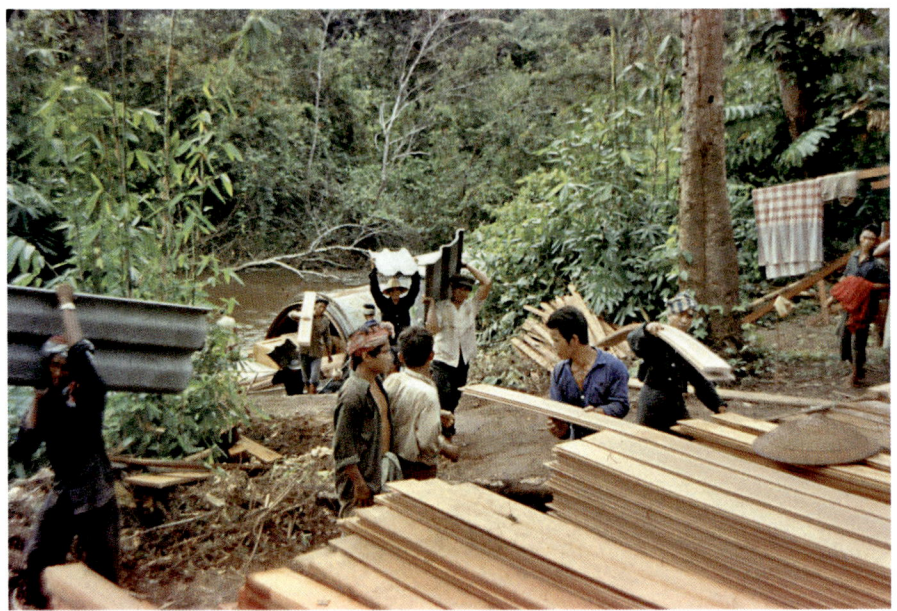

Unloading lumber and roofing from a barge that had been towed up-stream from Kanchanaburi. These were for the construction of the first two residences at what would become the Kwai River Christian Mission. (from Dr. Corpron)

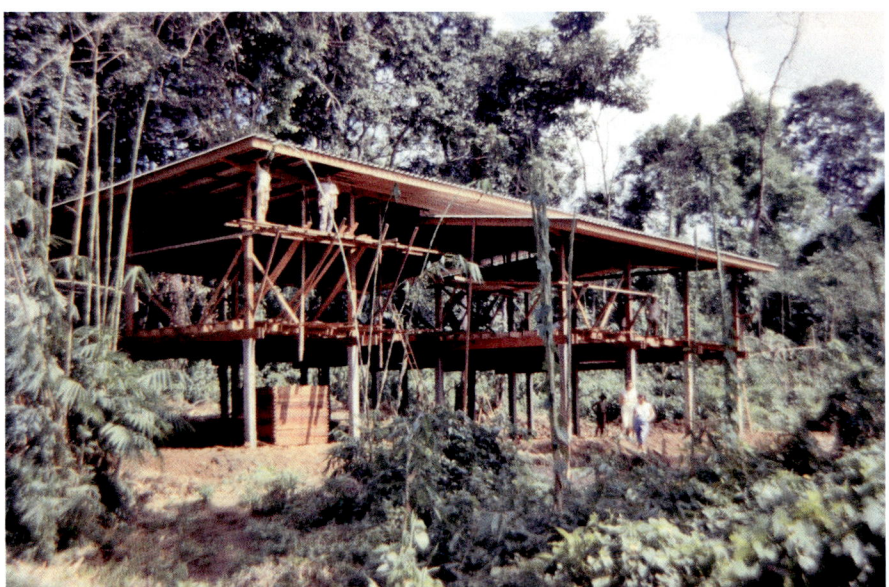

The doctor's house (also called the "Corpron House") under construction. This house—and one just like it for the Dodge family—was built by a team of builders from Kanchanaburi. (image from Dr. Doug Corpron)

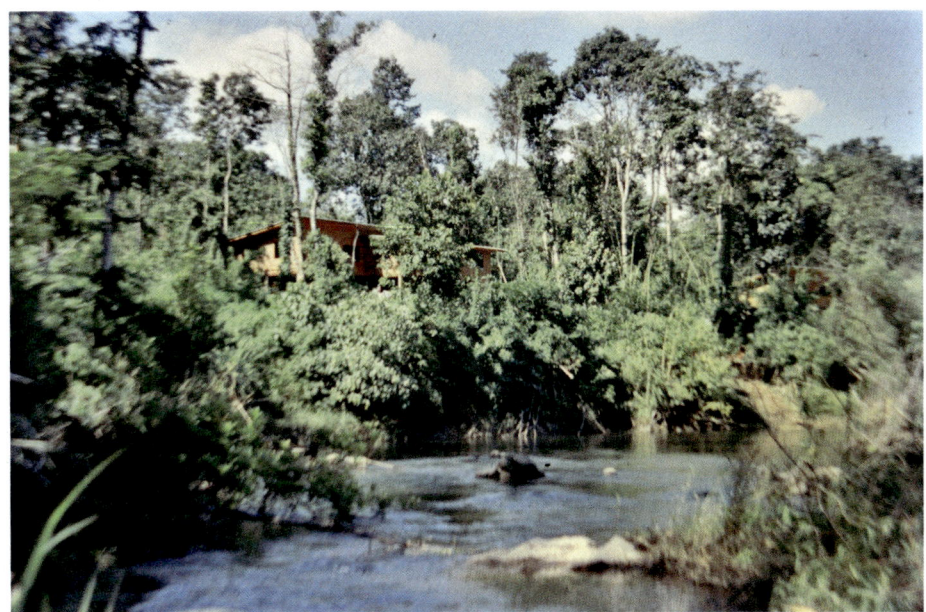

The Ranti River is flowing toward the viewer, past the newly built Dodge house (far right) and Corpron house (center), to join the River Kwai (River Khwae Noi) about 1 km downstream. (image from Dr. Doug Corpron)

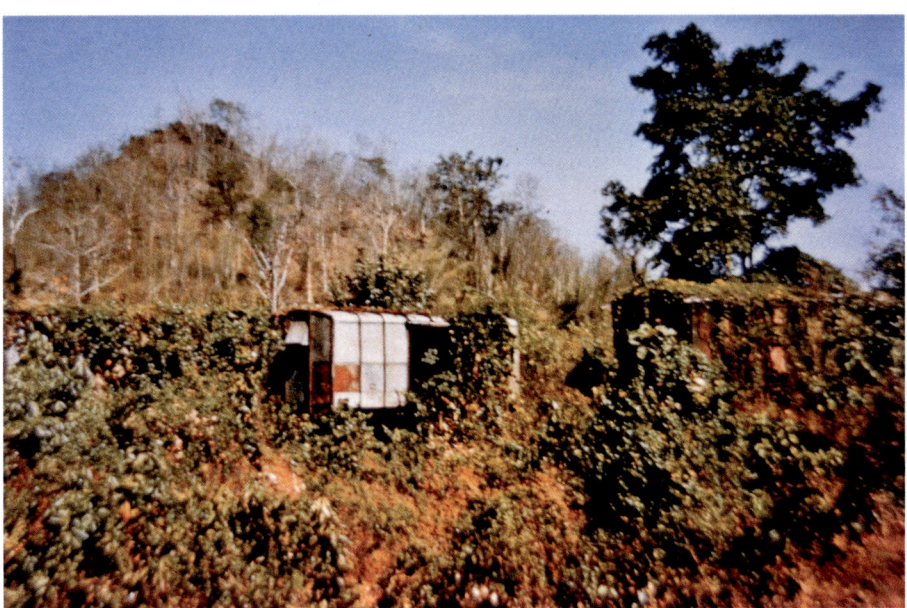

The jungle is taking over these long-abandoned railway cars from the "Death Railway" of WW II. The original site of the KRCH was a short walk from this deserted rail yard. (image from Dr. Doug Corpron)

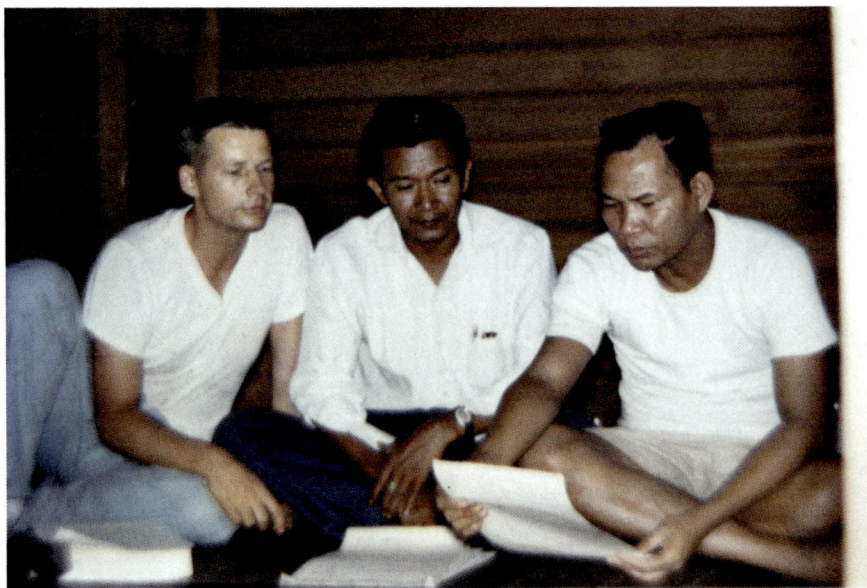

Dr. Douglas Corpron confers with two local government officials over paperwork related to the mission property. (image from Dr. Doug Corpron)

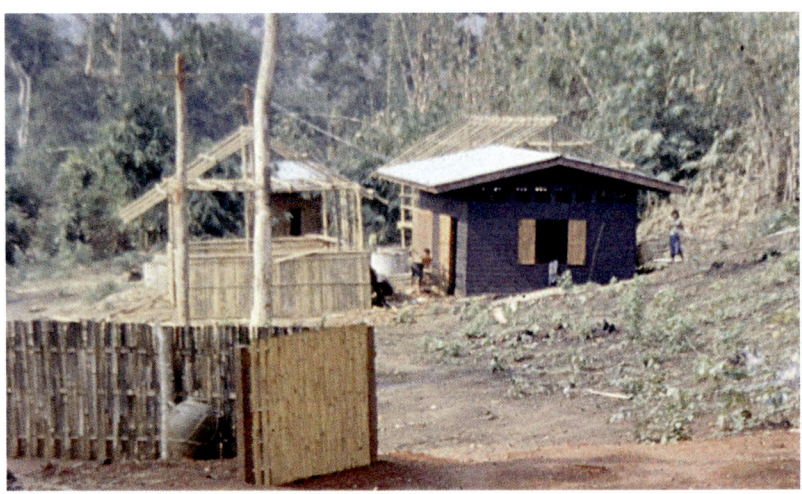

Before there was a hospital and before there was a dispensary, Dr. Corpron treated patients in the open space under his house (not shown). Mrs. Corpron was concerned about her children mingling with patients who might have TB. Completion of the hospital was still 2-3 years in the future. As a stop-gap measure, a storage shed (dark brown building above) was converted to a dispensary. The bamboo "sala" on the left became the waiting room. The structure behind the dispensary became a guest house for overnight patients. (image from Dr. Doug Corpron)

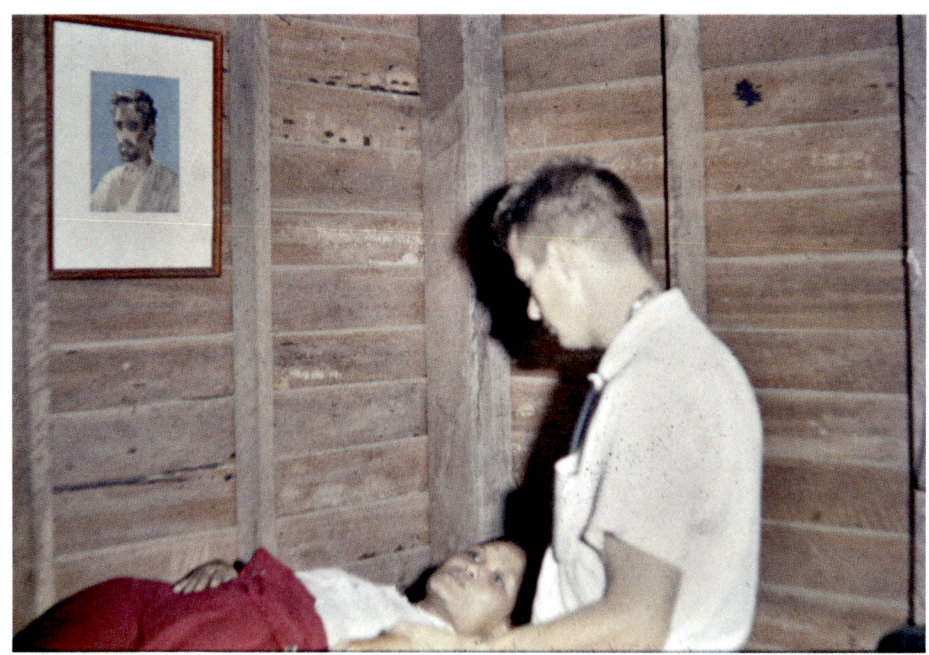

Dr. Doug Corpron examining a patient in the dispensary—a converted storage shed—in early 1960s. (image from Dr. Corpron)

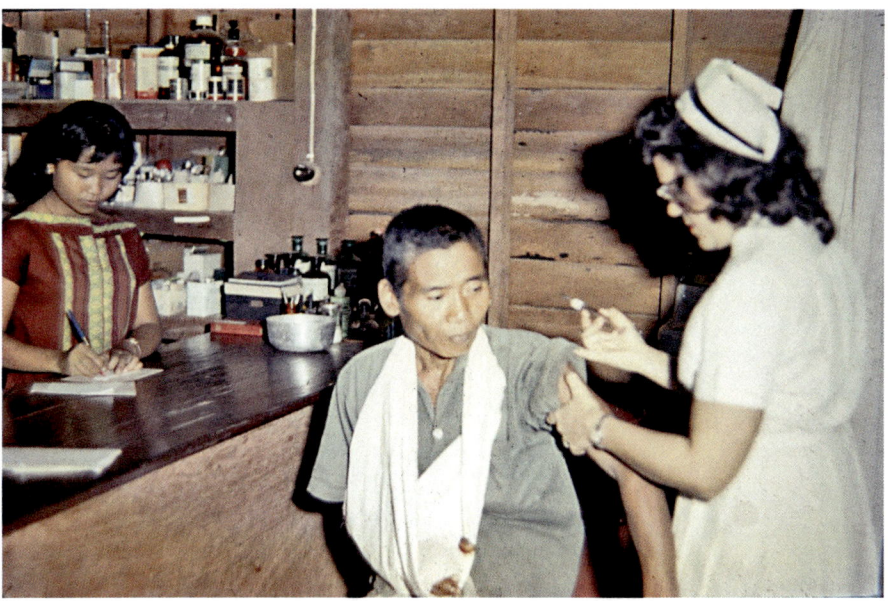

Inside the dispensary: (L to R) Sudah, patient, Winnie Dodge, RN. Sudah served as receptionist, translator for the Pwo Karen language, and general helper around the dispensary. (image from Dr. Corpron)

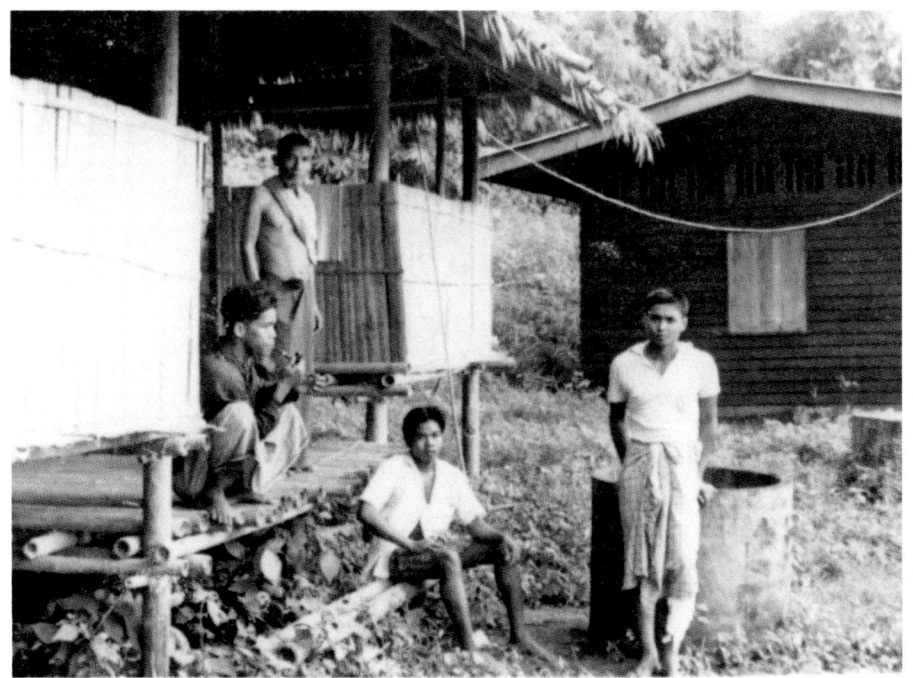

Overnight patients in bamboo-and-thatch guest house behind the dispensary.

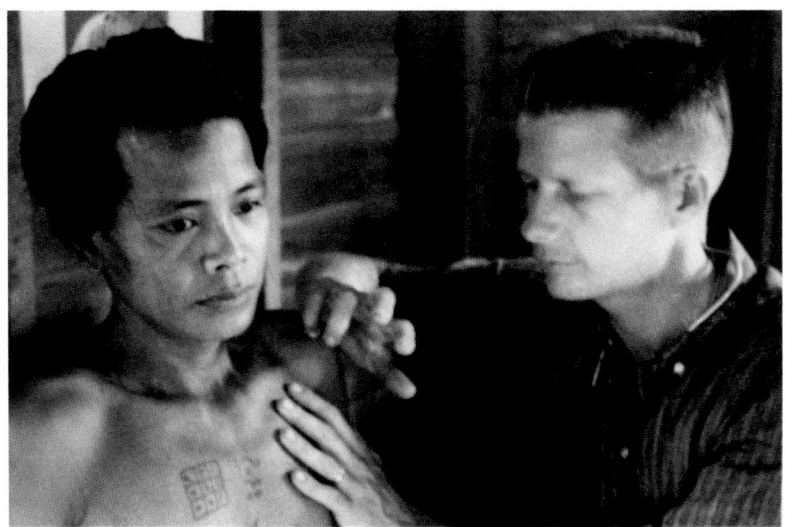

Dr. Corpron percussing the chest of a TB patient. (both images on this page from Rev. Paul Dodge)

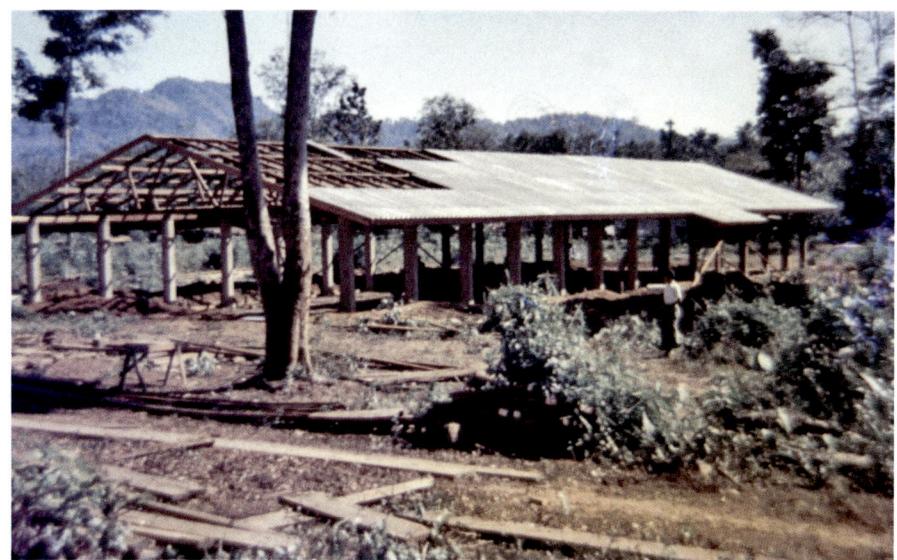

Original Kwai River Christian Hospital building under construction. Much of the building material had to be towed up from Kanchanaburi on barges. This added to expenses. Use of soil-cement blocks helped to reduce cost of construction.

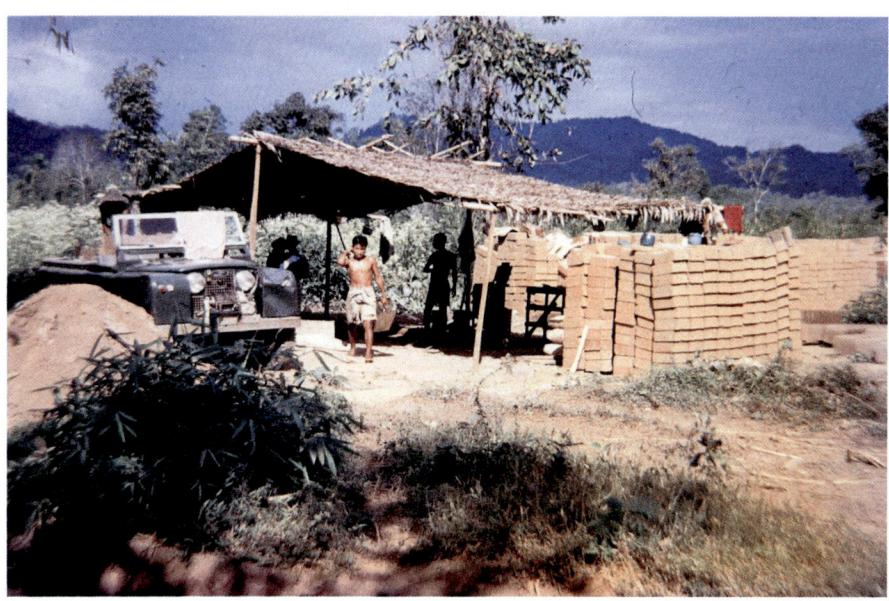

Soil-cement blocks were produced on site using a hand-operated compression device. Local laterite soil was combined with cement in a ratio of about 19-to-1 for these blocks. These held up well to testing in the river. (both images on this page from Dr. Corpron)

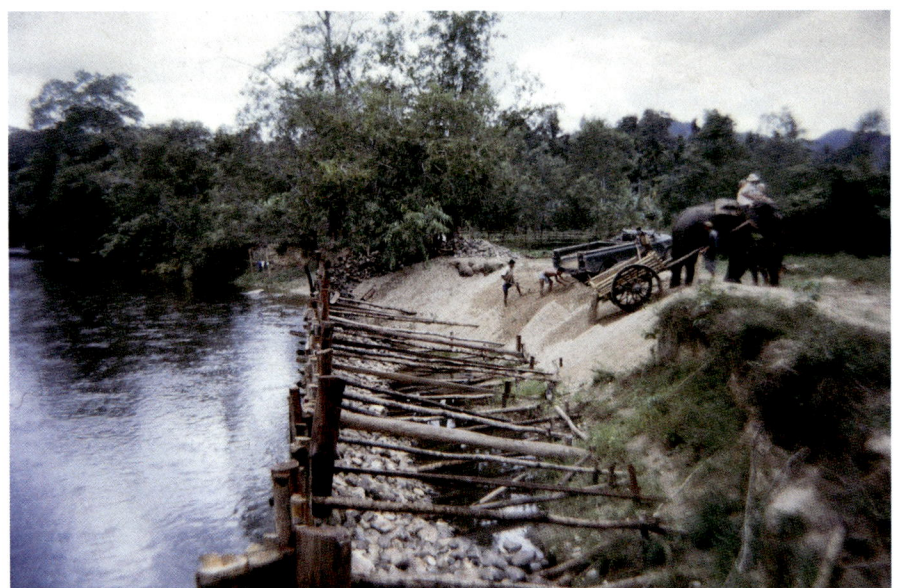

An embankment project was undertaken to prevent erosion of the mission property by the Ranti River. (image from Dr. Doug Corpron)

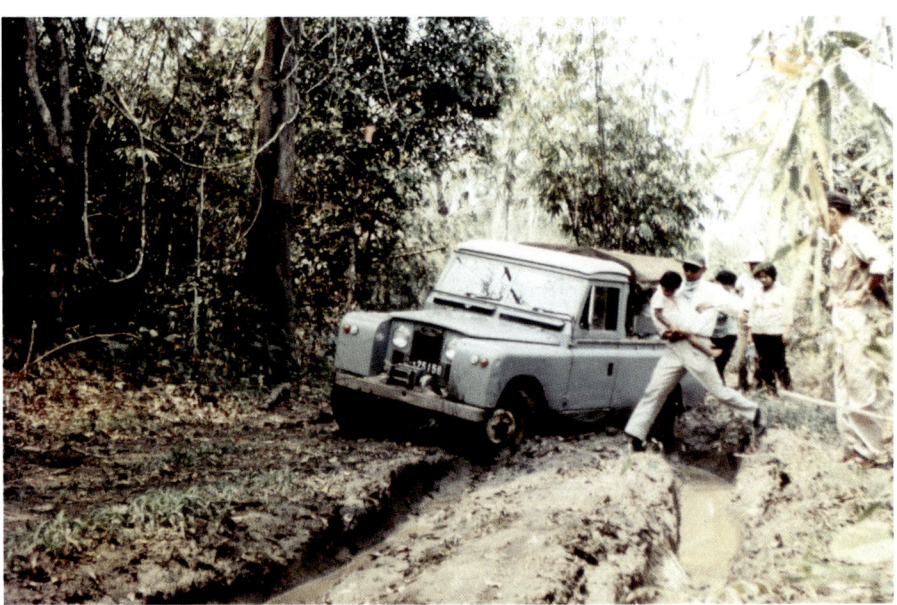

Travel was difficult and often dangerous in the early days of the Kwai River Christian Hospital. A trip from Bangkok to KRCH typically involved about 7 hours by train to Wangpo, another 7-8 hours by "long tail" boat to Takanun, and then 6-8 hours by Land Rover to Sangkhlaburi. (image from Rev. Paul Dodge)

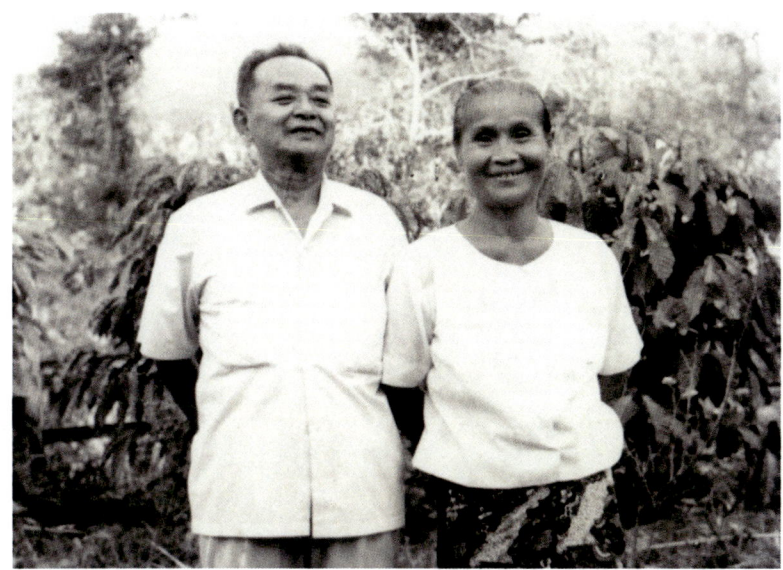

Olivepa (left) and Olivemo were key people in the history of the KRCM. They were evangelists, hostel parents, and Karen language tutors. Olivepa helped organize some of the early visits to the Telakhon (Talako). (image from Rev. Paul Dodge)

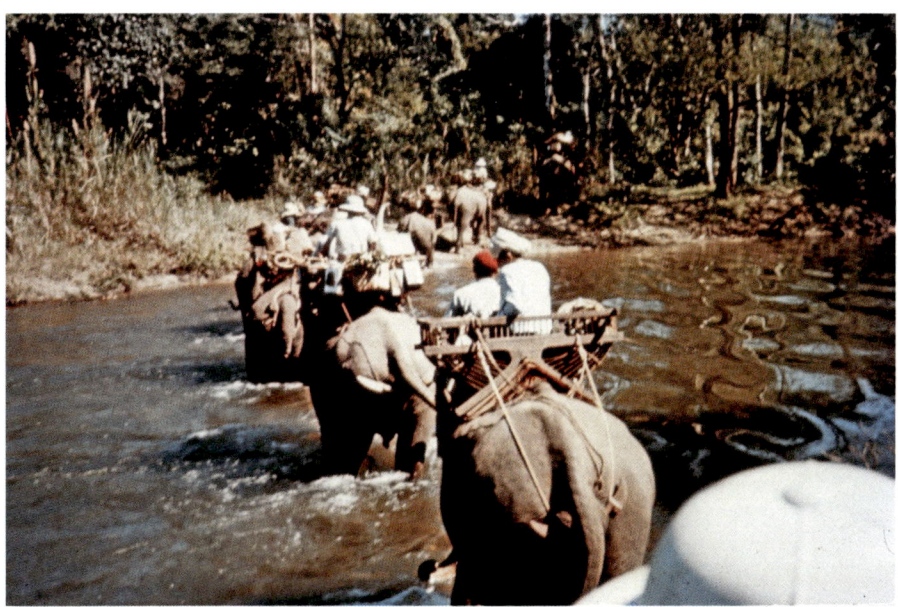

Trekking through the jungle on elephant back to visit the Talako. (image from Rev. Paul Dodge)

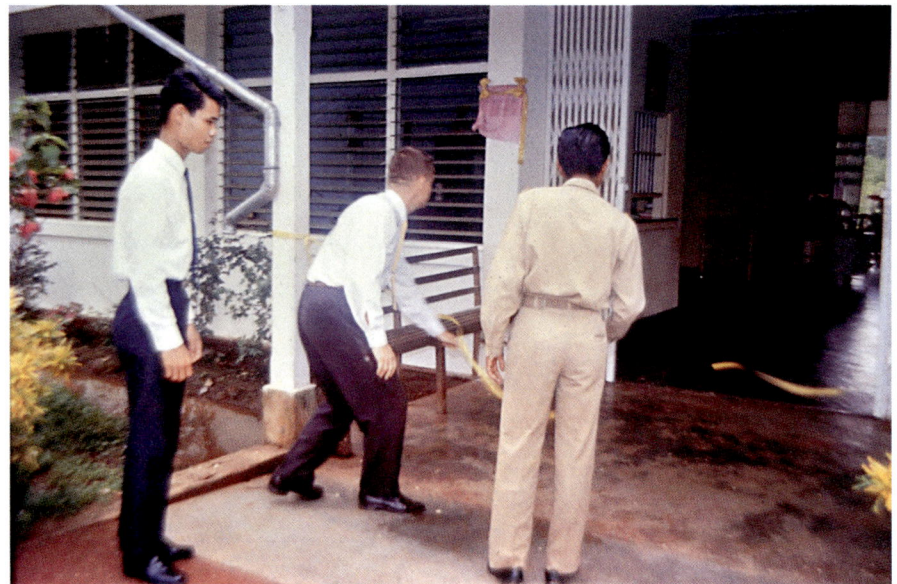

The original hospital building was officially opened on May 27, 1967, the same day that the Christian school was officially opened. The hospital building had already been in use about three years. (image from Dr. Corpron)

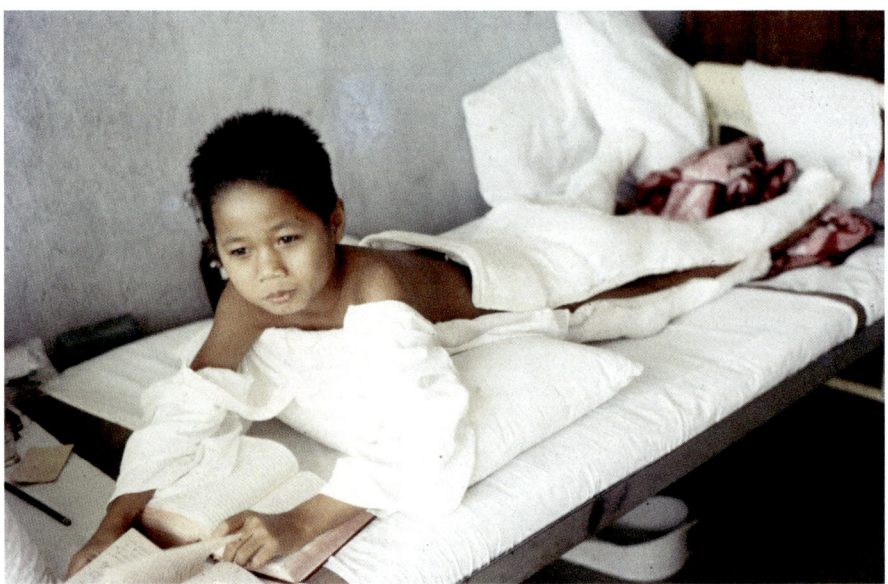

Narin in the Kwai River Christian Hospital as a boy. He had TB of the spine and was being treated in a body cast. Here he is studying the Bible and a hymnbook. (image from Rev. Paul Dodge)

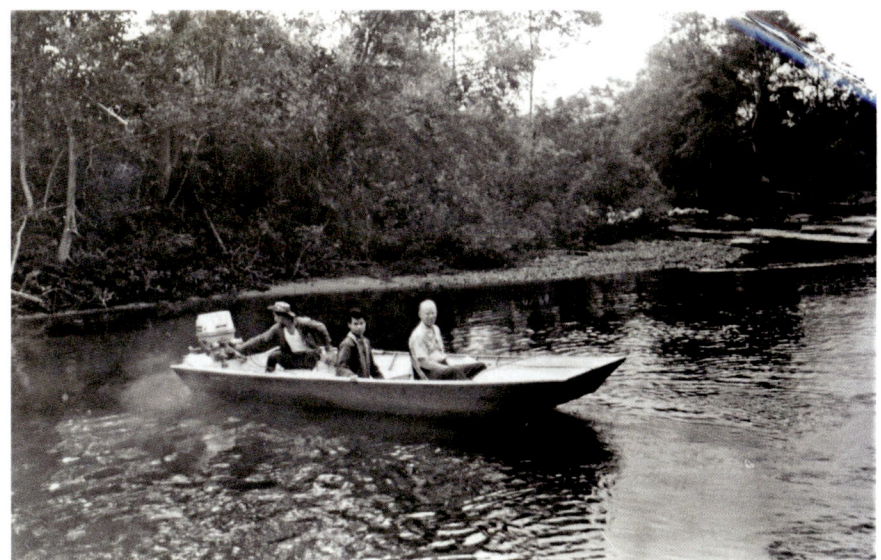

Dr. Ed McDaniel (in front) starting out on an ambulance trip while filling in for Dr. Corpron. The aluminum boat above was one of several boat types tried at the Kwai River Christian Mission. Over time, it became more cost effective to hire local "long tail" boats. (image from Rev. Paul Dodge)

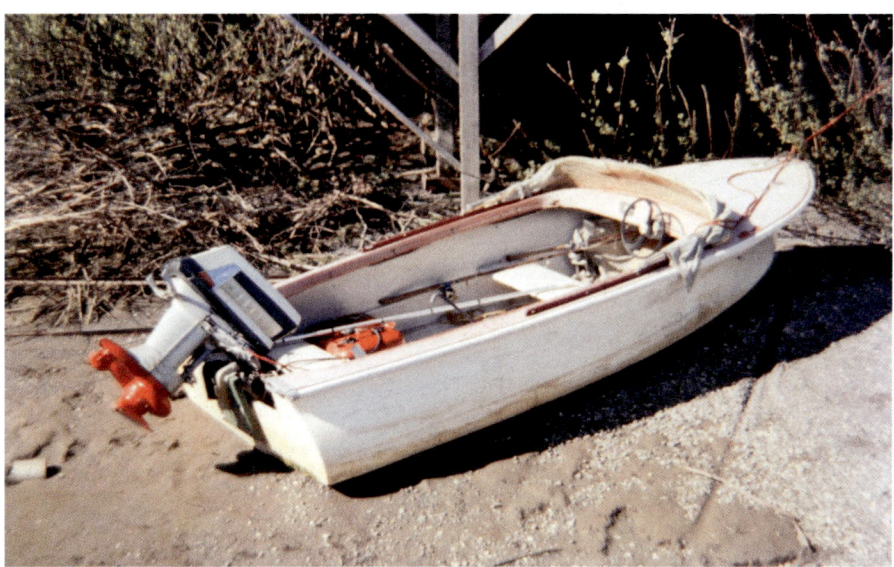

The outboard motor on this boat has been fitted with a jet pump (the red gadget where the propeller would normally be). A jet pump was less likely to be damaged by rocks than a conventional propeller. (image from Dr. Doug Corpron)

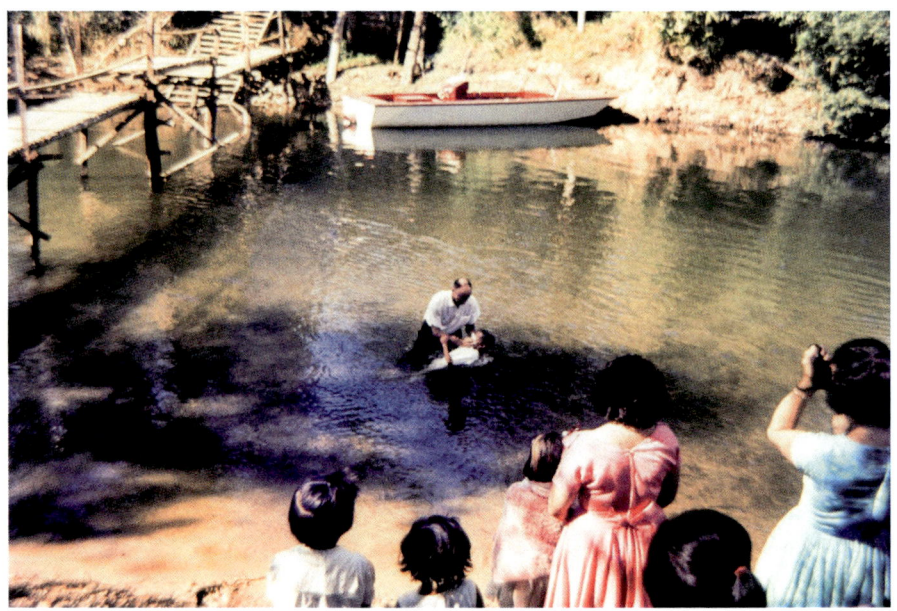

Rev Paul Dodge baptizing Oswald, the youngest child of Olivepa and Olivemo, in the Ranti River on Easter Sunday, 1966. Rogue River style jet boat in background. See chapter 2 for the story on that. (image from Dr. Corpron)

Rev. Paul Dodge (in red shirt) and friends ready to head out as a work team in the well-worn mission Land Rover.

The man on Paul's left is Rev. Nira Kamhaengsorn.

(image from Dr. Doug Corpron)

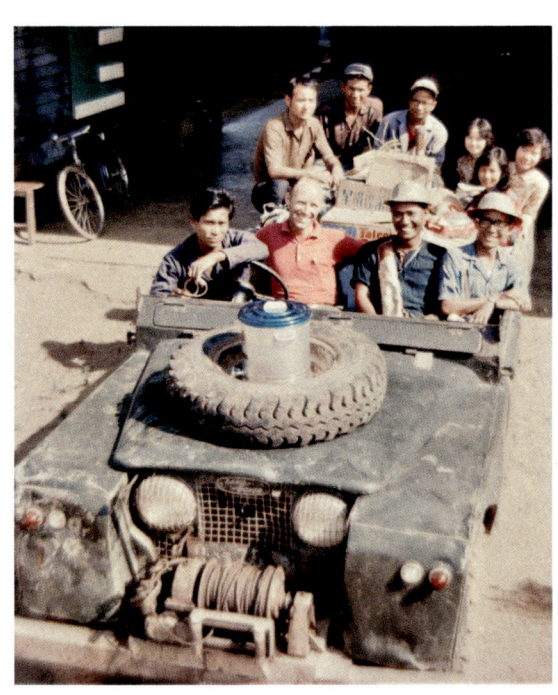

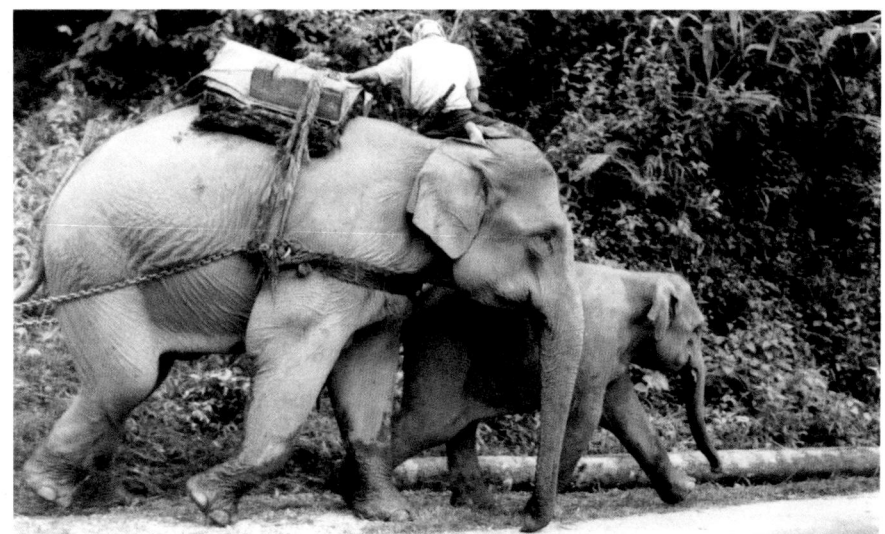
Elephants were used to haul logs to the saw pits on the mission compound. Here, a working mother and her baby. (image from Rev. Paul Dodge)

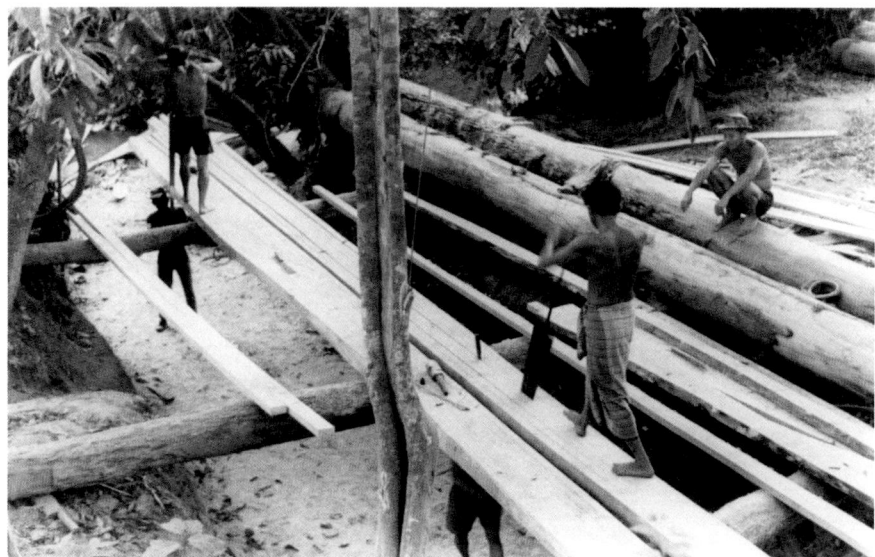
Locally harvested logs were sawn into lumber for building the boarding house, head teacher's house, and several other buildings in the early and mid-1960s. Work in these saw pits was exhausting and dangerous. (image from Rev. Paul Dodge)

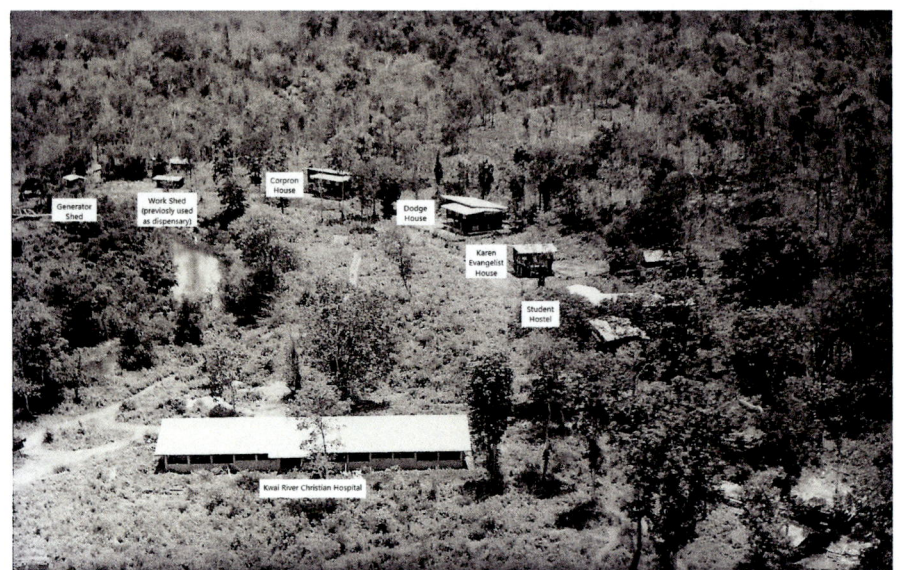

Kwai River Christian Mission: view from a helicopter, circa 1965. The Ranti River is on the left, water flowing away from viewer to join the River Kwai (Khwae Noi) about one kilometer from this site. (image from Dr. Corpron)

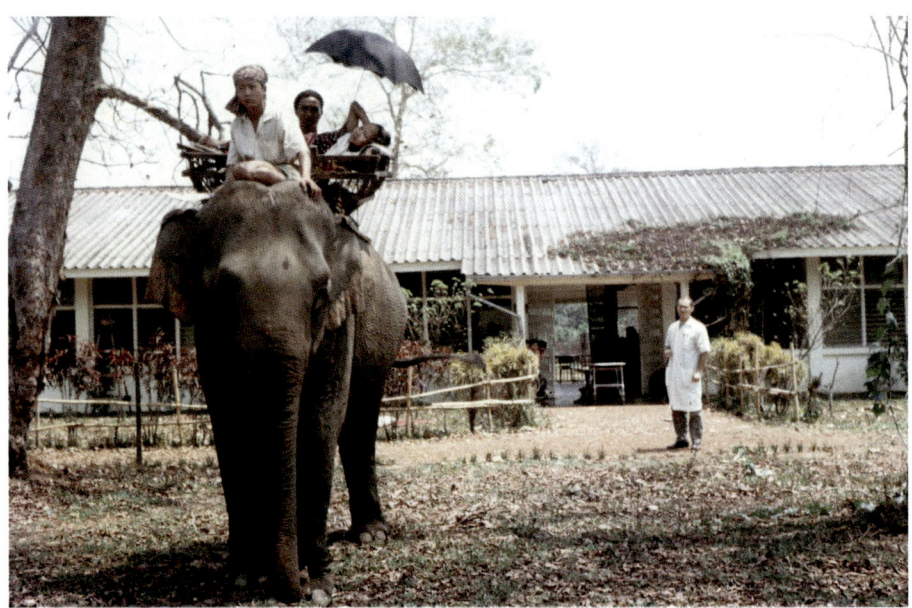

Patient (reclining on howdah) arrives in front of the hospital. Dr. Roy Myers in background. (late 1960s, original Lainam location of hospital) (from Paul Dodge)

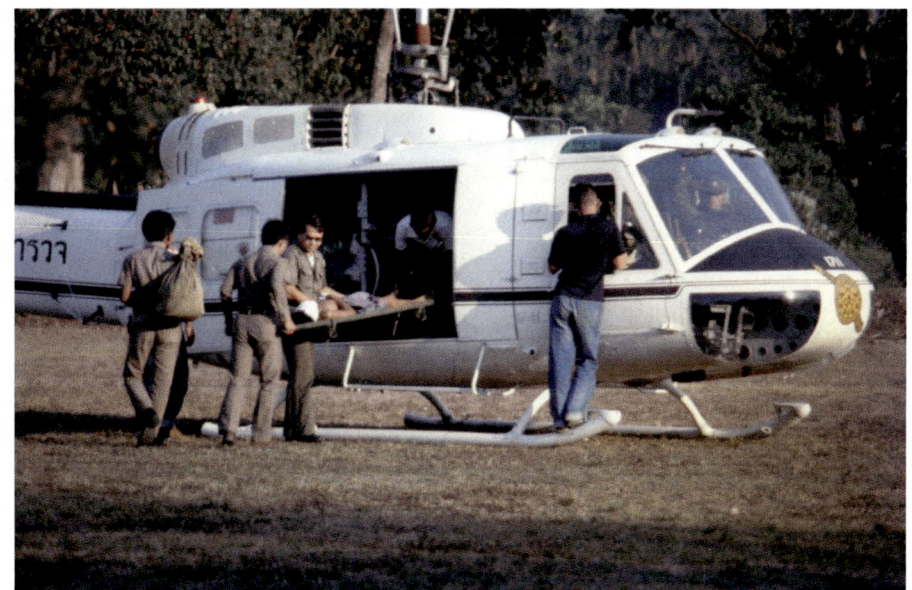

Severely injured patients were occasionally airlifted by helicopter to the provincial hospital, courtesy of the Thai border police. (photo by Dr. Ed McDaniel)

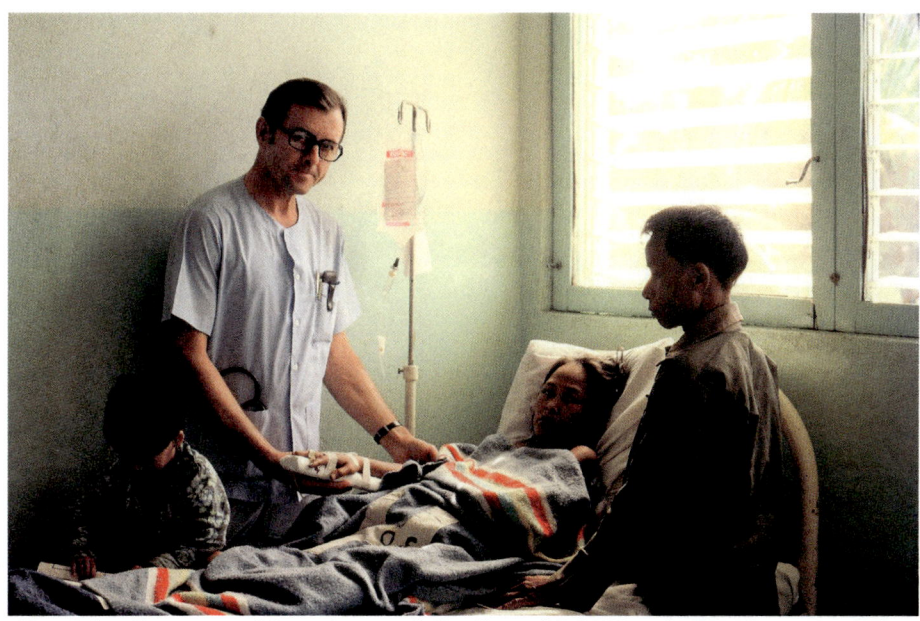

Dr. John Freeman with patient and family, mid 1970s. (image from Dr. John Freeman)

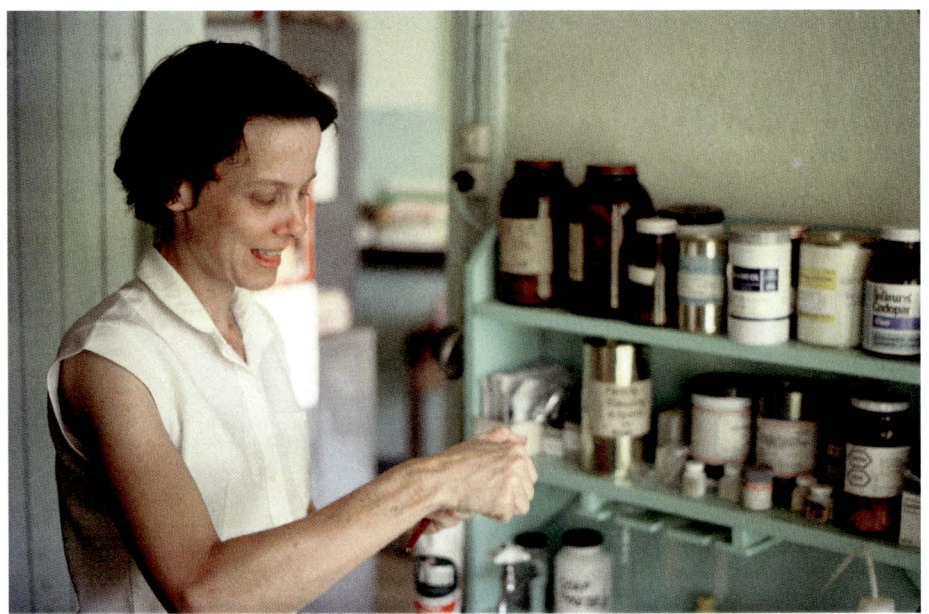

Nancy Freeman helping out in the pharmacy (image from Dr. John Freeman)

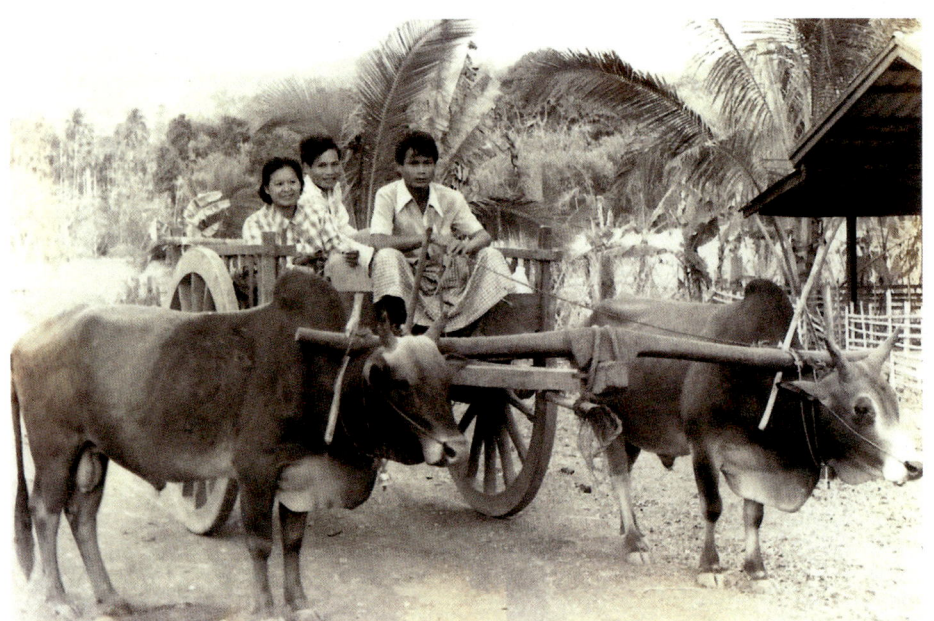

The mobile clinic team traveled to some villages on the circuit by oxcart in the 1970s and early 1980s. (image from Jan Yawan)

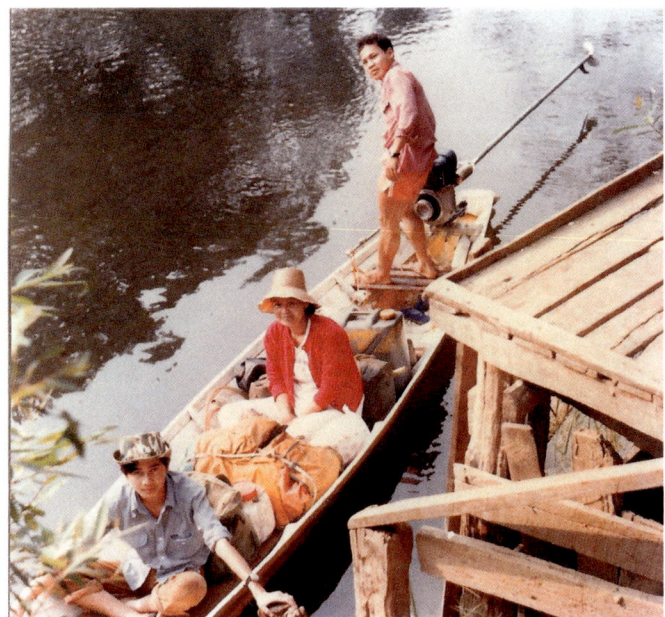

The team could reach some villages most efficiently using the mobile clinic's "long tail" boat. This could glide over fairly shallow water by raising the prop. Olivia (center) was leader of the village health team. (image from Jan Yawan)

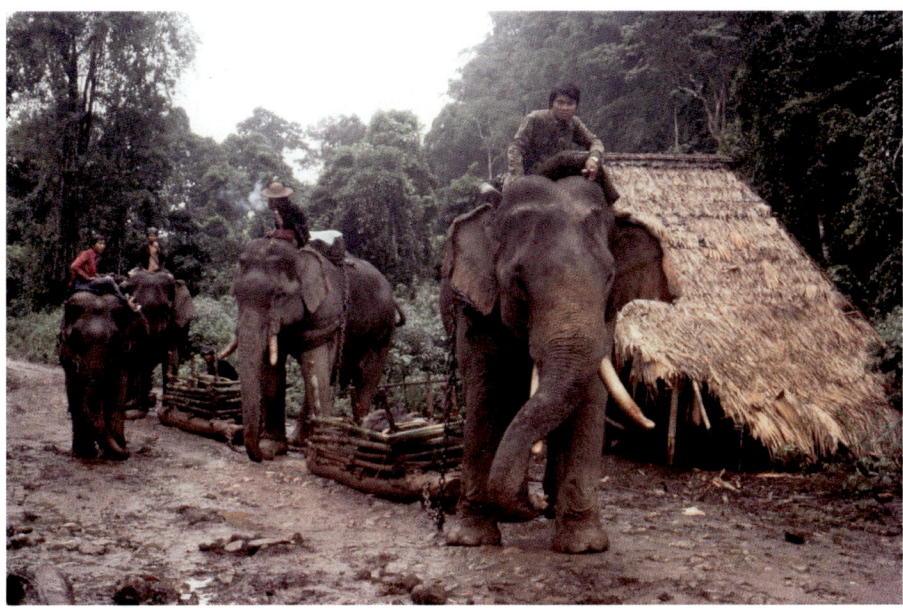

A cooperative elephant can perform useful heavy work. Unfortunately, an irritated elephant can inflict severe injuries on its mahout or bystanders. We saw many types of elephant-inflicted injuries at KRCH. (image from Dr. John Freeman)

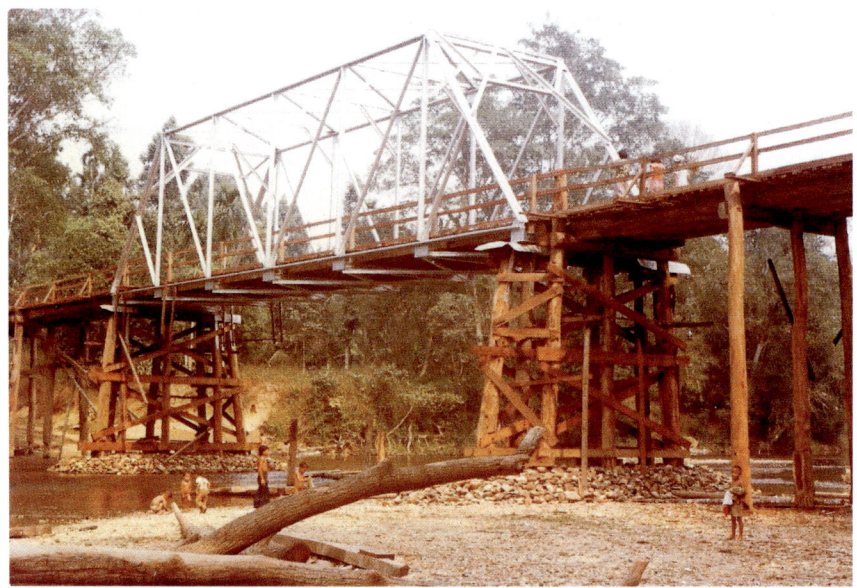

"Friendship Bridge," the brain child of Dr. John Freeman, was a cooperative effort with the area headman. The center section was built with straightened rails from the death railway. This photo was taken in the dry season. The water level could be well up the pylons in the rainy season. (image from Dr. John Freeman)

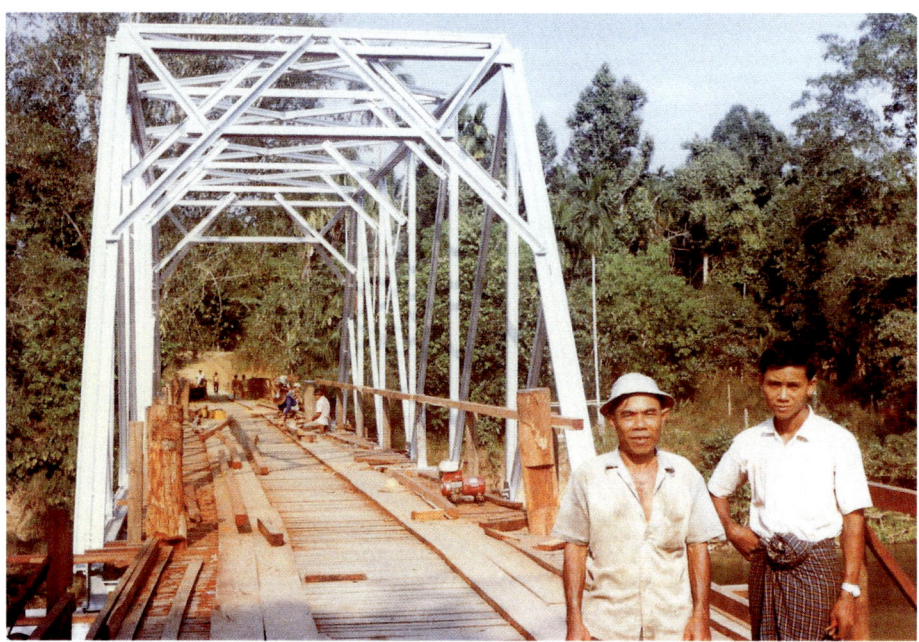

Left: Nai Chert, the blacksmith who straightened the crooked rails
Right: Nai Sanghlang, builder who oversaw the building of the middle section
(image from Dr. John Freeman)

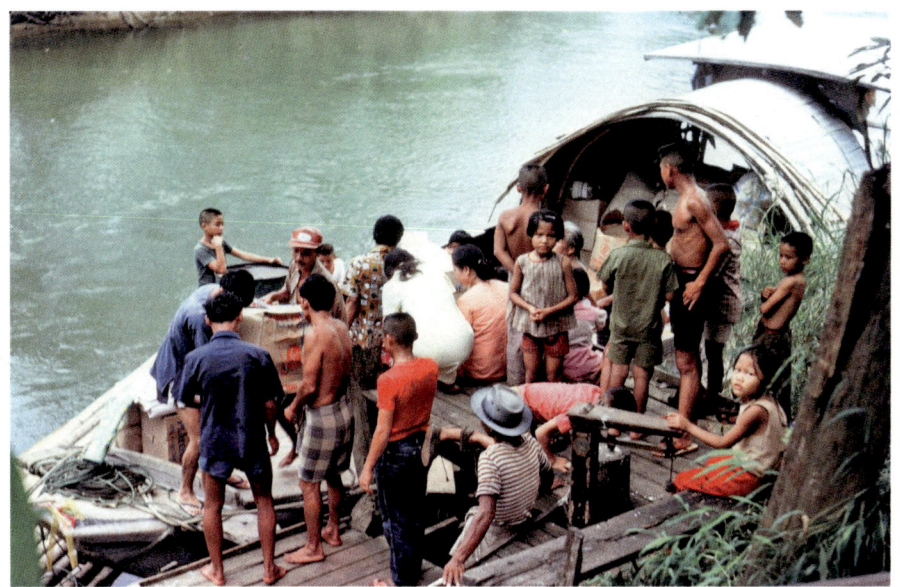

Unloading a big buy from a barge at the mission boat dock in front of the doctor's house. (photo by Dr. Phil McDaniel)

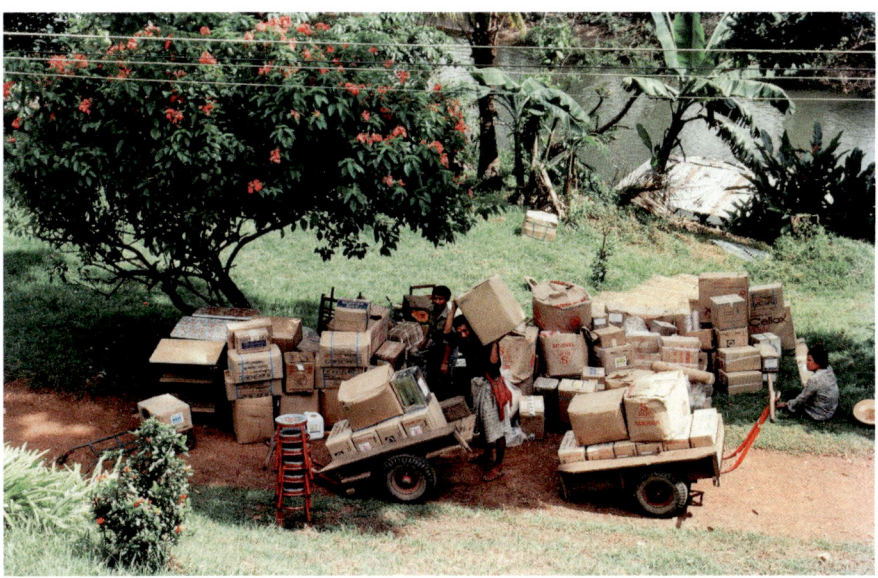

Off-loaded big buy goods ready for distribution to hospital, boarding house, and residences on the mission compound according to orders previously placed. (photo by Dr. Phil McDaniel)

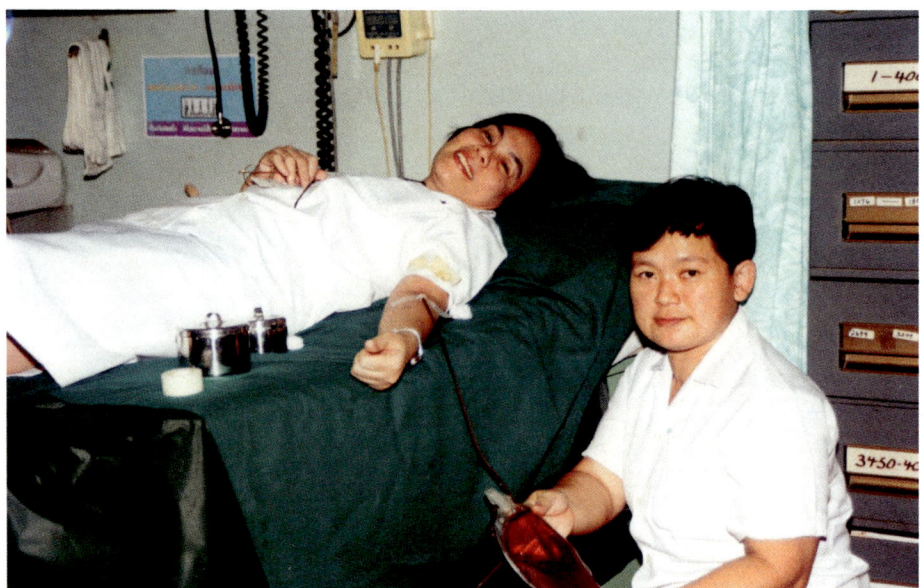

Both missionary and national staff occasionally gave blood when urgently needed if the family and friends of the patient were unable or unwilling to give. Here Lea Lindero, missionary nurse from the Philippines donates. (1980s, Huay Malai site; photo by Dr. Phil McDaniel)

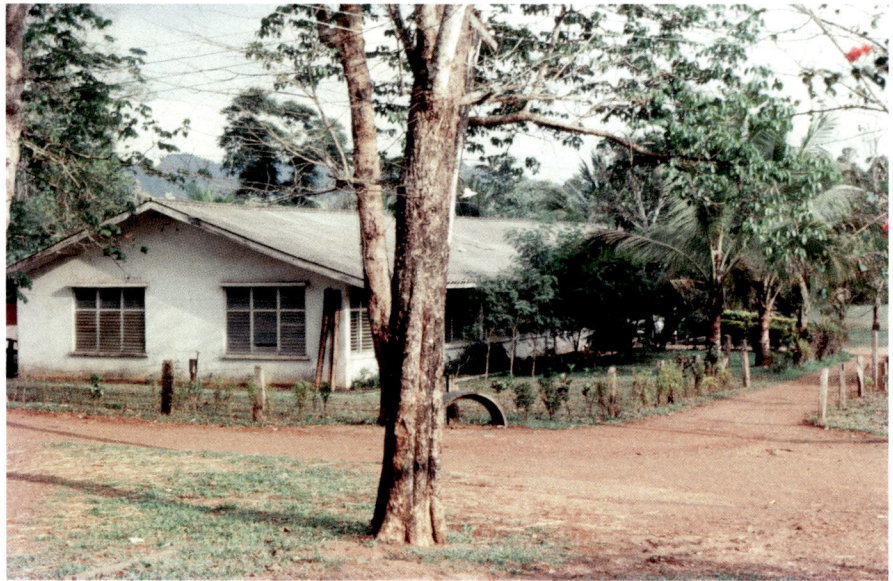

Main building of the Kwai River Christian Hospital, early 1980s, at the original Lainam site. (photo by Dr. Phil McDaniel)

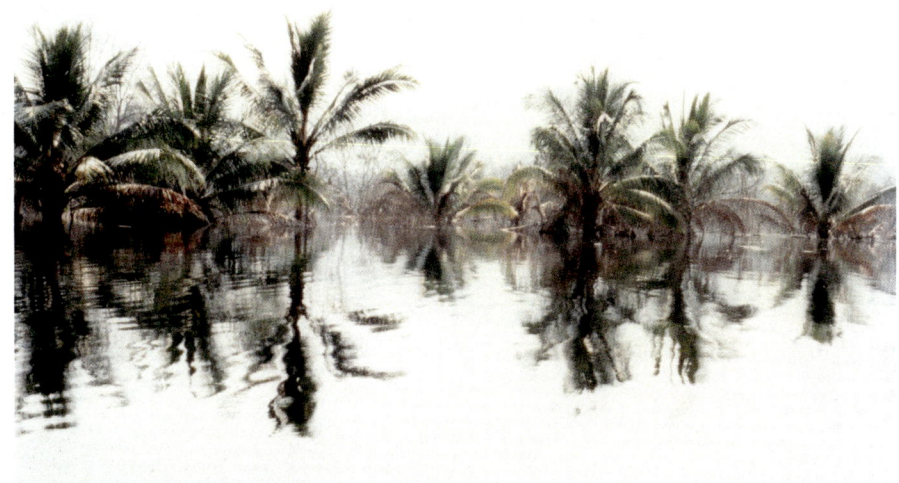

Somewhere under this water is the shell of the original hospital building. These coconut trees had been planted around the hospital in the 1970's. This photo was taken in the mid-to-late 1980s. (photo by Dr. Ed McDaniel)

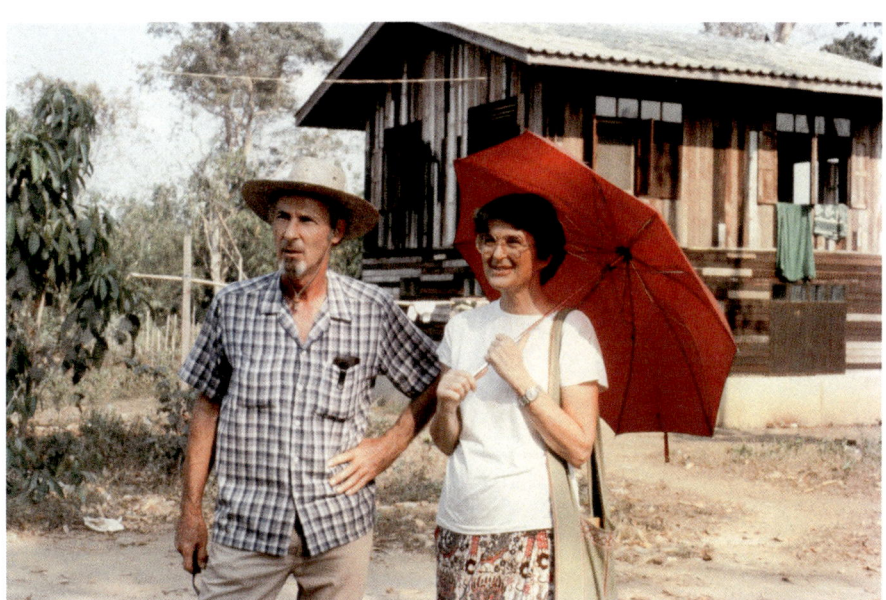

Ben and Doris Dickerson on the Huay Malai KRCH/KRCM compound. Note the patchwork of new and old, stained and unstained wood comprising the walls of the teacher's house behind them. (photo by Dr. Phil McDaniel about 1984 or 1985)

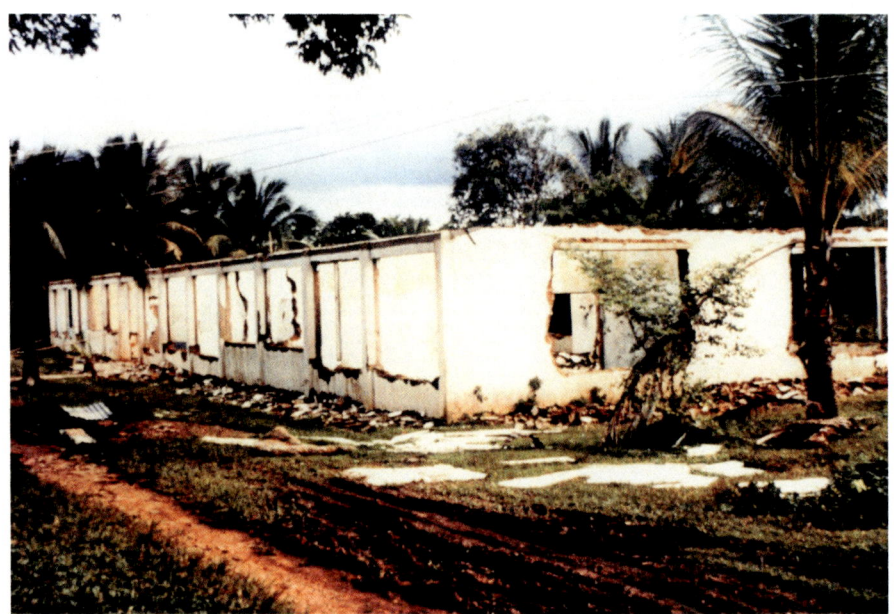

This is what remained of the original Lainam KRCH building after the roofing, window frames, and doorframes had been salvaged for use in the "new" KRCH building at the Huay Malai relocation site. (photo by Dr. Phil McDaniel)

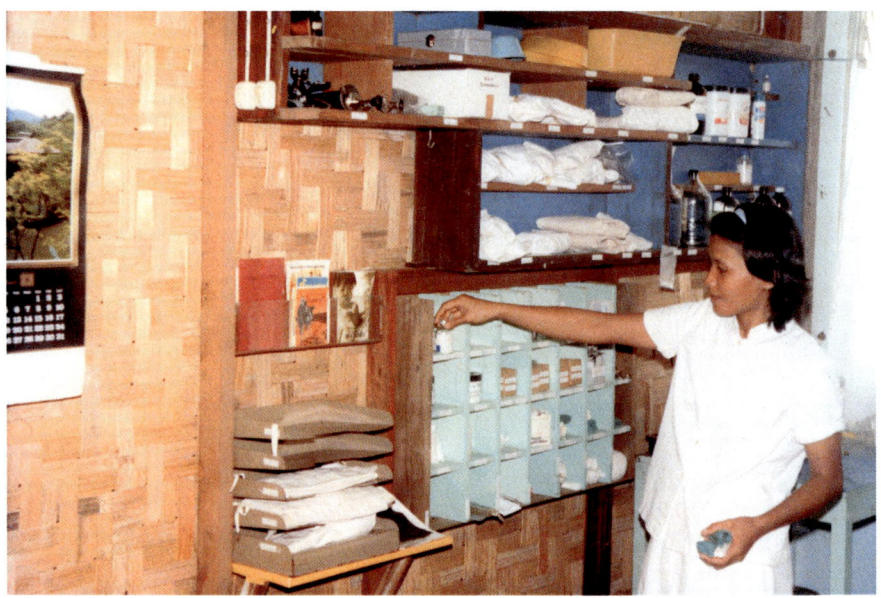

Nurse aide L'Ong reaching for a vial of local anesthetic in outpatient exam room. Note the woven bamboo forming the wall between room 1 and 2. This was a cost saving measure. (photo by Dr. Phil McDaniel about 1985)

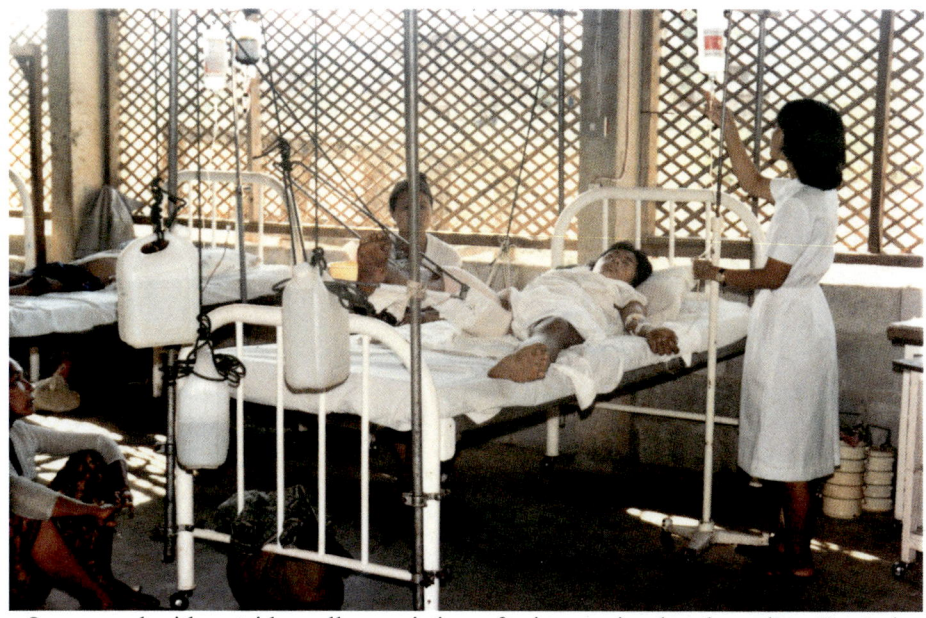

Open ward with outside walls consisting of crisscrossing bamboo slats. Dr. Lois Visscher had suggested that since the future of the hospital was uncertain, parts of it should initially be built "bambooish". (photo by Dr. Phil McDaniel about 1985)

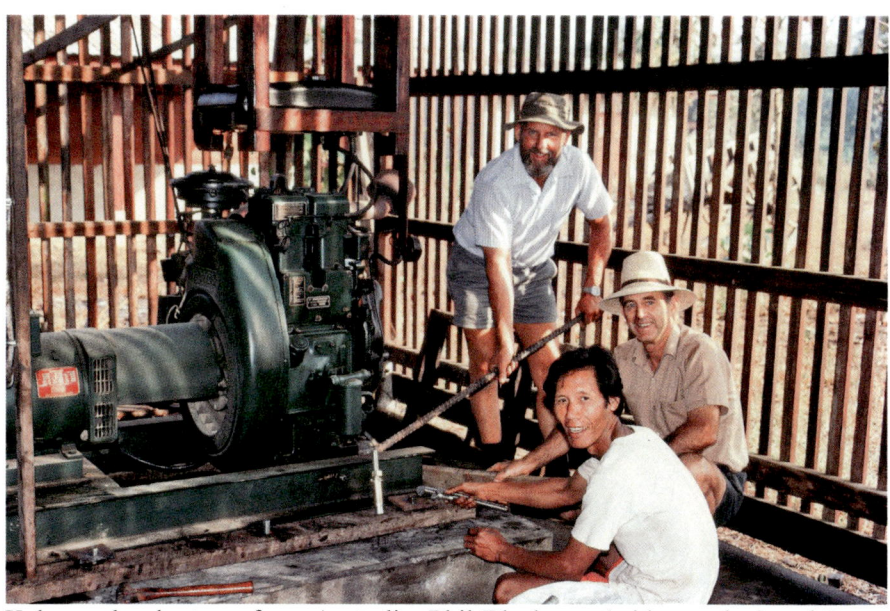

Kalay and volunteers from Australia, Phil Blackman (with crowbar) and Bruce Mills, levering 15 kVA Lister generator set into place, about 1984 or 1985. (photo by Phil McDaniel)

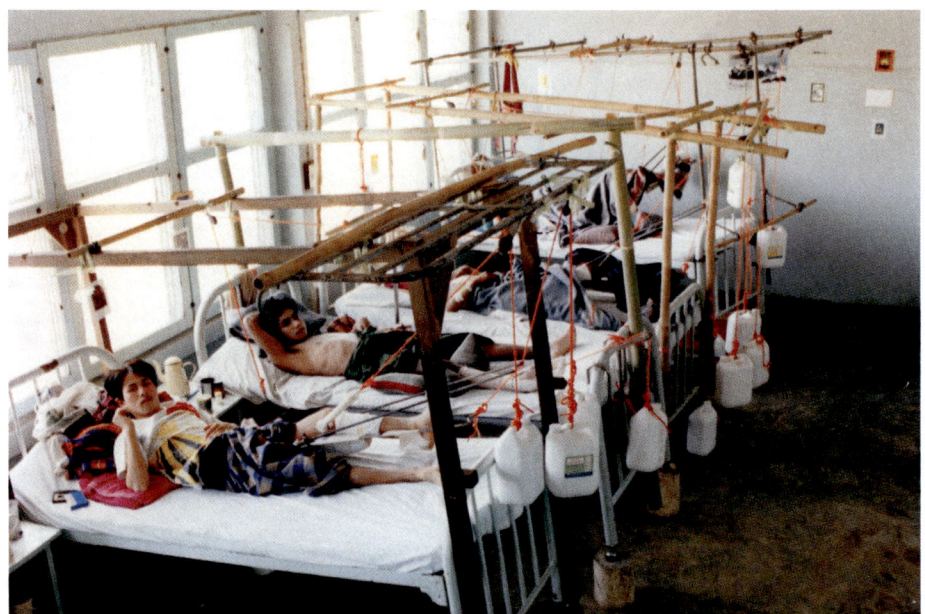

"Traction Row": Soldiers and civilians with (mostly) femur fractures. Note heavy use of bamboo (from hospital grounds) for traction frames and use of gallon containers from pharmacy as adjustable weights. (photo by Dr. Phil McDaniel)

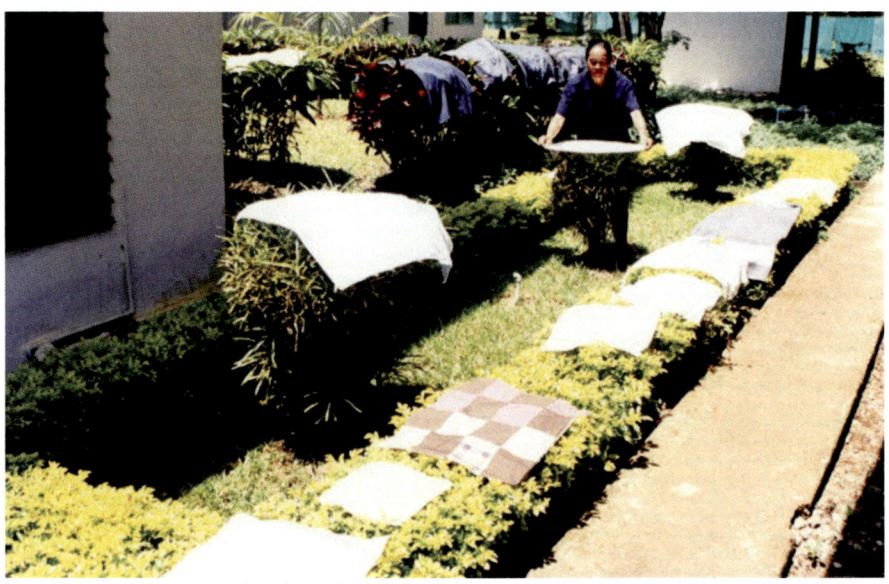

The hospital generated quite a bit of laundry. Ma Tin Aye, at times with a helper, did all the hospital laundry by hand. They usually managed to keep up with the washing, but drying sometimes required some ingenuity. (photo by Phil McDaniel)

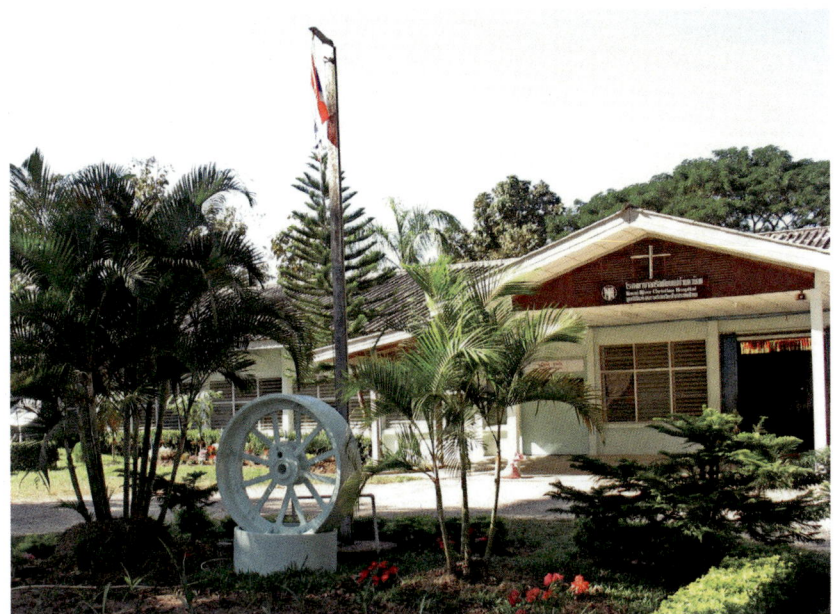

KRCH at Huay Malai in 2006. The flagpole is a rail from the Siam-Burma rail line ("Death Railway") of WW II. Wheels are from an abandoned rail yard that was a few minutes walk from the original Lainam hospital site. (photo by Phil McDaniel)

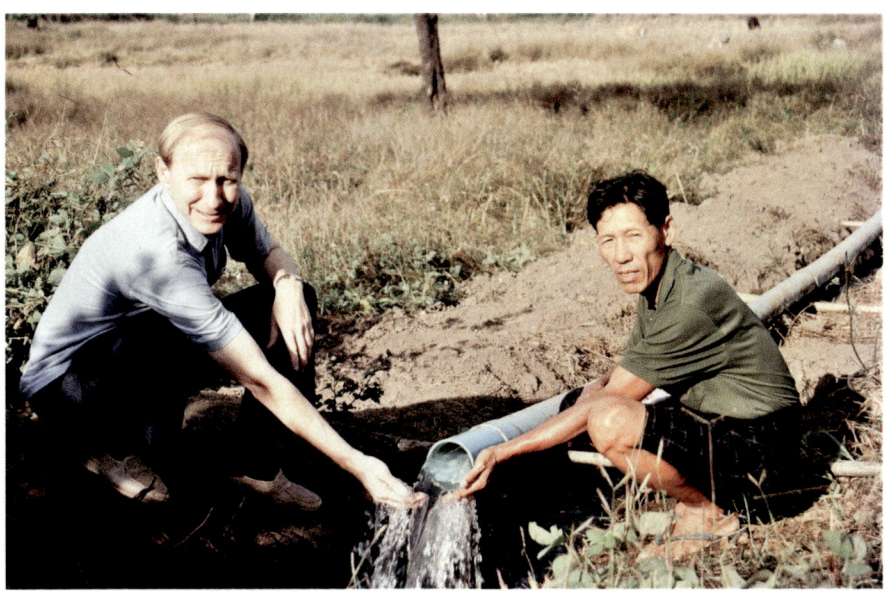

Running water vastly improves quality of life. The village health program was able—with funds from NGO's, expertise from Australian volunteers, and participation of the villagers—to install gravity-fed water systems in six villages. Left: Phil McDaniel, director KRCH; Right: Kalay, Village Health Program (photo by Dr. Phil McDaniel)

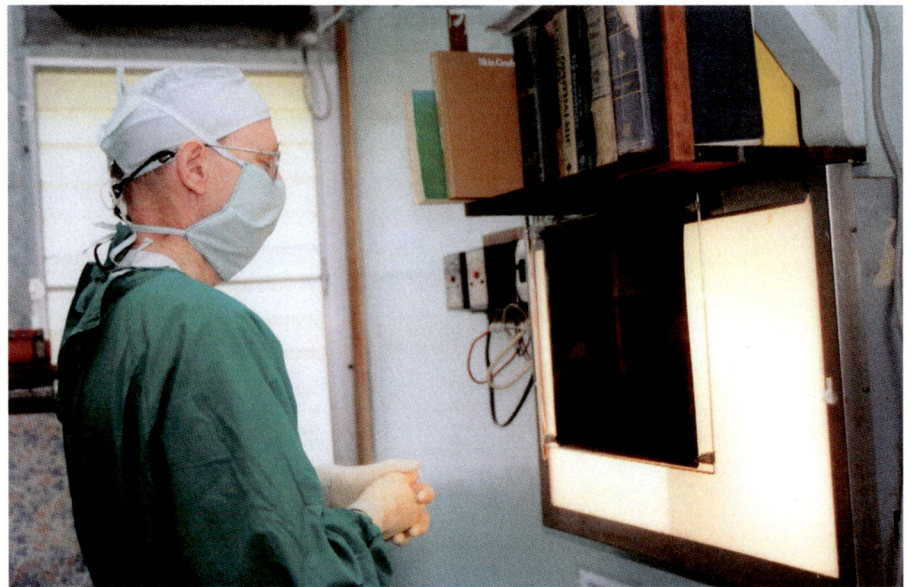

In the operating room there was an X-ray view box. Just above it was a shelf of books on anatomy and surgical technique. These were sometimes consulted during operations. (photo by Dr. Phil McDaniel)

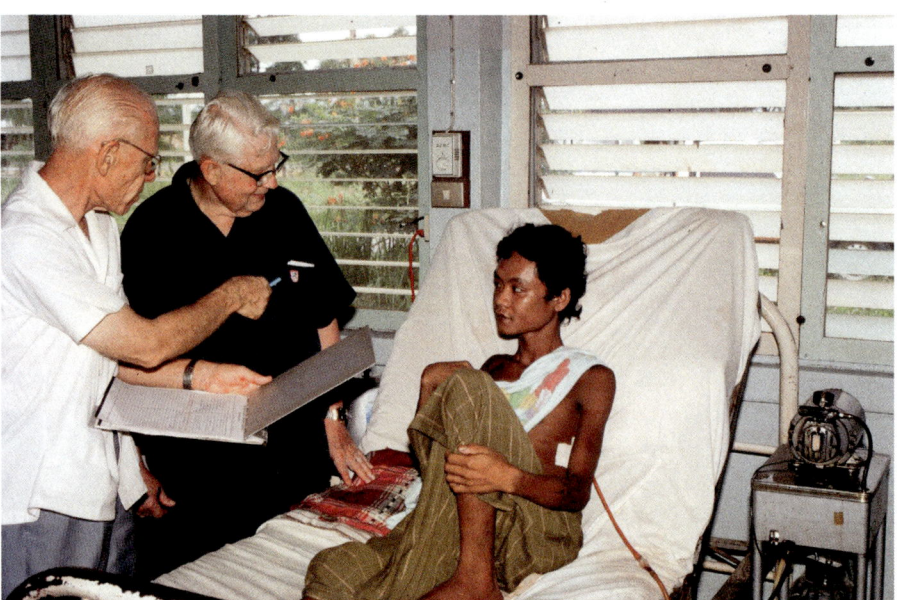

Dr. Ed McDaniel (L) and Dr. Frank Curry visit a patient in the "new" (relocation) hospital in Huay Malai. These two 70-year-old retired physicians covered the hospital on one of Dr. Phil McDaniel's furloughs. (photo by Phil McDaniel, 1987)

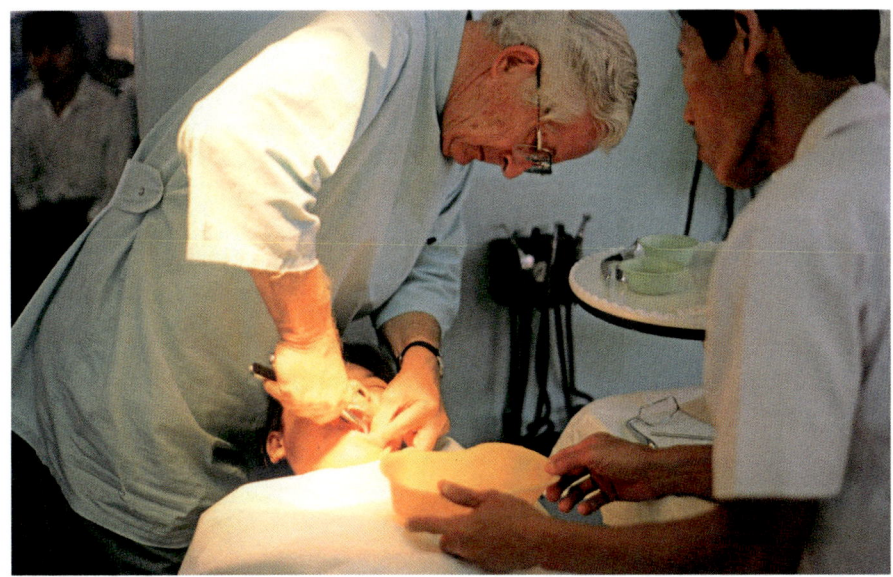

Dr. Phil Horton (dentist) made about 7 trips to KRCH to do both prevention and treatment. He stayed for about a month each time. On the right is Kalay, assisting and translating. (photo by Dr. Phil McDaniel)

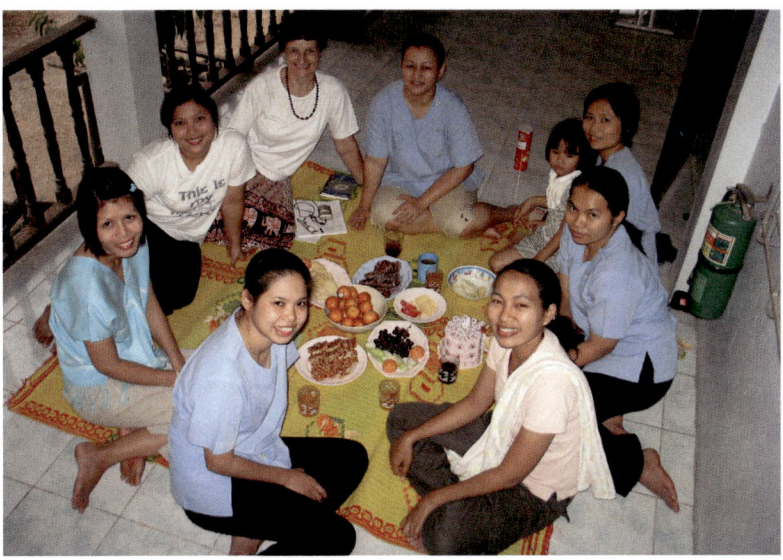

Except for the little girl in the back and Kathryn McDaniel (wearing a necklace), these ladies all graduated from McCormick School of Nursing in Chiang Mai. Kathryn was their informal guardian while they were students in Chiang Mai. Here they are having a little reunion at KRCH. (photo by Dr. Phil McDaniel)

Volunteer doctors, dentists, nurses, electricians, plumbers, accountants, teachers, and pharmacists have given of their time and talents to help the KRCH serve the people of Sangkhlaburi and beyond. These good-hearted people have come from Australia, the USA, the UK, Singapore, Germany, New Zealand, the Philippines, and Thailand. Here are just a few.

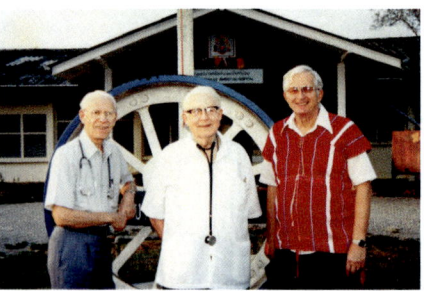

(L to R) Ed McDaniel, MD; Frank Curry, MD; Phil Horton, DDS

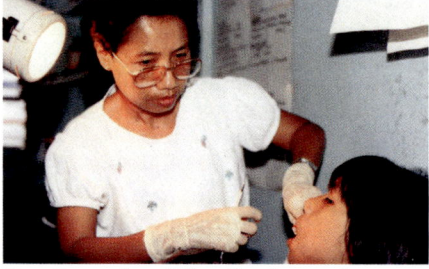

Dr. Rawadee Bitanilapin, volunteer dentist from Chiang Mai, Thailand

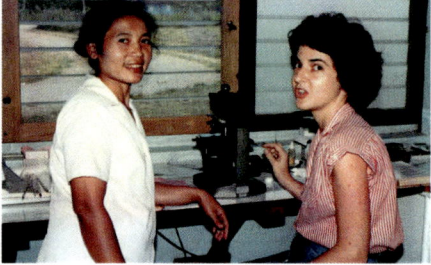

Dora with Marcia Dickerson (R), laboratory technologist from USA

Don Cross, electrician from Australia, did multiple volunteer stints at KRCM/KRCH.

(photos by Phil)

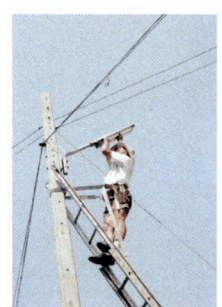

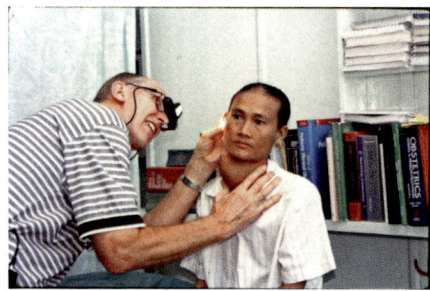

Jamie Rines, MD from USA

Jim Smith, MD, ear, nose, and throat specialist from USA

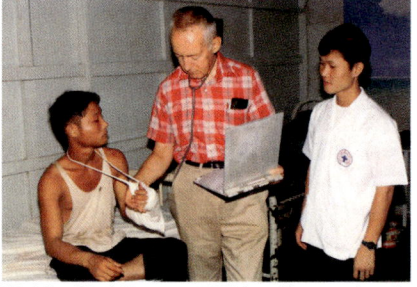

Keith Dahlberg, USA (formerly in Burma and in Maesariang, Thailand)

Appendix 1

KRCH Timeline for the first 24 Years

Editor's note: This timeline of events related to the Kwai River Christian Hospital is based on Emilie Ballard's undated manuscript, "16th District of the Church of Christ in Thailand," and supplemented by information from Doug Corpron, Paul Dodge, Jan Yawan, and Phil McDaniel. It covers events at the original (Lainam) site of the Kwai River Christian Hospital. Where sources differ on the date of an event, I have used the date of the source closest to the event. (For dates related to the school, boarding house, and evangelism, see Emilie Ballard's manuscript.)

1960

Second half of 1960

Start of construction of the first buildings of what would become the Kwai River Christian Mission: house for Corpron family, house for Dodge family, a generator shed, and a storage shed. (This latter was converted to a dispensary or clinic around March or April 1961.)

1961

February

Dodges moved to Sangkhla.

March

Corprons moved to Sangkhla.

Unspecified month

Sudah Yawan, a young Pwo Karen lady, was hired to help as a receptionist, bookkeeper, and translator.

Unspecified month

Surin, a Mon man translated for Mon speakers and carried out simple lab procedures.

Unspecified month (1961)

1st class clinic officially registered. [Also see Aug. 15, 1963; not clear how these differ—Editor] The clinic was a converted storage shed.

1962

Note from E. Ballard's outline: "In early 1962 Jut, one of the first operation cases at the hospital [a gastroenterostomy done in the dispensary—a converted storeroom] … was hired as an assistant to prepare and sterilize instruments."

June

Corprons left on furlough. Winnie Dodge carried the responsibility for the hospital [which was technically still a clinic].

1963

February

Clinic moved into the hospital building, which was nearing completion.

April

Nurse Esther Greenmun came to the Kwai River Christian Hospital from Maesariang Christian Hospital for several weeks in 1963 to be the midwife for the delivery of Brooks Dodge (who was born at the Dodge house on April 26, 1963) and to help with the clinic while Winnie was recovering from the delivery. (Corprons were still on furlough.)

July

Dodges left on furlough.

August 13

Corprons returned from furlough [arrived on site Aug 13 per Helen Corpron's memoir].

August 15 (1963)

The official permission was granted to establish the clinic.

Unspecified month (1963)

Hospital and hostel construction completed.

1964

January

Seater-Margaret Drever, American Baptist nurse, helped at the KRCH part of 1964.

July

Dodges returned from furlough.

1965

Unspecified month

Sometime during the year official permission was given to establish a 10-bed hospital.

1967

May

The new school building as well as the hospital building were officially dedicated on May 27. [Note that patient care had been going on in the hospital building since 1963.]

June (1967)

Drs. Roy and Gillian Myers from South Africa began work at KRCH.

Corprons finished their work at KRCH.

July (1967)

Esther Greenmun, an American Baptist nurse came to help at KRCH. She had come once before in April 1963 (see above).

Ebra Sanba, Karen nurse from Burma, joined staff.

1968

June

Dodges left for furlough in USA. On their return to Thailand, they were assigned to the Center for the Uplift of the Hilltribes (CUHT) and various other responsibilities in the Chiang Mai area.

September

Emilie Ballard arrived at Sangkhla to cover for the Dodges in their absence.

December

While visiting Chiang Mai, Roy Myers came down with severe viral hepatitis which kept him out of circulation for many weeks. After his recovery, he spent time honing his surgical skills with missionary surgeon Dr. Harold Hanson at McCormick Hospital in Chiang Mai.

1969

June

Esther Greenmun left for furlough.

July (1969)

Myers returned from Chiang Mai at the end of July.

1970

July

The hospital was officially closed as of July 20, after the Meyers left.

1972

Sometime before April

Josie Falla, missionary nurse from Australia, arrived in Thailand and began language study.

April

On April 1 the hospital was officially reopened as a lady doctor from Bangkok Christian Hospital agreed to take responsibility and go herself or send someone else to Sangkhlaburi every second month for several days each time. Emilie Ballard and Josie Falla were to be the two registered nurses required at the hospital.

June

Hospital closed again due to Emilie not on hand, Josie in language study, and only irregular visits by a doctor.

1974

March

Hospital reopened by Dr. John Freeman.

Unspecified month

Village Health program started by Dr. John Freeman shortly after starting work at the KRCH.

Unspecified month (1974)

Jan Stretton arrived in Thailand and began language study.

December (1974)

Jan Stretton took leave from language study to work at KRCH for a while.

1975

June

School health program started.

1976

January

Mobile clinic program funded with aid from the Baptist Union of Sweden and Church World Service.

Sometime in first half of 1977

Completion of Public Bridge #2, a joint effort between Dr. John Freeman and his team (who worked on the center span) plus the area headman and his team (who built the approaches). This was a fairly substantial bridge, which spanned the Ranti River and allowed safe and convenient access to the hospital by folks in town. The villagers called it "Dr. John's Bridge."

September

Josie Falla returned to Australia on furlough and remained there.

<h1 style="text-align: center;">1977</h1>

May 16

Dr. John Freeman and family left Thailand.

May 30

Jan Vertigan (later Yawan) arrived in Thailand. She went up to KRCH with Jan Stretton about 10 days later. She did language study on site at KRCH.

August

Loes de Vos (pharmacist from Australia) arrived in Thailand. She went up to KRCH after annual TBMF (Thailand Baptist Missionary Fellowship) conference. She did language study on site.

December

Jan Stretton left for her first furlough.

<h1 style="text-align: center;">1977-1978</h1>

Intermittent

Dr. Bina Sawyer and Dr. Keith Dahlberg made occasional (once every few months) visits to KRCH in order to keep the hospital open. The hospital was registered under Dr. Sawyer after Dr. John Freeman left. Dr. Ed McDaniel did a volunteer stint or two during this time as well.

1978

July

Shirley Burman (missionary evangelist from Australia assigned, with her husband, to the Kwai River Christian Mission) was killed in a two-boat collision on the River Kwai (Khwae Noi).

August

Dr. Phil McDaniel, Melba, and Linette arrived in Thailand. They started language study after TBMF annual conference and a brief orientation trip to the Kwai River Christian Hospital.

December

Jan Stretton returned to Thailand from Australia after her first furlough.

1979

April

Dr. Phil McDaniel began work at KRCH after about 6 months of language study in Bangkok and one month of OB training under Dr. Ed McDaniel at McCormick Hospital in Chiang Mai.

1980

December

Jan Vertigan went on her first furlough Dec. 1980 to Dec. 1981.

1981

Unspecified month

Loes de Vos went on one-year furlough. Did language study in Bangkok on return.

1982

June

Dr. Lois Visscher arrived at KRCH to cover the hospital while the McDaniels were on furlough. McDaniels left on furlough to USA shortly thereafter.

1983

June

McDaniels returned from furlough.

September 8

Dr. Lois Visscher was stabbed multiple times in her apartment by two unknown assailants. She was flown to Bangkok the following day by Border Police helicopter. She was treated at Bangkok Christian Hospital. (See "A Night of High Drama" in Jan Vertigan/Yawan's memoir for the rest of the story.)

December

Jan Stretton left on her second furlough.

1983–1984

The Kwai River Christian Hospital along with the Christian elementary school, student hostel, housing for teachers, housing for hospital personnel, hut for long term patients, house for TB patients, generator shed, fuel shed, and maintenance shed all had to be moved from Lainam Village to the Huay Malai area. This move was required to dodge flooding caused by the Vajiralongkorn (Khao Laem) dam. The new site was about 16 kilometers (10 miles) by road from the original site. This move was a defining moment in the history of the Kwai River Christian Hospital. Those of us involved in the move still sometimes speak of events as having happened "before the flood" or "after the flood."

Appendix 2

Talako Outreach Follow-up

Rev. Paul Dodge in chapter 1 and Dr. Doug Corpron in chapter 2 both mention the outreach to the Talako sect of Karen deep in the jungle as being one of the reasons for the establishment of the Kwai River Christian Mission in Sangkhlaburi. They both mention Allan Eubank and his tenacity in pursuing this outreach. Here is a brief account of the decades-long outreach to the Talako in Allan's own words.

From the 2015 version of his book, *Where God Leads…Never Give Up:*

In 1958 I felt called to the Talako sect of the Karen people. After graduating from seminary and studying Thai for a year, we made the first elephant trip to the Talako in 1962.

The Talako welcomed us as their long-lost brothers according to their ancient legends. But they expected us to give them political power and economic prosperity. All we had to give was Jesus. The remoteness and general political instability made the area difficult to visit. (Eubank, 2015, 353)

In a "Thai Lights" mission newsletter dated February 2017, Allan Eubank wrote:

After four visits [in the 1960's], the Communists came in and held the area many years. We were only able to return in 1988. On May 4, 1990 the Talako asked us to drink the water of covenant to always build up and never betray each other. The first baptisms only happened in 2008. Before each baptism the house and land were cleansed from spirits and they burned their spirit items. When we first came to this area in 1962 there were no Christians on the Thai side of the border as far as we knew. Now there are at least 13 churches, and we shared in planting eight of these.

Appendix 3

Relieving Physicians: A Lifeline

By Phil McDaniel

When I was still brand new at the Kwai River Christian Hospital, I stood one day on the path that ran from the doctor's house to the hospital and wondered how best I could do my part. I reflected on how difficult (often impossible) it had been to keep the hospital staffed with even one doctor and one nurse. It had already closed twice for lack of a doctor. I resolved to try to last as long as I could in order to provide stability. A huge help in this regard were the doctors willing to cover the hospital from time to time to give me a chance to go on furlough or to a conference or on a family vacation with a free conscience and without depriving the patients of doctor care. I owe a great debt of gratitude to the following doctors, who covered the hospital during my furloughs. These were all retired missionary doctors. They understood my predicament!

1982–83 furlough	**Dr. Lois Visscher**
1987–88 furlough	**Dr. Ed McDaniel and Dr. Frank Curry**
1990 Sept.–Dec.	**Dr. Tom Roberts**
1993–94 furlough	**Dr. Keith Dahlberg**

Some of these same doctors plus others (John Freeman, for instance) covered the hospital for shorter periods as well. Among the frequent returnees were Roy and Gill Myers, who had served as regular KRCH doctors in the late 1960's. In their retirement—after careers in trauma surgery (Roy) and public health (Gill)—they returned to the KRCH on multiple occasions to help out.

I returned as a KRCH relief doctor myself 11 times after moving back to the States in 2002. Each visit was for 2-4 weeks. I went, in part, to "pay forward" the gift of respite.

Appendix 4

Official Correspondence

Editor's note: This document (from the files of Dr. Doug Corpron) appears to be a summary of the rationale for establishing a Christian outreach in Sangkhlaburi District.

Churches of Christ Mission
Thailand
Karen Survey Summary
April, 1958

As a part of the total strategy of the Disciples of Christ to encourage and hasten the growth of the church by seeking out and working with more responsive groups, the Thailand Mission Group started some two years ago to investigate the location and responsiveness of Karens, Lao and other groups located within the area allocated to the Disciples by an early comity agreement. Work has already begun with the Lao and Lao Song groups as a result of this strategy policy. Investigation also revealed that the Karens had been one of the most responsive groups to Christianity in Southeast Asia. Several survey trips into the remote and underdeveloped sections of the assigned Disciple area indicated the presence of large numbers of Po and Sgaw Karens.

With the aid of Karen Christians from the northern part of Thailand, Christians from the Nakon Pathom area, and our own missionary staff, we have completed eight survey trips into areas where the Karen are located. Several of these trips have had as their chief purpose the gathering of more information about the Karens in northern Ganburi [Kanchanaburi] and southern Tak province. Although the presence of large numbers of Karens in this area was confirmed some time ago, considerable difficulty has been experienced in finding a satisfactory location from which to serve these people.

Geographically speaking, the Karens in northern Ganburi and southern Tak are isolated from outside communication and transportation facilities because of their location along the western slope of a long mountain range running just inside the western edge of Thailand. A road crosses this mountain range in the Tak-Maesod area, but an irregularity in the Thai-Burma border prevents reaching areas to the south from this location. The 6,000-foot mountain ranges to the east can be crossed by foot or elephant but would be too much of an obstacle to permit supplying a mission from this direction.

The Meklong [Mae Klong] River, which flows through Banpong, Tha Rua, and Ganburi reached up into this area from the south. Just north of Ganburi, the Meklong River divides into two main branches. The east branch has as its source, the area around Umphang, in southern Tak province. A trip up this branch revealed that one could not depend on this river for communication, since its flow is often over narrow, swift rapids. The western branch does not offer the same obstacles. Trips up this river indicate that it is both possible and practical to travel up into the Karen areas near the Ganburi-Tak border from this direction. [Editor's note: The eastern branch is now called the River Khwae Yai and the western branch the River Khwae Noi. The spelling "Kwai" as in "Kwai River Christian Hospital" is an alternative spelling of the word "Khwae."]

Near the upper reaches of the western branch [River Khwae Noi] of the Meklong, about three days by boat from Ganburi, is the town [Sangkhlaburi]. It is populated almost entirely by Karens. For some 50 miles to the south of this town, one finds Po Karen villages along the river banks. Near Sangkhla, the River divides, and it is possible to proceed to the West and South and reach other Karen villages by boat travel. Within 20 minutes' walk from Sangkhla, one can reach other Karen villages of about 40 houses. We have had universal agreement from the national and missionary workers that had visited this area, that this town of some 1,000 people would be the best location for beginning a mission to the Karens in the northern Ganburi, southern Tak area.

Historically speaking, Sangkhlaburi has been the traditional center for Karens from this section of Thailand. The headquarters of the old Pra Tu Wan Kingdom was at Sangkhla. This kingdom passed from existence some 25 years ago, at the time of the Japanese occupation. The Pra Tu Wan did not have any sons to take over the job of hereditary governor for the Karens in this area. The son-in-law Agoon is still living in Sangkhla, but he did not choose to be burdened with the huge administrative task his wife's family had carried for seven generations. Since this period, the Karens have been under a regular Thai system of government.

Travel to Sangkhlaburi:
Because of the great differences in the wet and dry season here, travel must be covered according to the seasons. The situation during the wet season

would be as follows: The distance of almost 200 km by River from Ganburi to Sangkhlaburi could be made in a motor type boat capable of drawing cargo boats in 3–5 days. The shorter time limit would be for travel downstream and the longer time for travel against the current. A 35-horsepower outboard motor boat with around six passenger capacity could make the trip in about 11 hours.

During the dry season, travel would have to be by land. A Dodge Power Wagon could leave the end of the rail line at Tha Saw, and make the trip to Sangkhlaburi in two days. The overland trip would be about 160 kilometers from the end of the rail line. Daily rail service from Bangkok, Nakon Pathom, Banpong, Ganburi, and Tha Saw would make the total trip not over three days in length.

Security:
The Thai police maintain a number of border police stations in this area. The headquarters for this area is in Sangkhla. According to information given by local residents, police, and government officials, there is absolutely no trouble from banditry in this area. A Karen Christian in the Maesod area indicated that he had known about the existence of a bandit type tribe in the area along the Tak-Ganburi border. He had not had any information on them in some 30 years and was not able to indicate as to whether they still continued to harass travel. The existence of a border police station in the area that had at one time been known to be the center of activities of this group would indicate that it is likely they have either changed their ways or moved from the area. We traveled to within 15 miles of the area where this group was known to have been located some 30 years ago and didn't hear anything of them.

Food and equipment:
The ability to transport large amounts of food and equipment from the Bangkok-Nakon Pathom area by motor drawn barge during the rainy season makes it possible to bring in the necessary supplies with no transportation difficulties. Rice, vegetables, some fruits, and some meats can be purchased locally. The meats would be limited to fish, pork, and chicken, but with occasional wild deer, buffalo, etc. from the forest. Sangkhla has several stores, and Tah Kanun, some 60 km away is a large market.

Medical facilities:
No medical facilities exist in this area. Malaria, typhoid, and tuberculosis are common. Due to the almost absolute lack of medicine, most of the people exercise a fatalistic attitude toward sickness. When we traveled through this area, Dr. Chen was called upon many times daily to examine patients. Our

medical kit has been in constant demand on the occasion of our travel through this area. On our last trip to Sangkhla, we distributed some 30,000 pills for control of malaria. These pills are available free from Church World Service, but would have cost $7,500.00 to these Karens if they had been purchased on the local market. The Nakon Pathom Mission Hospital is well known to most of the people in this area, although it is almost 300 km away. Dr. Chen and Dr. Chek-ling have treated many of the people's families, and through them our missionaries have a ready welcome in many of the villages.

Education:
A government school has been started at Sangkhla. It offers classes up to the sixth grade at this time. The facilities are very inadequate, but it does offer some opportunity for education for some of the local children. With the exception of one other extremely small school offering two classes, we did not find any education facilities open to the Karens in this area. Since the villages are so scattered, and often too small to support a school, it is likely that these people could best be served by a boarding school.

Present religious attachment:
A rather large Buddhist wat [temple] is to be found at Sangkhla; smaller wats are to be found in many of the villages. Indications are that the people are not strict Buddhists, but that they mix Buddhism with animism. The more remote the village area, the more this is true. In villages about half day walk from Sangkhlaburi, we found that chickens and pigs were not raised because they formed a part of the spirit worship of the people.

Indications of local interest:
During our survey trips into this area four Karens from northern Thailand traveled into this area with us. Each of them has been sufficiently impressed with the possibilities of this area that they have asked for an opportunity to work in this area if we open it. While visiting in one of the villages one of the Karens was asked to just stay and explain Christianity to them while she was there.

The manager of a mine at Tha Kanun [now called Thong Pha Phum], 60 kilometers to the south, offered to use his workers and his elephants to bring the trees out of the jungle that would be needed to build a school, boarding school [boarding house], and the hospital. He stated that this would be done at no cost to us, since the mine was interested in seeing these new facilities open to an almost completely undeveloped area. He also took a survey of the educational needs of his own area, and indicated that Tha Kanun could need places for 60 boarding students within a year after we could open the school.

The government officials have indicated that we should be able to get land and lumber tax-free for building school buildings, hospital, and boarding facilities. We might have to pay tax on lumber for mission houses.

Scores of local people have contacted us in the hope that we might be able to play a part in bringing education and medicine to this area.

Indication of Karen Christian support:
Not only the Karen workers that have accompanied us on these trips, but quite a number of other Karen leaders have indicated that they hope that we could open a Christian work among the Karens in this area. The Karens in the neighboring border area of Burma have expressed a similar hope. A former Karen school headmaster and his wife, who are registered Thai refugees, have indicated a desire to come and head up the school.

Possible relationship of the Sangkhla work to the Talakon sect:
Although not a major consideration at this time, the possible opportunity that exists in this area with the Ta-la-kon (or Ta-la-ku) sect should be mentioned. Because of the nature of this sect and the conditions surrounding it, the possibility of a mass movement developing through contact with it cannot be ruled out.

The seventh, and supposedly the last chief of the Ta-la-kon sect lives inside Thailand, some 4-5 days walk north of Sangkhla. He is located at Htee-maw, at the foot of a sacred mountain by the same name. Their tradition states that seven chiefs will reign, and at that time, the white man with the golden book (containing the teachings of God) and the silver book (containing the knowledge necessary for educating their people) will bring to the Ta-la-kon sect of the Karens a gospel of salvation. The present chief is a man in his 30s. He states that he believes that the Christian religion is the answer to their religious tradition, and that he is looking forward to the coming of the missionary to lead his people into a fuller knowledge of God. These people already worship one God, whom they hold to be the Creator of the world. The total adherents to this religion (it is officially registered as a separate religion in Burma) is unknown, but it has been estimated to have as many as 25,000 adherents, mostly in Burma. The Karen Christians in Burma are urging our missionaries to contact this man, since they feel that the next few years will be the critical time for this sect. By their [Talako] own admission, they are in the reign of their last chief, whose duty it is to lead his people to the true religion that has been kept for them by the white man from the West.

Official Correspondence

Nature of the mission needed to serve this area:
It seems that three things would be necessary to best serve the needs of this area. The order of listing does not indicate a priority, since all three of them would be needed to adequately serve the people.

1. A small well-stocked hospital staffed by a doctor and at least two nurses. The doctor should be free to travel some into the remote village areas during the dry seasons. Public health education is much needed.
2. A good school, supported by a large boarding school. Hundreds of villages have no school facilities. The school would offer opportunity for teaching Christianity to students from a large area. Any future church in this area would need to depend on leadership trained in our school.
3. An evangelistic program that could reach out into the mountain villages during the dry season, and along the river during the rainy season. Karen workers living in the remote areas could aid greatly in bringing the Christian message to the hundreds of villages located in an area within five days walk of Sangkhla. Special emphasis would need to be given to the Ta-la-kon [Talako] sect.

[Editor's note: in September 1965 the survey trip described below was made to evaluate the work of the Sangkhla Christian Mission (later renamed the Kwai River Christian Mission). This evaluation took place 5 years after the start of construction of the first buildings on the mission compound.]

October 12, 1965

Subject: Report and Recommendations of Sangkhla Survey Trip

At the instigation of the Sangkhlaburi Sub-committee of the Committee on National Missions of the CCT, a survey trip to the Sangkhla Christian Mission, Kanjanaburi Province, was made September 25th to 29th this year. Those participating on the survey team were Acharn Tongkam Pantupong, chairman; Acharn Charoon Wichaidist, Dr. Kenneth Wells, Dr. Pipat Trangratapit, Acharn Bamrung Atipat, Khun Sanong Purarak, Forrest Travaille, John Sams, and Richard Worley. This survey was in keeping with the proposal of the National Church meeting at Wattana to survey all of the work of the CCT both as to present work and future development.

The Sangkhla Christian Mission was established in 1961. [Editor's note: construction of the first buildings on the compound was started in the second half of 1960.] Since that time extensive capital has been invested and outreach has been made in evangelism, medical care, and education. There is now established the River Kwai Christian Hospital, with ten beds, and a combination school and hostel, presently with two classes in Prathom 1, but with permission to open grades to Prathom 7. Two resident missionaries and their families live in Sangkhla, Dr. and Mrs. Douglas Corpron and Rev. and Mrs. Paul Dodge. The rest of the staff consists of 1 person in evangelism, 1 boatman, 3 in the school, 3 in the hostel, and 10 in the Hospital, making a total of 18 on the staff.

The members of the survey team became oriented with the area before discussing the various problems in committees. As a result of these discussions, definite recommendations were made. These recommendations were made and agreed upon by the entire survey group. The recommendations are herewith enclosed, in turn covering the medical program, school program, evangelistic outreach, general recommendations, and recommendations for capital needs. Also enclosed are maps of the Sangkhla area and the station proper. It is hoped that the attached recommendations will be a guide to the

317

Sangkhla Station personnel, to the governing sub-committee, and to the Missions and Boards involved.

Sangkhla Sub-Committee

MEDICAL SURVEY REPORT AND RECOMENDATIONS

1. The charges for drugs and medicines at the hospital is in line with current price patterns at Bangkok Christian Hospital and McCormick Hospital. No change recommended.
2. The charge for shots should be increased from 5.00 Tcs [about 25 cents, US] to 10.00 Tcs per shot.
3. In cases where a long series of shots is indicated, a special rate can be adopted, but collections should be made whenever medication is given.
4. It was suggested that the registration fee for the hospital be set at 2.00 Tcs [about 10 cents, US] for each patient card issued.
5. It was recommended that an examination fee of 3.00 Tcs be set.
6. It was agreed that board and room charges should be held at the current rate for the present. It was suggested that if the overall economic potential of the community increased, that this rate should be adjusted accordingly.
7. It is strongly recommended that a down payment or deposit be received from those entering the in-patient care of the hospital. It was felt that in cases of elective surgery that financial arrangements should be worked out between the patient and the hospital prior to admittance.
8. The committee recommends that every effort be made to collect as much of every medicine and hospital bill as it is possible. It was pointed out that a full and continuing system of billing is maintained and that each patient with outstanding bills is consulted about this before further treatment is given.
9. After consideration by the full survey committee, it was voted that we should reaffirm that we consider the medical program at Sangkhla to be an essential part of the total missionary program in this area. We recommend further, that the emphasis be twofold: a local hospital program and village visitation

through itineration, with an emphasis on public health education in both areas.

10. After consideration by the full survey committee, agree that the medical program has reached a point where two doctors are essential in order to meet the total opportunity here.
11. Recommend that Dr. Piphat endeavor to recruit Thai medical staff personnel (physicians and nurses) for Sangkhla.
12. Recommend that scholarship funds be found and personnel recruited for training to prepare Thai medical workers for assignment to this specific program.
13. Request the Medical Committee of the Church of Christ in Thailand to again endeavor to furnish a doctor to fill in for Dr. Corpron during the trip to the Talekon area and during his vacation in 1966.
14. Recommend that, if possible, one person be appointed as nursing supervisor to look after cleanliness, food preparation, operating room, medical supplies, equipment preparation and the staff working in each of these areas.
15. Recommend, if possible, that someone be appointed as business manager to look after accounts, inventories, billing, collections, and local purchasing of food. Suggest that this person be trained locally, and that they be able to use the main languages of the community.

Editor's note: *Tcs* is an abbreviation for *tical*, which is an old name for the unit of Thai currency, the baht. I believe that around the time this report was written, one *tical* (baht) was equal to about 5 cents, US.

Appendix 5

Informal Correspondence

From Dr. Ed McDaniel to his Children from the Kwai River Christian Hospital in Huay Malai toward the end of a volunteer stint as relief doctor to cover the hospital so that son Phil could go on a family vacation.

Huay Malai
20 April, 1986

Dear Ed and Julia, Carol and Jeff, and Julia [Julie],

I write this as the first big rainstorm of the season is abating and the sun is trying to shine through clouds over the nearby hills.

Just before the storm began, I finished our fourth C. Section of our time here. I say "our" because this time Dr. Steve Morse, a D.O. from Oklahoma, is here with me, doing a lot of the work! I don't know what I would have done without him—or how Phil manages to survive working here as the only doctor most of the time, month-by-month and year-after-year. It surely takes a special kind of devotion and patience. And that goes for the expatriate nurses and pharmacist here, too, as well as the national staff.

Phil and Melba and Nathan are due back from their vacation in four more days. I can hardly wait to turn over the patients to Phil. Several of them are waiting for his more expert care and experience. One has a collapsed lung, cause undetermined. One has a bad fracture of the wrist, sustained when he fell off a scaffolding while helping to build a local temple. One is a Mon (rhymes with "gone") fighter who took a Burmese mortar fragment to his right leg, shattering the bone badly. He was brought in eleven days after the injury! (The pain was such that he could not be carried very far in a day, and the fighting took place quite far away.)

—In the bed next to him is a Karen soldier who blew away part of his left hand trying to defuse one of his own land mines! Phil did a skin flap from the abdomen to cover what was left, and will detach his hand from the abdomen (where it has been for the past 3 weeks) soon after he gets back. [This was a transfer flap and it "took" fine.]

—In the next bed is a young chap who severed a couple of tendons in the back of his left hand when the big knife he was using to clear a field slipped. Steve and a volunteer American male nurse (son of a missionary [probably Chris Gage]) spent several hours putting things back together again yesterday.

—Just another bed down the row in the men's ward is a little boy who looks fairly well but is passing deeply red urine—probably the so-called "blackwater fever" of falciparum malaria, a type quite commonly found here; though he may instead be suffering the untoward effects of medicine taken before he came to us yesterday. Steve has just started him on high doses of prednisolone.

—In the end bed of the same room is an elderly man suffering from a bout of severe gastroenteritis.

—In the women's ward are three C. Section cases, one of them having bled profusely from a placenta previa before arriving at hospital. Because of her rather poor condition, despite a couple of units of blood, we did her whole operation under local anesthesia. She is making a good recovery. The baby had already been dead for a day or two before the mother came to us.

—This morning (Sunday) another full-term pregnant woman came to hospital with the baby lying transverse in the womb, with an arm about to prolapse. So, we sectioned her. She is making a good recovery.

—In the same room is a baby recovering from pneumonia and a little girl recovering from malaria. Another patient in this room is recovering from malaria and P.I.D. (pelvic inflammatory disease).

—One of our most interesting patients is a little premature girl who weighed just 700 grams (1 lb. 10 oz.) when born 6 weeks ago. A lot of loving care has now brought her up to a weight of 1,100 grams (2 lbs. 8 oz.). No longer does the hospital generator have to run day and night to power "Jenny's" incubator!

—In the "sala" (shed) just behind the hospital is a man undergoing treatment for pulmonary TB.

—Patients not admitted to hospital are often interesting too. Yesterday a teenage girl came in after running a three-inch splinter of wood into her foot. She had been running with open, rubber sandals. Also yesterday was a woman in for her second course of Methotrexate to treat her chorioepithelioma, a cancer developing along with her molar pregnancy, and discovered by Dr. Dick Schroeder, the visiting 0B/GYN specialist who came up here with me a few weeks ago.

Not all hospital patients leave the way we would like them to. Recently a C. Section case on whom many of us labored to save her life, ran away one early morning without paying anything at all on her bill! A couple of days ago we lost a man who had been stabbed by a friend in a drunken brawl. After extensive surgery to close stab wounds in his stomach and liver, his condition went bad; and he didn't survive an extensive re-exploration. We are still trying to get over the disappointment and shock of that one.

Not all has been direct patient care for me. I have had fun exploring how very useful.... (Hold everything! Needles of fire! I just put an arm into one sleeve of a shirt which had been hanging in my clothes closet only to be met by sudden fire all over my arm and shoulder! And just as I threw the shirt down in fright, out ran a scorpion! It disappeared. Later: Steve and I found it again inside my bed sheets, shook it loose on the floor and crushed it with one blow of Linette's big book on Energy! ... Three and a half hours later, and one spot on my arm still feels like it's being slowly burned! The local saying about scorpion bites is "You only cry three days") ... [Note from Phil McDaniel: My recollection of this saying is: "If you get stung by a scorpion you only cry for three hours; if you get stung by a centipede, you cry for three days—we had some big ugly centipedes in Huay Malai!]

Well back to the "useful" X-ray. Since the bigger machine went off to Bangkok for repair with Phil three weeks ago, I have learned how much can be done with a little old 15 milliamp army surplus portable machine. Calculating thickness-exposure charts for the more commonly used procedures has taken a lot of time and effort, but is rather fun.

I have also succeeded in reviewing 104 stereo colposcopic teaching slides and am through the "S's" in my little English-Thai 5,000-word dictionary—a great way to enlarge one's vocabulary and to finally learn of mistakes in pronunciation which one has made for the past 35 years! The Thai are usually too polite to tell one!

There has been good opportunity to worship with the hospital staff every morning and with the English-speaking staff and volunteers after "community supper" Sunday evenings.

With Steve here doing much of the work, I've also managed to squeeze in reading the fascinating and inspiring stories of the lives of

Elizabeth Blackwell, the "First Woman Doctor", and the Wright brothers.

Languages can slow down and complicate communications between doctors and patients. We use Thai, Karen, Mon, Burmese, and a little bit of English.

Fortunately, a capable interpreter is never far away.

Most importantly, a young man [Kyin Tun] has just returned from Bible school in Burma and has now become the new hospital evangelist. He speaks Thai, Karen, Mon and Burmese [and English]. He is greatly needed here!

[Dr. Ed McDaniel]

Bibliography

Ballard, Emilie M. "16th District of the Church of Christ in
Thailand." undated manuscript

Dahlberg, Keith. *Bridge Ahead: A Medical Memoir.*
Bloomington: iUniverse, 2008

Eubank, L Allan. *Where God Leads…Never Give Up.* Chiang
Mai: Pan Rak Foundation, 2015

Freeman, John D. *Jungle Episodes: A Missionary Doctor in
Thailand.* Columbia, SC: 2018

Hovemyr, Maria. *A Bruised Reed Shall He Not Break: A History
of the 16th District of the Church of Christ in Thailand.*
Chiang Mai: Office of History of the CCT, 1997

"Ministry to the Least," a pamphlet prepared by the staff of the
Kwai River Christian Hospital for the celebration of 50
years of medical ministry in Sangkhlaburi, 2010

"Vajiralongkorn Dam." Wikipedia, Wikimedia Foundation, 29
July 2019,
https://en.wikipedia.org/wiki/Vajiralongkorn_Dam

Abbreviations

ABM: American Baptist Mission (Later, this became the Thailand Baptist Missionary Fellowship.)

AFRIMS: Armed Forces Research Institute for Medical Sciences, a cooperative effort between the medical arms of the Thai army and US army to do research into detection, treatment, and prevention of tropical diseases. The diseases of particular interest to AFRIMS were often the diseases of particular interest to KRCH as well.

APM: American Presbyterian Mission

CCT: Church of Christ in Thailand, a non-denominational church body

KRCH: Kwai River Christian Hospital, historically one of the ministries of the Kwai River Christian Mission

KRCM: Kwai River Christian Mission, comprised of a hospital, a school, a student hostel, and an evangelism program

SCM: Sangkhla Christian Mission, an earlier name for the Kwai River Christian Mission

SEATO: Southeast Asia Treaty Organization

TBMF: Thailand Baptist Missionary Fellowship, a cooperative body comprised of Baptists from the USA, Australia, Sweden, Japan, the UK, and other nations.

UCS: United Christian School, historically part of the Kwai River Christian Mission

UCMS: United Christian Missionary Society, the mission arm of the Christian Churches (also called Disciples of Christ)

USIS: United States Information Service